Physical Diagnosis
for the
Chiropractor

Edward Brown, DC, DABCI
Professor
Parker College of Chiropractic
Dallas, Texas

Physical Diagnosis
for the
Chiropractor

Copyright © 2005 – All Rights Reserved
Dr. Edward Brown

Photo credit p. 295: www.holmbergphotography.com

ISBN 1-59196-345-1
(Fourth printing August 2005)

Dedication and Acknowledgments

This book is dedicated to my wife Nancy. Without her love, kindness, and support over the years I would not have been able to write this book.

We are each indebted to the excellent instructors that have paved the way for us, and I have had many. Three deserve special mention. Doctors John Amaro and Michael Cessna are two of the most outstanding post-graduate instructors I have had the privilege to learn from. Their selfless dedication to the chiropractic profession will be felt for years to come in the work of their many students.

Dr. Richard Brouse and I practiced together for many years in Oregon. Dick is a unique individual who combines the qualities of an intellectual curiosity for learning, a kind and gentle heart, and a razor sharp mind. I am fortunate to be able to include him among my mentors.

Table of Contents

1 – Introduction to Physical Diagnosis

Diagnosis is the process of generating hypotheses regarding the cause of your patient's complaints. It often employs specialized laboratory and radiographic procedures. However, the most fundamental diagnostic technique is 'physical' diagnosis, using the senses of sight, sound, smell, and touch to assess your patient.

Diagnosis is one of the most important courses you will take during your professional training. Today, approximately 80% of health care dollars go toward treatment of chronic degenerative disorders, such as heart disease, high blood pressure, arthritis, cancer, etc. These conditions are referred to as *'diseases of civilization'*. Most physicians agree that the first remedy for these conditions should be diet, exercise, and lifestyle modification. It is estimated that 50% of the deaths in the US can be traced directly to lifestyle factors:

- o   cigarette smoking
- o   lack of exercise
- o   poor eating habits
- o   excessive alcohol intake
- o   abuse of drugs & medications
- o   prolonged stress
- o   negative mental attitude

Look at the common thread running through each of these causes - No drug or treatment can change these factors. Our profession quite rightly promotes itself as preventive health care. However, if we are truly interested in preventing chronic disease in our patients, in addition to their spinal health, we must actively work to optimize their health in these areas. Of all health care professionals, who has the best training in diet, exercise, and lifestyle modification? You do! The next time you are at the magazine counter pick up a Ladies Home Journal or McCalls magazine. Note how often you find articles on natural remedies for PMS, headaches, or various common complaints. The public is clamoring for sensible advice in natural health care. We can fill this role if we choose to. However, excellent examination and diagnosis skills are essential if you are going to treat chronic degenerative disease.

One way of conceptualizing the new patient encounter is to visualize the stages a young couple might pass through prior to marriage. The initial interview where you record the chief complaint and past health history represents your *'first date'*. As you proceed with the examination, you and your patient are *'courting'*. Finally, the report of findings represents the *'marriage ceremony'* where you explain your commitment to your patient's health recovery and ask your patient to agree to the recommended course of treatment. At each step in this process, while you are gathering the information necessary to determine what type of care your patient needs, your patient is also checking you out, deciding if you possess sufficient skill and knowledge to be '*their doctor*'.

A helpful practice management concept is the '*leaky bucket*' analogy. If a water bucket has many small holes in the bottom, we must continually pour in more water if the bucket is to remain full. The amount of water in the bucket represents the financial security of your practice. Which makes more sense: continually pouring more water into the bucket (recruiting new patients), or repairing the holes in the bucket (keeping existing patients)? Any businessman will tell you it costs much more time and money to generate a new client than to keep an existing one.

How you conduct the initial workup of your new patient is the key to repairing the holes in the bucket. You should approach every new patient with the attitude that they will pick you as their doctor until one of two things happens: they are no longer living, or you retire from practice. A thorough history and comprehensive examination, and possessing excellent diagnostic skills are the foundation of this lifelong relationship.

Dr. John Amaro once remarked, "*It is not necessarily the patient you get well who refers others to your practice, it is the patient you impress.*" Imagine you are just preparing to close your office Friday evening and a truck driver comes in asking you to 'crack his neck'. You perform a brief exam and render the needed chiropractic treatment. While he leaves your office feeling better and is satisfied with your care, he may never return or refer others to your practice.

On a different day you have a new patient who has been experiencing headaches of increasing severity. This patient receives a thorough history and comprehensive examination. The patient may even remark, "*That is the most thorough examination I have ever received.*" A few weeks later, this patient is in church and a new member asks, "*Do you know a good chiropractor?*" Who do you think they will recommend?

Key Points in Diagnosis

A study in the British Medical Journal (2:486-489, 1975) found:

> 82% of diagnoses are made from the history
> 9% are from the physical examination
> 9% are from laboratory examination

For this reason, please do not short change the time you take for the history. If you find you are taking substantially less time on the history than you are with the examination, you are probably not spending enough time on your history. At the end of the history, you should have a good idea of what is causing your patient's complaints. Usually the examination only confirms what you suspect from your history.

While you must ask specific questions to gather the facts needed to understand your patient's specific health problems and general health status, listening is the key to taking a good history. Sir William Osler, considered to be the father of modern medicine, once remarked, "*If you listen to your patient long enough, he will tell you what is wrong with him.*" If your patient feels rushed during the interview, they may not volunteer important information you neglected to ask. Likewise, when the interview is comprehensive, the patient will be at ease, and may remark, "*Finally, I found someone who understands my problem!*"

If this is not sufficient motive for you to become proficient with history taking, there is another reason. Your Part IV national boards are comprised of many stations where you have five minutes to perform a set of tasks. Three of those stations will be taking a chief complaint history. The elements you need to cover must be second nature to you. If they aren't, you may not pass those stations.

Open Ended Questions *You DONT WANT TO PUT WORDS IN YOUR PATIENTS MOUTH*

When possible, give your patient the opportunity to answer 'in their own words'. For example, ask "*Can you describe the quality of your pain?*", rather than, "*Is that a sharp or dull pain?*" Sometimes your patient is not specific enough and you may have to offer them choices. They say their pain is, "*Every now and then.*" You may have to elaborate, "*Are we talking about once an hour, once a day, once a week?*" However, in general, it is best to try the open ended question first.

Present Time Consciousness

When your patient is talking, *LISTEN*. Your patient is paying for your time and they have every right to expect your full attention. If your mind is wandering to personal problems or the last patient you saw, snap out of it and focus on the patient in front of you now. While you must take notes to record the history, you should maintain frequent eye contact with your patient throughout the interview. When your patient is discussing sensitive information, put your pen down to give full attention to what they are saying. It is a hallmark of successful doctors that they make the patient feel like the most important person in the world. For the brief time you are with them, they <u>are</u> the most important person in your world.

Personal Appearance

You are a professional and should dress and act accordingly. Read John Malloy's book <u>Dress for Success</u>. One guideline is that you should dress as well as your **best** dressed patient. Patients want to go to successful doctors. However, you should refrain from an overly flashy display of wealth, such as expensive jewelry.

While there is room for individual styles of dress, there is no excuse for a doctor having poor hygiene. In practice, you may find it too restricting and warm to wear a clinic jacket while adjusting. However, it makes a good first impression if you wear one during the initial interview, examination, and report of findings.

Avoid Jargon

You have spent a great deal of money on your chiropractic education. A part of this process is gaining new vocabulary, which is essential to learn anatomy and physiology. Just remember that most of these words are literally another language to your patient. Imagine you are conversing with a Russian immigrant and every tenth word you hear is in Russian. This is the same difficulty your patient has when you use technical words. It may be appropriate to use technical words, after you have first taught your patient their meaning. However, when in doubt use the more common lay terms, for example:

Technical term	Lay term
cervical spine	neck
thoracic spine	mid back
lumbar spine	low back
glenohumeral joint	shoulder
thorax	chest

Over-familiarity

You may be an outgoing person and like to call everyone Buddy. This is not necessarily bad. Friendly doctors are successful doctors. However, always remember to treat your patients with respect. The person in front of you may be older than your parents. When you first meet, is it really appropriate to greet them by their first name? Instead say, "*Mrs. Jones, I am Dr. Brown. Thank you for coming in. How may I help you?*" Once you gain their confidence and establish rapport it may be appropriate to switch to a first name basis.

Never Speak Ill of Other Doctors

Many times we see patients who are 'medical failures', meaning they have tried orthodox medical care and it was unsuccessful. They may speak poorly of their MD. Even if this line of talk began with your patient, don't ever run down another doctor. It makes you look petty, and is a no-win situation. Keep in mind we are seeing a self-selected group of patients. If they had received good results with the MD, these patients might not have come to you. By the same token, MD's may see individuals who did not get relief under chiropractic care. Is it fair for the MD to form an opinion of chiropractic based on that small group of patients? We should each be humble and realize that every doctor is trying to do their best for

4

the patient based upon their training and experience. No doctor can achieve 100% success.

Pertinent negatives "FLEXION / DESTRACTION TABLE"

When documenting your patient's history, we sometimes wonder how much is too much to record. Some symptoms are important enough that we refer to them as pertinent negatives. While there are no specific rules as to what constitutes a pertinent negative, they are danger signals of serious illness. For medico-legal reasons, it is important to document both your question and the answer. Suppose you asked about bowel and bladder dysfunction, but because the answer was 'no problem', you didn't record anything. Later your patient developed neurological deficit from a cauda equina syndrome. Without documentation that you performed a thorough history and examination, you may be vulnerable to a claim of 'failure to diagnose'.

Dead Doctor's Rule

During your clinical training, you will be working in a multi-doctor clinic. You must document your history well enough that a doctor taking over for you can learn what you know about the case. Specifically, the questions you asked and the answers given. This also means that if your handwriting is not legible, you should PRINT. After you graduate, even if you practice alone, the rule still applies. Two to three months may lapse from the time you take your initial history until you are asked to write a narrative report. You will have seen many similar patients over that time. Unless you have a truly remarkable memory, what is on the paper is your memory.

Differential Diagnosis

Prior to beginning your physical examination, it is useful to create a differential diagnosis list. Even when your skills are good, a complete physical examination may take 30 minutes. Many new patients need a focused examination, rather than a comprehensive examination. However, you have the challenge of deciding what procedures are essential, and what to leave out. The differential diagnosis list helps you make those decisions. It is a mental brainstorming session where you visualize the range of possibilities that might account for your patient's symptoms.

Once you have created your DDx list, look at each item and decide which examination procedures will help you narrow the list to the most likely cause of your patient's complaints. This process helps you perform a much more focused and coherent exam. With practice, you will shift to doing the list mentally rather than writing it down, however until you gain that experience, write your DDx list.

General Examination Guidelines

With a few exceptions, it is a good principle of examination to begin with the least invasive procedures, leaving the most stressful procedures for last. This gives your patient the opportunity to say, 'Ouch!', and alerts you to the need to proceed more slowly in that area. Another important principle is when dealing with bilateral structures, examine the uninjured or well side first. This provides you with a baseline of normal to compare against, as well as letting your patient know what you will do next on the painful side.

The historical information you gain from the initial interview is considered *subjective:* symptoms that are perceived by only one person. Information obtained from examination is considered *objective:* signs that can be perceived by an observer. Physical examination relies on four techniques: inspection, palpation, percussion, and auscultation.

Inspection

Initially, you may wonder if inspection is all that valuable. With experience, you will learn it often yields more information than the other three techniques. Inspection begins when the patient first walks in your office. Do they have any abnormalities of gait or posture? What is the texture of their hair and skin? Are the lenses of their eyes clear? Does the individual exhibit any tics or alterations of speech? Although not literally a part of inspection, sometimes we observe (smell) body odors that provide clues to metabolic disease.

With an experienced doctor, it may appear that he or she is spending very little time with inspection. In reality, the doctor is taking in and processing a great deal of information that is not readily apparent to the casual observer. When no abnormalities are seen, inspection may proceed quickly. However, when something unusual is apparent, the doctor will shift focus, and devote much more time to inspection of all the visual clues of the condition. Sometimes these clues are detected during the history, prior to the examination. This visual information may help account for the very high percent of diagnoses made via history.

Palpation

As chiropractors, you will gain a great deal of information from your superior palpatory skills. The tips of your fingers enable you to detect the size, shape, consistency, mobility and tenderness of body structures. Use the back of your hands and fingers, where the skin is thinner, to assess temperature. The fifth metacarpal bone or metacarpophalangeal joints of your hand are best to assess vibration. To test this for yourself, touch a vibrating tuning fork first to your fingertips, then to the bones of your hand.

6

Percussion

Percussion involves tapping an area and listening to the sound it produces. With indirect percussion (sometimes called mediate percussion), you place your middle finger firmly on the skin, then strike your own finger with the middle finger of your dominant hand. Your striking finger is called the *plexor,* while the finger laid on the body surface is the *pleximeter.* A second method, direct percussion (sometimes called immediate percussion), involves striking the body surface directly, without the intervening pleximeter finger. The sound emitted gives us information about the relative density of underlying structures. Try this for yourself: listen to the sound emitted when you percuss over your lungs, stomach, and thigh bone. In addition to assessing the relative density of body structures, percussion helps us map out the size and borders of underlying structures. Examples of the five percussion tones are:

Tone	Underlying Tissue
Resonant	Normal lung parenchyma
Hyperresonant	Emphysematous lung tissue
Dull	Liver
Flat	Bone
Tympany	Bowel gas

Auscultation

Auscultation involves using a stethoscope to listen to sounds produced by the body. The stethoscope does not magnify the sound produced, rather it helps you to focus on a small area and block out room sounds. For this reason, it is important to keep room noise to a minimum while listening with the stethoscope. The diaphragm of the stethoscope is used to listen to higher pitch sounds, such as sounds produced by the heart and lungs, and abdominal bowel sounds. Use the bell of the stethoscope to listen to lower pitch sounds such as vascular bruits or heart murmurs. (Note: Bruit is the French word for 'noise', and is pronounced brew-EE, with the T silent.)

Clinical Impression

When your history and examination are complete, you must analyze the available data to determine the cause of your patient's complaints. Consider the most likely possibilities first. The scientific principle of Occam's razor teaches that if two hypotheses explain the facts equally well, then the simpler hypothesis is preferable. Stated another way,

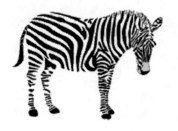

"When you hear the sound of hoofbeats, think of horses, not zebras."

However, always keep in mind that humans are complicated beings and it is very possible that your patient is suffering from two or more, possibly unrelated, conditions.

Study Guide Objectives

- Know why preventive health care is important.
- Know some examples of 'diseases of civilization' and how these chronic degenerative conditions are prevented.
- Know the purpose and importance of a complete health history.
- Approximately what percentage of the clinical diagnosis comes from the history? From the physical examination? From x-ray and laboratory examination?
- What is the most important technique you use to gain information during the interview?
- Why are open ended questions helpful during the chief complaint history?
- Know when and why we create the differential diagnosis list.
- Know the general guidelines related to the sequence of examination.
- Know examples of objective vs. subjective information.
- Know the four main techniques used during the physical examination and why each is important.
- Know which parts of the hands are best for which type of palpation.
- Know the two types of percussion and how each is performed.
- Know the characteristics and examples of the five percussion sounds.
- Know the purpose of the good stethoscope and when to use the bell vs. the diaphragm.
- Know how to modify the health history and physical examination for different types of patients, such as children or the elderly.

2 – Interview and Health History

The interview and health history is your patient's *'first impression'* of you. Your demeanor and confidence are critical to establishing rapport with your patient. *"You never get a second chance to make a good first impression."* You should approach every new patient with the attitude that they will pick you as *'their doctor'* for the rest of their life. Excellent examination and diagnostic skills are the foundation of a successful practice, and the keys to cementing a lifelong relationship with your patient.

The health history is comprised of the following areas:

- o Presenting or chief complaint
- o Past health history
- o Family health history
- o Personal and social history
- o Review of Systems

Chief Complaint History

The chief complaint covers the reason the patient is seeking care, which is sometimes referred to as the iatropic stimulus. After introducing yourself, begin your initial conversation with an open ended question such as, *"How may I help you?"* or *"I see you are having headaches, tell me about them."* Then let your patient talk for several minutes before you interrupt. They may not have been to a doctor for several years, and have been rehearsing what to say. If you interrupt 30 seconds into their narrative with, *"Is that in the morning or the evening?"*, you in effect *'rain on their parade'*. Most people will not take that long, but if they want to, let them speak uninterrupted for several minutes. After your patient has told their initial story, ask follow up questions to fill in the details. You may choose to record "in quotes" the exact words the patient uses to describe their condition.

Very rarely you might have a patient who will talk for ten minutes non-stop if you let them. If that happens, you must very tactfully interrupt. You might say, *"This is very important information you are telling me and I want to discuss it with you in greater detail later on, however in order for me to treat you today, we need to cover some other areas."*

There are many areas you must cover in your chief complaint history. The *Bates' Guide to Physical Examination and History Taking* refers to seven attributes of a symptom:

- o Location - Where is it? Does it radiate?
- o Setting - Also referred to as Onset. What factors, activities, or circumstances contribute to the complaint?

- o Timing - Details the chronology of symptoms, i.e. When did it start? How long does it last? How often does it come?
- o Quality - What is it like?
- o Quantity or severity - How bad is it?
- o Modifying factors that make the complaint better or worse.
- o Associated symptoms

We have different mnemonics to help us to remember the key areas. The OPQRST mnemonic is used by many chiropractors. The initials stand for:

Onset: When did the problem begin? Is there a known cause? Did the problem begin gradually or suddenly? What does the patient think might be the cause of the problem?

Provocation: What makes the pain worse?

Palliation: What makes the pain better? Is the patient using any over the counter or home remedies, such as heat or ice?

Persistence: How long do these complaints last?

Progression: Overall are your symptoms getting better, worse, or staying the same?

Prior: Have you had similar complaints before?

Quality: Is your pain dull, sharp, throbbing, etc?

Quantity: On a scale of 0 to 10, how would you rate your pain?

Radiation: Does your pain travel down your arms or legs?

Restrictions: Does your pain interfere with your daily activities?

Region: Where is your pain?

Site: Where is your pain? Can you point to it?

Severity: If you did not rate the pain under Quantity, use S to rate severity.

Sequela: Do you have ongoing problems from previous conditions?

Symptoms (associated): Do you have any other symptoms that you feel are related to this problem?

Timing: Is your pain constant or intermittent? If it is intermittent, what is the frequency and duration of your symptoms? Is there a daily pattern to your symptoms? T also refers to previous treatment.

While the OPQRST scheme covers all the needed areas, the sequence of the flow can be improved upon with a little rearranging. The LOCQSMAT mnemonic presents an alternative order for the questions. Whichever scheme you use, the order you choose is not as important as ensuring that all areas are covered.

L - Location / radiation. Have the patient point to their pain. They may say, "*My hip hurts bad!*", but they point to their SI joint. Record the anatomical structures they point to, for example:

® SI pain rad to ® glut msl & ant groin

With spinal complaints the location of the pain may be misleading, due to the diffuse pattern of referred pain. However, with extremity complaints the patient may be able to put a single finger over the precise anatomical structure that is damaged. Visceral pain may generate more diffuse referred pain. Be sure to ask about radiation of pain. "*Does your pain stay right in that area, or does it radiate up or down from that point?*"

O - Onset. "*When did you first notice this pain?*" Was the onset sudden or gradual? When there is a sudden precipitating event, you must detail the mechanism of injury. Ask specific questions such as, "*What direction did the impact come from?*", "*Did you notice any popping or snapping sounds?*", "*Was the pain immediate?*"

Follow your patient's symptoms for 12-24 hours after the initial injury. "*So what happened next, did you go to the hospital?*", "*As time when on, did your pain worsen, or did you experience any additional symptoms the next day?*"

If the onset is non-traumatic and gradual (sometimes referred to as insidious), try to determine the cause. "*Do you have any idea what might have brought your symptoms on?*" Probe for changes in work, home activities, exercise, etc. that may have contributed to their complaints.

TYPES OF PAIN

C - Chronology & Timing. "*Is your pain all the time, or does it come and go?*" If constant, is it 24 hours a day? Does it prevent sleep? If intermittent, what are the frequency and duration of episodes? Frequency and duration of painful episodes are helpful markers to monitor improvement at subsequent re-examinations. Is there a known cause for the flare-ups, or are the episodes associated with any specific activities?

Is there a daily pattern? Morning pain and stiffness that improves with activity suggests chronic inflammation and edema, typical with rheumatoid arthritis. The American Rheumatism Association defines seven criteria for the diagnosis of RA. First on their list is "*Morning stiffness lasting longer than 1 hour before improvement.*" Pain and stiffness that improves with rest and increases with activity is more indicative of osteoarthritis. In discussing osteoarthritis, the American Academy of Emergency Medicine states, "*The pain may get worse with overuse and may occur at night. With progression of this arthritis, the pain can occur at rest.*" Pain that is not affected by rest or activity usually indicates bone pain. "*Do you experience night pain?*" Night pain in a patient with cancer may indicate metastasis to bone. According to Haldeman in <u>Principles and Practice of Chiropractic</u>, "*Spinal pain in cancer patients should be considered evidence of metastasis until proven otherwise.*"

Is the condition progressive? "*Overall, is your condition getting better or worse since it first came on?*" Your exit question before leaving chronology is, "*Has this ever happened before?*" If so, detail chronology and timing of prior episodes.

The following graphic may help provide a visual reminder of some of the important questions you must cover under chronology and timing:

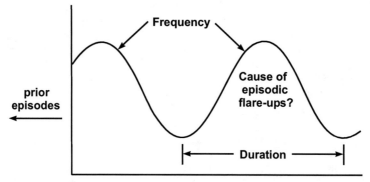

Q - Quality. "*Can you describe the quality of your pain?*" Different anatomical structures generate different types of pain. Throbbing pain suggests a vascular problem. The pain from a fracture is sharp, severe, and does not improve with rest. Muscle pain is cramping, dull and achy. Nerve pain is sharp and shooting, and may have an electric quality. If the description is unusual, record the patient's exact words.

S - Severity. Ask your patient to rate their pain. Use a numeric pain scale (0-10), or mild, moderate, severe. You should also assess the affect on activities of daily living (ADL). Quantify the impairment with time or distance measurements, such as "*How long do you sit before your pain gets bad?*" or "*How far can you walk before you experience pain?*"

M - Modifying Factors. "*Is there anything that makes your pain better or worse?*" Document any medications (Rx or OTC) or home remedies (heat, ice, etc.) your patient is using to treat their pain.

A - Associated Factors. Start with an open-ended question such as, "*Are you experiencing any other pain or symptoms you think might be related to this injury?*" Even when the answer is no, follow up with specific questions that are danger signals for the area of concern, such as numbness, tingling, or weakness, and changes in bowel or bladder function, etc. As previously discussed, a 'pertinent negative' is a danger signal for a potentially serious health problem, and it is important to document the questions asked and the patient's response. This can be quickly charted as: Ø NTW, Ø Δ B/B.

T - Treatment History. It is important to document previous treatment. If previous diagnostic imaging is available, you will want to send for the results. If this is a chronic complaint, your patient might be able to tell you what treatments have worked well or poorly for them.

It is also helpful know your patient's goals for treatment. You might ask, "*What made you seek treatment at this time?*" or "*Is there anything you would like to do, but are unable to because of your pain?*" Don't assume your goals for treatment are the same as your patient's. With chronic degenerative complaints, you might ask, "*How long has it been since you felt really good?*" It is always good to close with the question, "*Is there anything else you would like to add that I neglected to ask?*" You might be surprised at the answer.

Past Health History — ON PIECE OF PAPER , BUT WE NEED TO KNOW PG.19 MANUAL

After you have completed your chief complaint history, you will shift to past health history, family health history, and personal/social history. You might say to your patient, "*I would now like to ask a few questions about your general health status.*"

With each item on the past health history, document <u>what</u> or <u>why</u>, <u>when</u>, and the <u>outcome</u> for each incident. For example, under surgeries you might chart: *Surg: Tonsils removed, 1972, NRE.*

An example of incomplete charting might be: *Surg: tonsils.* It is not unreasonable to assume the tonsillectomy was in childhood, however tonsils are occasionally removed in adults. When the chart does not show the age or year of surgery, the record is incomplete. It is also probable that the patient recovered with '*No Residual Effects*', however can you be sure of that? If you don't ask, your patient might not volunteer information such as, "*I almost died from a post-operative infection.*" Don't assume your patient knows what information is important.

The categories you should cover in past health history are:

- o   Serious illnesses
- o   Previous accidents or injuries
- o   Hospitalizations

- Surgeries
- Medications (current and past medications, Rx and OTC)
- Allergies

Family Health History

A detailed family health history entails asking about the health of specific family members one at a time. For each family member, document their current age (or age of death), and current health status (or cause of death). This obviously can take some time. In practice you may find it more convenient to ask, "*I am interested in diseases that sometimes run in families. With your parents, grandparents, brothers, sisters, and your children, do any of them have or have they ever had:*"

- Heart disease
- High blood pressure
- Stroke
- Diabetes
- Arthritis
- Cancer
- Tuberculosis
- Blood disorders

Personal/Social History

Personal/social history factors may have a strong influence on your patient's ability to recover. It is important to maintain a neutral, non-judgemental manner when asking questions that may be sensitive to your patient.

- Family situation
- Occupation
- Exercise
- Diet
- Sleep patterns
- Bowel and urinary patterns
- Alcohol, tobacco, recreational drugs
- Stress

If you suspect your patient has an alcohol substance abuse problem, consider asking the CAGE questions:

C – Have you ever felt the need to **C**ut down on your drinking?
A – Have you ever felt **A**nnoyed by criticism of your drinking?
G – Have you ever felt **G**uilty about your drinking?
E – Have you ever felt the need for a morning **E**ye-opener drink?

Review of Systems

The interview and health history concludes with a review of systems. Usually, you look over a check-off form filled out by the patient. When you find an unexpected item, ask specific questions to fill in the details (what or why, when, and outcome). If you do not have the benefit of the review of systems form, verbally ask about the individual systems. Prompt with a few examples appropriate to each area. For example, "*I want to make sure you don't have any additional health problems I should be aware of. Do you have or have you ever had trouble with...?*"

- EENT
  - o Changes in vision
  - o Difficulty hearing
  - o Sinus congestion
  - o Nosebleeds
  - o Toothache
  - o Frequent sore throats

- Heart and lungs
  - o Difficulty breathing
  - o Coughing up blood
  - o Chest pain
  - o Rapid or irregular heart beat

- Gastrointestinal
  - o Indigestion
  - o Nausea, vomiting
  - o Food intolerance
  - o Constipation
  - o Diarrhea

- Urinary
  - o Frequency, urgency
  - o Painful urination
  - o Difficulty voiding
  - o History of kidney, bladder or prostate problems

- Endocrine
  - o Thyroid problems: unexplained weight change, heat or cold intolerance
  - o Diabetes: polydipsia, polyuria, polyphagia
  - o Menstrual: painful menses, heavy flow, absent flow, last menstrual period (LMP)

- Immune
  - o Unusual bleeding or discharge
  - o A lump or thickening in the breast or otherwise
  - o A sore that does not heal
  - o Persistent hoarseness or cough

- Skin
  - o Itching, dryness
  - o Bruising
  - o Change in a wart or mole

The character of Sherlock Holmes was patterned after Dr. Joseph Bell, an English surgeon who taught Arthur Conan Doyle during medical school. Synthesizing the various bits of information obtained from the history is very similar to the deductive reasoning process that the detective Sherlock Holmes used to solve his cases.

The precise and intelligent recognition and appreciation of minor differences is the real essential factor in all successful medical diagnosis. - Joseph Bell (1890)

Study Guide Objectives

o   Know the categories of information that comprise the complete health history and the specific items you cover in each category.
o   Know the seven factors you must document for the chief complaint symptom.
o   Know what questions you ask for each of these factors.
o   Know what items are covered under OPQRST.
o   Know the types of questions used to investigate the mechanism of injury.
o   Know the daily pain pattern of osteoarthritis vs. rheumatoid arthritis.
o   Know quality of pain patterns for vascular, bone, muscular, and nerve structures.
o   Know why a functional assessment (activities of daily living) is important.
o   Know which type of information is considered to be a 'pertinent negative' history item and why.
o   For each of the components of the past health history (such as surgeries), know the three items of information that should be documented.
o   Know the family health history conditions you should document.
o   Know the type of questions related to alcohol abuse, eg CAGE questions.
o   Know why we perform a review of systems.
o   Know examples of questions used during the review of systems.

3 – General Survey & Vital Signs

General Survey

Most narrative reports have a few introductory sentences at the beginning of the examination section that provide a general overview of the patient. These sentences cover elements such as:

Physical appearance
- Age
- Sex
- Level of consciousness
- Signs of distress

Body structure
- Apparent state of health
- Posture

Mobility
- Gait
- No involuntary movement

Behavior
- Mood and affect
- Dress
- Personal hygiene

Sample Documentation

Mrs. Jane Doe presents as a tall, thin, white female who is employed full time as an office manager. She is well groomed and appears younger than her stated age of 45. She is alert, oriented, and responds appropriately to questions. She is in no apparent distress and moves about without difficulty or abnormality of gait.

Vital Signs

Height *SHOULD BE TALLER IN THE MORNING. DISC'S SOAK UP FLUID*

- Height is usually recorded with shoes off. If not, subtract your estimate of heel thickness to obtain height without shoes, or record height as taken with shoes on.
- Quite often your patient will question the reading, *"That's not what my driver's license says."* Some loss of height is a normal consequence of aging, however unexpected loss of more than an inch of height suggests a vertebral body fracture. This highlights the importance of periodically measuring your patient's height.

Weight

- Weight is usually recorded with your patient in a gown, which weighs less than a pound. If you weigh your patient with street clothes on, have them remove any heavy coats, and record your findings appropriately, e.g. 130 pounds (dressed).
- Obesity is defined as greater than 120% of ideal body weight. Obesity increases the risk of hypertension, diabetes, and hyperlipidemia, each of which increases the risk for heart attack and stroke. If your patient is 20-30% overweight they have a 20-40% increased mortality risk, and if they are 50-60% overweight they have a 150-250% increased mortality risk.
- Body mass index is the calculated value of weight in kilograms divided by the square of height in meters. A BMI between 21-24 is normal. A BMI within 25-29 is considered to be overweight. A BMI greater than 30 is obese, and a BMI of greater than 40 is morbidly obese. On the other hand, if a person's BMI is between 18-20, they are underweight and if they are severely undernourished, the BMI is less than 16. When using pounds and inches the formula is:

$$(weight \times 703) / (height \times height)$$

- A quick and efficient way to assess body fat status is with infrared body fat testing (http://www.futrex.com). From a practice management point of view, gadgets are good. While the main purpose is to provide additional diagnostic information, they have the added benefit of helping to promote your practice. You should strive to deliver services over and above the 'average' chiropractor. If you practice just like every other DC in your community, why should a patient choose your service, versus an office that might be closer to their home?

Temperature

- Oral temperature is easy to take, with either an electronic or glass mercury thermometer. Rectal temperature is reserved for cases when the patient might bite the thermometer, such as with infants or unconscious patients. The newer tympanic thermometers have many advantages. They work in just a few seconds, and because the ear canal is not a mucous membrane, there is less chance of cross contamination between patients.
- Some chiropractors do not measure the temperature directly. Instead they use the back of their fingers to assess temperature as NTT (normal to touch). However, with the low cost of tympanic thermometers which only take a few seconds, why take this short cut?
- Temperature is an indirect measurement of body metabolism. Increased temperature suggests inflammation or infection. Decreased body temperature may indicate a hypothyroid tendency.

Pulse

- Using the tips of your index and middle fingers, palpate the radial pulse near the styloid process of the radius. While looking at the second hand of a clock or your watch, count the number of beats. If the rhythm is regular, you may count for 15 seconds and multiply by 4. However, when the rhythm is not regular you should count for a full minute.
- When charting your findings we usually record three variables: rate, amplitude, and rhythm. This might translate as: "*Pulse was 60, strong, and regular.*"
- Normal pulse for an adult is 60-100. Values lower than 60 are considered bradycardia, and values over 100 are tachycardia.
- In patients with a fast heart rate, counting the apical heart rate is more accurate than the radial pulse rate. The radial apical pulse is a technique where one examiner listens to the apical heart rate while another examiner counts the radial pulse for 60 seconds. When the apical heart rate is greater, this is referred to as a pulse deficit, traditionally associated with extrasystole and atrial fibrillation.

Respiration

- To assess respiration, you should <u>not</u> announce, "*I need to check your breathing*", as this will undoubtedly alter the rate you are seeking to measure. While still holding the radial pulse, glance at the individual's chest and count each chest rise with full inspiration. Normal respiratory rate is 12-20. While it is acceptable to count for 15 seconds and multiply by 4, it is more precise if you count for 30 seconds and multiply by 2 to obtain the respiratory rate.

Blood Pressure

- When assessing blood pressure on a new patient, <u>first</u> take a palpatory systolic reading. With this rough estimate of the target systolic pressure, inflate the cuff to 20-30 mm Hg above the palpable systolic pressure. This graphic shows the relationship between the Korotkoff sounds and the phases of blood pressure. While deflating the cuff slowly (2 mm Hg per second is about right), use either the bell or diaphragm of your stethoscope to listen for the appearance of Korotkoff sounds (phase 1). As the cuff continues to deflate, listen for the sounds to muffle (phase 4), and then disappear (phase 5). Most of the time

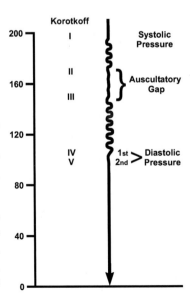

phases 4 and 5 occur almost simultaneously. If so, record only the lower number, e.g. 120/80. However, if there is more than a difference of 10 mm Hg, record both values, e.g. 160/90/78.

- The auscultatory gap is the loss and reappearance of the pulsatile sound while listening with the stethoscope during cuff deflation. It is caused by the vascular stiffness that results from atherosclerosis, and is seen primarily in the elderly. The possibility of a falsely low systolic pressure reading is the primary reason for taking a palpatory systolic reading prior to listening with the stethoscope. A summary of this phenomenon can be found in: <u>Ann Intern Med</u> 1996 May 15;124(10):877-83.

- Many factors can lead to blood pressure measurement errors, such as: 'white coat hypertension', the patient's back not supported, the arm not level with the heart, etc. However, probably the most important factor you must control for is the correct cuff size. You should have three cuffs to attach to your sphygmomanometer: pediatric, adult, and the extra large or thigh cuff. When in doubt, use a larger cuff. Other technique errors include wrapping the cuff too loosely, and deflating the cuff too fast or too slow.

- Pulse pressure is the difference between the systolic and diastolic pressure, normally about 40 mm Hg. Large differences, such as 80 mm Hg, may be caused by aortic regurgitation allowing blood to flow from the aorta back into the heart.

- All new patients should have blood pressure taken in both arms. If there is a difference of greater than 10-15 mm Hg in the systolic value, there may be arterial occlusion, such as a subclavian steal syndrome, on the side with the lower reading.

- <u>Pulsus paradoxus:</u> Due to decreased intrathoracic pressure, systolic pressure decreases during inspiration and increases during expiration. This difference is normally less than 10 mm Hg. If the fall during inspiration is greater than 10 mm Hg, this suggests constrictive pericarditis or emphysema.

- If postural hypotension is suspected, take supine, then standing blood pressure readings (Ragland's test). When you stand, your blood initially falls toward your legs. However, as your body senses this, your adrenal glands secrete epinephrine to constrict your blood vessels and compensate for this pooling of blood in your legs. As first described by Dr. Ragland, the normal test result is for blood pressure to rise 5-10 mm Hg when you stand up. At the very least your blood pressure should not fall. However, as the population becomes sicker, orthostatic hypotension is now defined as a systolic drop of greater than 20 mm Hg when moving from supine to standing.

- A diagnosis of hypertension is never made on the basis of a single reading. NIH guidelines are to take at least two readings on each of three separate days.

- If the systolic and diastolic readings place the individual in different severity of hypertension categories, your recommendations should be based upon the highest category.

The Seventh Report of the Joint National Committee on Prevention, Detection, Evaluation, and Treatment of High Blood Pressure (http://www.nhlbi.nih.gov/guidelines/hypertension/jncintro.htm) was released in 2003 with new categories and recommendations. First look at the previous 1997 guidelines: 140/90 = HYPERTENSION

Sixth JNC Blood Pressure Guidelines (1997)

Category	Systolic	Diastolic	Recommended follow-up
Optimum	< 120	< 80	None
Normal	< 130	< 85	recheck within 2 years
High normal	130-139	85-89	recheck within 1 year
Stage 1 hypertension	140-159	90-99	confirm within 2 months
Stage 2 hypertension	160-179	100-109	confirm or refer within 1 month
Stage 3 hypertension	= or > 180	= or > 110	refer immediately

Seventh JNC Blood Pressure Guidelines (2003)

Category	Systolic	Diastolic	Recommended follow-up
Normal	< 120	< 80	No antihypertensive drug indicated
Prehypertension	120-139	80-89	No antihypertensive drug indicated
Stage 1 hypertension	140-159	90-99	Thiazide-type diuretics for most
Stage 2 hypertension	= or > 160	= or > 100	Two-drug combination for most

While the new categories are indeed more simple and easy to remember, it is unfortunate that the guidelines are trending toward greater pharmaceutical intervention. For example, the Sixth report stated, "*A patient in Risk Group A with stage 1 hypertension (140-159 systolic and 90-99 diastolic) with no cardiovascular disease, organ damage, or other risk factors would try lifestyle changes for 1 year before taking drugs.*" Under the new guidelines these same individuals are now advised to take Thiazide diuretics. As a conservative health care doctor, you may want to consider using the 1997 recommendations as a safer guideline for your patients.

The Canadian recommendations for the management of hypertension can also be found online: http://www.cmaj.ca/cgi/reprint/161/12_suppl/s1.pdf

Sample Documentation

> Height: 68 inches
> Weight: 130 pounds
> Temperature: 98.8° F (tympanic)
> Pulse: 72
> Respiration: 16
> Blood Pressure: 132/80 L arm (sitting), 134/82 R arm (sitting), 130/78 R arm (supine)

Study Guide Objectives

o   Know the elements that comprise the general survey portion of the physical exam.
o   Know the importance of increased or decreased body temperature.
o   Know the advantages of the tympanic thermometer.
o   Know what variables are documented when recording the pulse.
o   Know the factors that lead to blood pressure measurement errors.
o   What is the significance of a large difference in blood pressure readings between the two arms?
o   Know how the Korotkoff sounds relate to the phases of blood pressure.
o   Know the cause and significance of the auscultatory gap.
o   Know the cause and significance of pulsus paradoxus.
o   Know the definition of orthostatic hypotension.
o   Know how to perform Ragland's test.
o   Know the NIH hypertension categories for: Normal, Stage 1 hypertension, and Stage 2 hypertension.

4 – Skin, Hair, and Nails

Anatomy & Physiology

The skin is the largest organ of the body, comprising about 20% of the body's weight. The primary function of the skin is to serve as a waterproof mechanical barrier that protects the underlying structures. This barrier serves to keep fluid within the body and microorganisms out. The skin is able to regulate body temperature by evaporation and conduction of heat from the body. The skin is richly supplied with sensory receptors that detect pain, temperature, touch, and pressure. The skin on the palms of the hands and soles of the feet is devoid of hair. These areas, referred to as glabrous skin, have greater tactile sensation than skin covered by hair. Another very important function is the ability of the skin to synthesize Vitamin D when exposed to sunlight. It is interesting to note that the chemical composition of sweat is similar to that of urine. When the body is toxic, the skin can provide an alternate route of excretion. While it is not strictly speaking a function of the skin, emotional states can manifest on the skin as blushing or blanching.

The skin is comprised of two layers, the epidermis and dermis, which rest upon a subcutaneous layer of adipose tissue, referred to as the hypodermis. The dermis forms about 95% of the skin thickness. This highly vascular layer contains the sweat glands, hair follicles, and nerve sensors. The dermis is comprised primarily of collagen which gives this connective tissue its tough elastic strength. The thin epidermis constitutes about 5% of the skin thickness. The epidermis is avascular and receives its nutrition from the underlying dermis. The lower basal cell layer of the epidermis is the stratum germinativum, which forms new cells. These cells are formed primarily from keratin, a tough fibrous protein. This layer also contains melanocytes which generate skin pigment. As the cells of the stratum germinativum migrate outward, they die and flatten out into a horny cell layer, the stratum corneum. This is a constant regenerative process, whereby the entire epidermis is shed and replaced every 3-4 weeks. Hair, sebaceous glands, eccrine and apocrine sweat glands, and nails are considered to be epidermal appendages, formed by epidermal cells that have invaginated into the dermis.

Nature of the Patient

Conditions such as impetigo, cradle cap, rubella, and rubeola are typically childhood infections. Acne vulgaris infection is usually associated with the teenage years. However, conditions such as psoriasis, lupus, scleroderma, dermatitis herpetiformis, pemphigus vulgaris, and skin cancer are usually considered chronic degenerative disease and thus rare in children. Many autoimmune disorders such as lupus, scleroderma, and dermatomyositis are more common in women.

Key History Questions

Do you have a history of previous skin problems?

- It is always important to learn what previous skin problems the individual has experienced and how the conditions were treated. Of special importance is family history, as many common skin conditions, such as eczema and psoriasis have genetic tendencies.

Have you noticed any recent changes in your skin?

- Pruritis – Itching can be caused by a number of underlying conditions, such as dry skin, allergies, drug reactions, and pest infestation.
- Rashes – Many skin conditions present with erythema or an inflamed red skin discoloration.
- Changes in a mole – Fifty percent of malignant melanoma arises from melanocytes contained in moles. This is why it is so important that changes in a mole be thoroughly investigated.
- Sores that don't heal – Skin lesions that do not heal are indicative of an underlying immune or vascular insufficiency.

Where are the lesions located?

- While eczema manifests at flexural and intertriginous surfaces, psoriasis tends to affect extensor surfaces. Acne occurs primarily on the face, neck, and upper back. Seborrheic dermatitis is a condition of the face and scalp. Pityriasis rosea manifests primarily on the torso. Obviously, sunburn and skin cancer are more likely in sun exposed areas.

What medications are you taking?

- In addition to causing urticaria or contact skin reactions, many medications can trigger a phototoxic sunburn-like reaction upon sunlight exposure.

Have you experienced recent hair loss or changes in hair consistency?

- While hair loss is common in aging males, dramatic changes in hair can be a sign of poor health status.
- Changes in hair consistency, either thick and coarse, or fine and thin, may indicate thyroid dysfunction.

Have you noticed any changes in your fingernails or toenails?

- According to <u>Bedside Physical Diagnosis</u> by DeGowin & DeGowin, "*With the exception of the eye, there is no region of comparable size in the body in which so many physical signs of generalized disease can be found."*

Examination

A chiropractor typically treats his or her patient on a more frequent basis than the MD and we usually observe the skin during the course of treatment. As such, we may be the first health care professional to observe a suspicious skin lesion. The health of the skin is a good indicator of the general health status of the individual, and many skin conditions respond to conservative nutritional and chiropractic care.

Skin conditions can manifest several different characteristics at once. However, for classification purposes, lesions are considered:

- Primary – arising from previously healthy skin.
- Secondary – resulting from a change in the primary lesion, such as from scratching or an infection.

Primary skin lesions

- Macule – a flat, nonpalpable spot < 1 cm diameter, e.g. freckle.
- Patch – a macule > 1 cm diameter, e.g. café au lait spot.
- Papule – a palpable, elevated bump < 1 cm diameter, e.g. mole.
- Nodule – a papule 1-2 cm diameter, e.g. small lipoma.
- Tumor – a nodule > 2 cm diameter. Strictly speaking, a tumor may be benign or malignant. However, to the lay person a tumor equals cancer, so be cautious about using this term in front of your patient.
- Vesicle – a palpable, fluid filled bump < 1 cm diameter, e.g. herpes simplex.
- Bulla – a vesicle > 1 cm diameter, e.g. blister.
- Pustule – a vesicle that is filled with pus, e.g. acne.
- Cyst – similar to a pustule, but typically larger and deeper, e.g. sebaceous cyst.
- Plaque – a flat, plateau-like, slightly elevated lesion, e.g. psoriasis.
- Wheal – a temporary elevation of the skin due to edema, e.g. insect bite, urticaria (hives).

Secondary skin lesions

- Crust – a dried residue of blood or pus, e.g. scab, impetigo.
- Scale – flakes of exfoliated skin, e.g. psoriasis, dandruff.
- Fissure – a linear crack that extends into the dermis, e.g. athlete's foot.
- Erosion – erosion of part of the epidermis, usually moist but not bleeding and heals without scarring, e.g. ruptured vesicle.

- Ulcer – like an erosion, but deeper into the dermis, may bleed, and heals with a scar, e.g. decubitus pressure ulcer or 'bed sore'.
- Excoriation – a superficial abrasion, often the result of scratching an intense itch, e.g. scratching with chicken pox.
- Lichenification – prolonged scratching may cause the epidermis to become rough and thickened, similar to a plaque, e.g. atopic dermatitis.
- Scar – when an injury to the dermis heals it is replaced by fibrotic connective tissue. Scars are initially thin and pink, later they are pale and atrophic, e.g. striae, healed surgery scar.
- Keloid – a hypertrophic elevated scar, e.g. some burns form keloids.
- Induration – sclerosis or hardening of tissue, e.g. scleroderma.
- Maceration – softened epidermis due to prolonged moist conditions, e.g. otitis externa (swimmer's ear).

Vascular skin lesions

- Petechiae – small hemorrhages < .5 cm diameter, e.g. intravascular defect such as idiopathic thrombocytopenia (ITP).
- Purpura – hemorrhages > .5 cm diameter. When purpura is caused by trauma it is referred to as ecchymosis, e.g. bruise.
- Telangiectasia – fine, irregular red lines due to dilated capillaries, e.g. spider angioma.

Pattern of skin lesions

- Annular – circular or ring shaped, e.g. ringworm.
- Target – also referred to as iris, circle within a circle, e.g. erythema multiforme.
- Confluent – lesions that run together, e.g. urticaria.
- Gyrate – also referred to as serpiginous, or snakelike, e.g. cutaneous larva migrans.
- Zosteriform – forms a linear pattern along a nerve dermatome, e.g. shingles.
- Intertriginous – found between folds of skin, e.g. athlete's foot.

Common Skin Conditions

Sebaceous and apocrine disorders

Acne vulgaris (ICD: 706.1)

A common inflammatory disease of the pilosebaceous glands characterized by comedones, papules, pustules, inflamed nodules, superficial pus-filled cysts, and (in extreme cases) canalizing and deep, inflamed, sometimes purulent sacs. (Merck Manual, p. 811)

- Acne is a very common condition affecting approximately 70% of the population. It is most common after puberty affecting an estimated 30% of teenagers. The lesions are found on the face, back, and chest. Accumulations of sebum within the pores are referred to as comedones. Initially the comedones are closed and present a whitehead appearance. As the pores open and become filled with dark material they are called blackheads. While comedones are noninflammatory, the lesions may become inflammatory if they progress to pustules or cysts. Conservative treatment should be directed to keeping the skin clean and avoiding the buildup of excessive sebum. Topical application of benzoyl peroxide or tea tree oil can limit bacterial overgrowth. Dietary changes should include avoiding refined carbohydrates and supplementation with vitamin A.

Rosacea (ICD: 695.3)

A chronic inflammatory disorder, usually beginning in middle age or later and characterized by telangiectasia, erythema, papules, and pustules primarily in the central areas of the face. (Merck Manual, p. 813)

- While rosacea has been called acne rosacea, it is unrelated to acne and has a different presentation. Rather than teenagers, this condition affects primarily females in the 30 to 50 year age range. Because it affects individuals of Northern European ancestry, it has been called the *'curse of the Celts'*. While there may be pustules, there are no comedones, and erythema and telangiectasia are more common. Marked hyperplasia of the nose (rhinophyma) may occur. Avoidance of factors that contribute to facial flushing (alcohol, spicy foods, and excessive heat or sun) may help to limit outbreaks.

Hydradenitis suppurativa (ICD: 706.9)

Painful local inflammation of the apocrine glands resulting in obstruction and rupture of the ducts. (Merck Manual, p. 800)

- The apocrine glands are specialized sweat glands located primarily in the axilla, groin, and genital region. These glands favor the growth of bacteria which create the characteristic odor of perspiration. When comedones or pustules manifest in these regions, hydradenitis suppurativa should be suspected. A 'double comedone' lesion, a large blackhead with two or more surface openings, is characteristic. These lesions may require surgical incision and drainage.

Eczema and urticaria

Eczema (ICD: 691.8)

Chronic, pruritic, superficial inflammation of the skin, frequently associated with a personal or family history of allergic disorders (eg, hay fever, asthma). (Merck Manual, p. 788)

- Eczema is also known as atopic dermatitis. Atopy refers to an inherited or genetically caused state of hypersensitivity. The lesions display erythema, edema, and intense itching (pruritis). The condition typically progresses to the formation of weeping vesicles and superficial scaling desquamation. Eczema usually begins in infancy and many of these children also have a history of asthma. In infancy the lesions usually manifest on the face or scalp. In later life the distribution of the lesions tends to favor flexural surfaces, such as the antecubital and popliteal fossae. Nutritional management of food allergies may be the key to providing symptomatic relief.

Contact dermatitis (ICD: 692.9)

Acute or chronic inflammation, often asymmetric or oddly shaped, produced by substances contacting the skin and causing toxic (irritant) or allergic reactions. (Merck Manual, p. 786)

- Contact dermatitis appears similar to eczema, but is caused by a cutaneous reaction to an external substance, such as poison ivy. The condition can occur at any age and is more common in families with a history of allergy. The main treatment is avoidance of the allergenic substance.

Urticaria (ICD: 708.0)

Urticaria is local wheals and erythema in the superficial dermis. Angioedema is a deeper swelling due to edematous areas in the deep dermis and subcutaneous tissue and may also involve mucous membranes. (Merck Manual, p. 1054)

- Urticaria or hives is a transient (usually less than 24 hours) edema reaction to a substance, such as ingestion of a drug or an allergic food. The condition is relatively common affecting about one-quarter of the population at some point in their life. Urticaria is more common in atopic individuals. When stroking the skin causes a wheal surrounded by intense erythema, this is referred to as Darier's sign. Dermatographism is considered to be a variant manifestation of urticaria. When larger areas of the dermis and subcutaneous tissue are affected, the condition is referred to as angioedema. Again treatment must be directed at avoiding the allergen. Severe cases of angioedema may require medical intervention with antihistamines or corticosteroids.

Psoriasis and other papulosquamous disorders

Psoriasis (ICD: 696.1)

A common chronic, recurrent disease characterized by dry, well-circumscribed, silvery, scaling papules and plaques of various sizes. (Merck Manual, p. 816)

- Psoriasis is caused by too rapid replication of epidermal cells. This accumulation of cells manifests as silvery scales on a red plaque. It tends to run in families, usually manifesting in the 20-40 age range. Koebner's phenomenon refers to formation of lesions at the site of physical trauma. As such, psoriasis lesions are much more common on the extensor surfaces of the knees and elbows. Auspitz sign refers to pinpoint areas of bleeding when the scales are picked off. While psoriasis has a strong genetic component, sunlight and nutritional supplementation with vitamin D and EPA fish oil has documented benefit. Bowel detoxification and liver support are also indicated.

Seborrheic dermatitis (ICD: 690.10)

An inflammatory scaling disease of the scalp, face, and occasionally other areas. (Merck Manual, p. 789)

- Seborrheic dermatitis is a relatively common condition, affecting about 5% of the population. It manifests primarily in areas of greater sebaceous activity: scalp, face, and intertriginous body fold regions. The lesions are similar to eczema, but the scaling may have a greasy consistency. As with most conditions, the cause is multifactorial, however a yeast, *Pityrosporum ovale* is usually present. On the scalp of adults seborrhea causes dandruff. When it occurs in infants, it is referred to as 'cradle cap'. Medical treatment may involve antifungal creams or shampoo that contains selenium (Selsun blue). Nutritional supplementation with B vitamins, especially biotin, B6, folic acid, and B12 has documented benefit.

Pityriasis rosea (ICD: 696.3)

A mild inflammatory skin disease of unknown cause characterized by scaly lesions and a self-limited course. (Merck Manual, p. 818)

- Pityriasis rosea initially manifests as a 'herald patch', a 2-10 cm salmon colored oval lesion on the trunk. About one week later, a pattern of multiple smaller scaling plaques appear. The lesions may itch and have white 'bran-like' scales. The condition is self-limiting and resolves in 1-2 months. Calamine lotion or corticosteroid cream may help when the itching is severe.

Lichen planus (ICD: 697.0)

A recurrent, pruritic, inflammatory eruption characterized by small discrete polygonal flat-topped violaceous papules that may coalesce into rough scaly patches, often accompanied by oral lesions. (Merck Manual, p. 819)

- Lichen planus is an itching hyperkeratosis of unknown etiology. The lesions are most common on the wrists, shins, and mouth. The irregular polyangular papules are flat topped, violaceous, and crisscrossed with white lines (Wickham's striae). The condition is usually self-limiting within 8-12 months. Symptomatic treatment may include antihistamines and corticosteroid creams.

Ichthyosis vulgaris (ICD: 757.1)

Dry skin. (Merck Manual, p. 831)

- Ichthyosis vulgaris is characterized by dry skin (xerosis) resembling fish scale, hence the name ichthyosis. This autosomal dominant genetic condition usually appears in early childhood. The lesions, most common on the shins, spare the flexor surfaces and intertriginal regions. The condition typically improves in humid climates and as the child ages. Applying lanolin containing lotion after bathing helps the skin to retain moisture.

Vesicular and bullous diseases

Dermatitis herpetiformis (ICD: 694.0)

A chronic eruption characterized by clusters of intensely pruritic vesicles, papules, and urticaria-like lesions. (Merck Manual, p. 830)

- Dermatitis herpetiformis, first described in 1884 by Louis Duhring, is sometimes referred to as Duhring's disease. The condition manifests as pruritic vesicles on the trunk and extensor surfaces. It is rare in children and favors males over females in a 2:1 ratio. Dermatitis herpetiformis is associated with gluten sensitive enteropathy. As such, treatment must include a gluten free diet.

Pemphigus vulgaris (ICD: 694.4)

An uncommon, potentially fatal autoimmune skin disorder characterized by intraepidermal bullae and extensive erosions on apparently healthy skin and mucous membranes. (Merck Manual, p. 829)

- Pemphigus vulgaris is a rare autoimmune disorder that can be fatal if untreated. The condition is characterized by blisters on the trunk and upper legs which rupture easily. This fragility is demonstrated by Nikolsky's sign: pressure on intact blisters causes the fluid to expand the blister laterally. The condition manifests primarily in the 40-60 year age range and is more common in Jewish ancestry. The trunk lesions are usually preceded by oral lesions. Management of this life threatening condition usually requires presnisone.

Bacterial infections

Impetigo (ICD: 684)

Impetigo (impetigo contagiosa) is a superficial vesiculopustular skin infection. Ecthyma is an ulcerative form of impetigo. (Merck Manual, p. 2319)

- Impetigo is a common bacterial infection that manifests primarily in children as honey yellow crusted vesicles on the face. The infective organism is usually *Staphylococcus aureus* which is part of the 'normal flora' of the nasal passages. When the condition is caused by Group A beta-hemolytic streptococcus, the child is at risk for a concomitant acute glomerulonephritis infection. The condition usually responds to over the counter triple antibiotic ointment. Streptococcal infections may require oral antibiotics.

Folliculitis (ICD: 704.8)

Superficial or deep bacterial infection and inflammation of the hair follicles, usually caused by S. aureus *but occasionally caused by other organisms such as* P. aeruginosa *(hot-tub folliculitis).* (Merck Manual, p. 799)

- Folliculitis is inflammation of a hair follicle. *Staphylococcus aureus* is the usual infective organism. Shaving may cause superficial trauma that initiates the infection. When this occurs, the individual should refrain from shaving until the infection resolves.

Furuncles and carbuncles (ICD: 680.9)

Furuncles: *Acute, tender, perifollicular inflammatory nodules resulting from infection by staphylococci.* (Merck Manual, p. 799)

Carbuncles: *A cluster of furuncles with subcutaneous spread of staphylococcal infection, resulting in deep suppuration, often extensive local sloughing, slow healing, and a large scar.* (Merck Manual, p. 800)

- When folliculitis spreads from the hair follicle into the surrounding dermis, this is a furuncle, more commonly called a boil. A carbuncle is a deeper infection comprised of a group of connected furuncles. Warm moist compresses may help to bring the infection to a head, allowing drainage of the infectious material. More severe lesions that are not responsive to conservative care may require surgical incision and drainage.

Cellulitis (ICD: 682.9)

Diffuse, spreading, acute inflammation within solid tissues, characterized by hyperemia, WBC infiltration, and edema without cellular necrosis or suppuration. (Merck Manual, p. 794)

- Cellulitis is a diffuse infection of the dermis and subcutaneous tissue, characterized by edema, erythema, and pain. Group A beta-hemolytic streptococcus is the usual infective organism. This condition may be caused by trauma, or it may be a manifestation of an underlying blood borne infection. Erysipelas, also known as St. Anthony's fire, is an acute, inflammatory form of cellulitis with a lymphatic infection, manifesting as a red streak. When infants develop a systemic *Staphylococcus aureus* infection, the diffuse erythema and exfoliative dermatitis are referred to as 'scalded skin syndrome'. Severe cellulitis may require hospitalization with IV antibiotics.

Scarlet fever (ICD: 034.1) (Merck Manual, p. 1152)

- Scarlet fever, which occurs primarily in children, is uncommon since the advent of antibiotics. When a group A beta-hemolytic streptococcus infection becomes systemic, it may manifest erythema and punctate petechiae on the skin. When the lesions occur in a body fold, the linear red streak is referred to as Pastia's lines. In addition to the skin rash, the child may manifest a bright red tongue with prominent papillae, or 'strawberry tongue'. Medical management is usually oral penicillin.

Sexually transmitted infections

Gonorrhea (ICD: 098.0)

Infection of the epithelium of the urethra, cervix, rectum, pharynx, or eyes by Neisseria gonorrhoeae, *which may lead to bacteremia and result in metastatic complications.* (Merck Manual, p. 1324)

- In addition to causing inflammatory lesions in the genital tract, untreated systemic gonorrhea can manifest arthralgia, tenosynovitis, and hemorrhagic pustules on the arms and legs.

Syphilis (ICD: 094.0)

A contagious systemic disease caused by the spirochete Treponema pallidum, *characterized by sequential clinical stages and by years of latency.* (Merck Manual, p. 1327)

- Primary syphilis manifests as a painless ulcer (chancre) at the site of initial contact. If the initial infection is not treated, the spirochetes spread via the bloodstream to every part of the body. Secondary syphilis manifests a variety of findings including arthralgia, photophobia, and a skin rash, particularly on the palms of the hands and soles of the feet. These skin lesions may mimic a variety of other skin disorders, such as pityriasis rosea or an allergic drug reaction. The moist, flat, pink lesions of secondary syphilis are referred to as condyloma lata.

Lymphogranuloma venereum (ICD: 099.1)

A sexually transmitted chlamydial disease characterized by a transitory primary lesion followed by suppurative lymphadenitis and lymphangitis and serious local complications. (Merck Manual, p. 1336)

- Lymphogranuloma venereum is a sexually transmitted disease caused by *Chlamydia trachomatis*. The primary stage is characterized by superficial painless ulcers on the genitals. As the condition progresses to the secondary stage it manifests painful enlargement of the inguinal lymph nodes.

Molluscum contagiosum (ICD: 078.0)

A poxvirus infection characterized by skin-colored, smooth, waxy, umbilicated papules 2 to 10 mm in diameter. (Merck Manual, p. 811)

- Molluscum contagiosum is caused by a DNA poxvirus, similar to the smallpox virus. While the transmission is usually via sexual contact in adults, the condition can manifest in children on the face, trunk, and extremities. The lesions manifest as multiple flesh colored papules that are centrally umbilicated. While the condition is self-limiting, cryosurgery may used to remove the lesions. The individual should avoid scratching the lesions, which may spread the infection to other areas of the body.

Condyloma acuminata (genital warts) (ICD: 078.11)

Hyperplastic lesions of the skin or mucous membranes of the genitalia caused by human papillomaviruses. (Merck Manual, p. 1338)

- Condyloma acuminata are soft flesh colored genital warts caused by the human papilloma virus (HPV). In females this infection is of concern as it is the same virus implicated in cervical cancer. Management may include cryosurgery. While the condition usually resolves without treatment in a few months, recurrence is common.

Kaposi's sarcoma (ICD: 176.9)

A multicentric vascular neoplasm caused by herpesvirus type 8 that has three forms: indolent, lymphadenopathic, and AIDS-related. (Merck Manual, p. 846)

- Kaposi's sarcoma is a malignant skin lesion usually associated with HIV infection. The lesions manifest as purple red macules that may progress to plaques. There is no cure for Kaposi's sarcoma. Treatment is given to improve the quality of life for the remaining lifespan.

Viral infections

Verruca (warts) (ICD: 078.10)

Common, contagious, epithelial tumors caused by at least 60 types of human papillomavirus. (Merck Manual, p. 808)

- Verruca or warts are benign skin lesions caused by an HPV infection of keratinocytes. Initially the lesions are smooth and flesh colored, which progress to a gray-brown domed lesion with black dots on the surface. The lesions are most common on the hands, elbows, and knees. When the lesions occur on the soles of the feet, they are referred to as plantar warts. While most warts disappear spontaneously without treatment, preparations such as Compound W may speed remission.

Herpes simplex (ICD: 771.2)

An infection with herpes simplex virus characterized by one or many clusters of small vesicles filled with clear fluid on slightly raised inflammatory bases. (Merck Manual, p. 1293)

- Herpes simplex in the oral region is referred to as herpes labialis, also known as a 'cold sore' or 'fever blister'. In the genital region, the lesions are referred to as herpes genitalis. In general, oral herpes is caused by HSV1, and genital herpes is caused by HSV2. The condition manifests as a painful cluster of vesicles on an erythematous base. After several days, the vesicles burst and form a red healing scab. Antiviral medication or nutritional supplementation may shorten the duration of the lesions.

Varicella (chickenpox) (ICD: 052.9)

An acute viral infection, usually beginning with mild constitutional symptoms that are followed shortly by an eruption appearing in crops and characterized by macules, papules, vesicles, and crusting. (Merck Manual, p. 2330)

- Varicella or chickenpox is a highly contagious viral infection that occurs primarily in children. The incubation period is about 2 weeks. During this prodromal period the child may experience malaise, headache, anorexia, and fever. The initial rash begins on the trunk and spreads to the face and extremities. Within a few hours the rash progresses to red papules that become umbilicated vesicles. The infectious period slightly precedes the appearance of the rash and continues until the lesions crust over. The lesions are very pruritic and calamine lotion may help control itching. While the child will have lifetime immunity to chickenpox, the virus remains dormant in spinal and cranial nerve ganglia and may manifest as shingles in later life.

Herpes zoster (shingles) (ICD: 053.9)

An infection with varicella-zoster virus primarily involving the dorsal root ganglia and characterized by vesicular eruption and neuralgic pain in the dermatome of the affected root ganglia. (Merck Manual, p. 1294)

- Herpes zoster or shingles is caused by reactivation of the varicella virus, most commonly after age 55. The lesions which are similar to the vesicles of herpes simplex, appear along a spinal or cranial nerve dermatome. While the lesions usually clear within a few weeks, post herpetic neuralgia may last for months to years.

Rubella (German measles) (ICD: 056.9)

A contagious exanthematous viral infection, usually with mild constitutional symptoms, that may result in abortion, stillbirth, or congenital defects in infants born to mothers infected during the early months of pregnancy. (Merck Manual, p. 2327)

- Rubella, also known as German measles, is a benign childhood infection caused by a RNA virus. Toward the end of the 2-3 week incubation period, the prodromal period is usually mild consisting of malaise, headache, and lymphadenopathy. The pink to red macules and papules begin on the face and neck and quickly spread to the trunk and extremities. The lesions resolve in three days, which is why rubella is also called 'three day measles'. Rubella is differentiated from rubeola by milder symptoms and the absence of Koplik's spots. If a pregnant woman becomes infected with rubella during her first trimester, her child is at risk for birth defects.

Rubeola (measles) (ICD: 055.9)

A highly contagious, acute viral infection characterized by fever, cough, coryza, conjunctivitis, enanthem (Koplik's spots) on the buccal or labial mucosa, and a spreading maculopapular cutaneous rash. (Merck Manual, p. 2320)

- Rubeola or measles is a paramyxovirus infection spread via respiratory droplets. It is a more serious condition than rubella, with a shorter incubation period (1-2 weeks) and longer lasting infection ('nine day measles'). During the prodromal period the only diagnostic feature may be Koplik's spots: tiny white spots on the buccal mucosa. Other prodromal symptoms may be cough, coryza, conjunctivitis, and photophobia. The maculopapular rash typically begins near the ears and spreads to the trunk and extremities in 1-2 days. At the peak of the infection, the fever may exceed 104° F. Treatment is primarily symptomatic to comfort the child. However, in third world countries having poor nutrition and sanitation, measles is often life threatening with 1-10% mortality, causing 1.5 million deaths per year.

Fungal infections

Candidiasis (moniliasis) (ICD: 112.9)

Infections of skin (usually of moist, occluded, intertriginous areas), skin appendages, or mucous membranes caused by yeasts of the genus Candida. (Merck Manual, p. 804)

- Candida albicans is part of the normal flora of oral, vaginal, and intestinal mucous membranes. When the balance of normal flora is altered, usually as a consequence of antibiotic medication, an abnormal overgrowth of candida can occur. When this occurs in the mouth, the white plaques are referred to as thrush. In the vaginal region, the infection appears as a white cheesy discharge. Candida does not normally grow on intact skin. However, when the skin is warm and moist, such as in intertriginous areas or an infant in diapers, candida infection can take hold. Cutaneous candidiasis manifests as erythema, papules, and marginal scaling. Treatment is directed at keeping the area clean and dry, and possibly the use of antifungal creams.

Tinea versicolor (ICD: 111.0)

An infection characterized by multiple, usually asymptomatic, scaly patches varying from white to brown and caused by Pityrosporum orbiculare. (Merck Manual, p. 805)

- Tinea versicolor is also called pityriasis versicolor because it is caused by the *Pityrosporum orbiculare* yeast. The lesions are small round macules manifesting primarily on the upper trunk. The color of the lesions will vary with the individual's skin color: light brown on untanned skin, white on tanned skin, and may be either hypopigmented or hyperpigmented on dark skinned individuals. While the condition usually resolves without treatment, selenium containing shampoo applied to the skin for 20 minutes a day for one week may hasten healing. Unfortunately, recurrences are common.

Dermatophyte (tinea) infections (ICD: 110.9)

Infections caused by dermatophytes–fungi that invade only dead tissues of the skin or its appendages (stratum corneum, nails, hair). (Merck Manual, p. 802)

- Tinea is a fungal skin infection with three common molds: *Microsporum, Trichophyton,* and *Epidermophyton.* The lesions, commonly referred to as 'ringworm', manifest as a flat, scaly, inflamed spot with a raised border. As the border spreads outward in a ringlike fashion, the center becomes hypopigmented. The infection is named for the region of the body affected:

  tinea corporis = body
  tinea capitus = scalp
  tinea barbae = beard
  tinea manuum = hands
  tinea unguium = nails
  tinea cruris = 'jock itch'
  tinea pedis = 'athlete's foot'

The individual should avoid scratching which can spread the infection. Treatment includes keeping the area clean and dry and topical application of antifungal creams (Lotrimin, Desenex, etc.).

Infestations and insect bites

Scabies (ICD: 133.0)

A transmissible ectoparasite infection, characterized by superficial burrows, intense pruritus, and secondary infection. (Merck Manual, p. 806)

- Scabies is an infestation with the *Sarcoptes scabiei* mite. It is transmitted by direct contact, such as sexual contact or contact with infected clothing or bed linens. The mite burrows underneath the skin creating a tan or skin colored ridge with a small papule or vesicle at the end of the burrow. The females lay eggs in the burrows which hatch in 3-4 days. At times the burrows are not visible, but the individual manifests secondary erythema and scaling from scratching due to intense itching, especially at night when the female mites are burrowing. The lesions are typically found in the groin area, hands, feet, and intertriginous regions. Treatment is with medicated shampoo and lotion (Kwell). Other family members may also need treatment, and clothing and bed linens should be washed in hot water to prevent reinfection.

Pediculosis (lice) (ICD: 132.2)

Infestation by lice. (Merck Manual, p. 807)

- Pediculosis, commonly referred to as 'crabs', is infestation with lice. In adults, *Pediculosis pubis* is the most common form, while *Pediculosis capitis* is more common in children. Infestation on the body is *Pediculosis corporis.* The lice lay eggs which are cemented to the hair shaft, referred to as 'nits'. The lice may be difficult to visualize as they move to evade detection. The skin may manifest excoriated areas due to the individual scratching the intense itch. Treatment requires a permethrin or pyrethrin shampoo. Unfortunately, Kwell shampoo may no longer work as the lice have evolved resistance to this medication.

Cutaneous larva migrans (ICD: 126.9) (Merck Manual, p. 808)

- Cutaneous larva migrans, seen most often in the feet, is caused by infestation with a nematode, commonly referred to as hookworm. The larvae enter the skin when the individual walks in infected sand or soil. As the hookworm migrates underneath the skin it creates the characteristic snakelike or serpiginous red lesion. While the condition is self-limiting and the organism will die in 2-8 weeks, antihelmintic drugs may be used to speed this process. Topical steroids may be needed to control the itching.

Lyme disease (ICD: 088.81)

A tick-transmitted, spirochetal, inflammatory disorder causing a rash (erythema [chronicum] migrans) that may be followed weeks to months later by neurologic, cardiac, or joint abnormalities. (Merck Manual, p. 1189)

- Lyme disease is a multisystem infection caused by *Borrelia burgdorferi*, a spirochete that is transmitted via a bite from a deer tick. At the site of the tick bite a red papule forms with an expanding annular ring and an area of central clearing. During stage I – localized infection, the individual may experience flu like symptoms in addition to the skin rash. Months after the bite, the infection may progress to stage II – disseminated infection. In this stage, the individual may show multiple smaller annular lesions as well as other symptoms such as heart irregularities, headaches, and arthritic joint pain. If the condition progresses to stage III – persistent infection, the individual may display generalized erythema and experience chronic arthritic joint pains and possibly neurologic symptoms (paresthesia, radicular pain, and mood, memory, or sleep changes). Treatment such as tetracycline or amoxicillin is most effective when begun in the early stages of the infection.

Rocky Mountain spotted fever (ICD: 082.0)

An acute febrile disease caused by Rickettsia rickettsii *and transmitted by ixodid ticks, producing high fever, cough, and rash.* (Merck Manual, p. 1230)

- Rocky Mountain spotted fever is a systemic illness caused by a tick that transmits rickettsial bacteria. While the infection was first recognized in the Rocky Mountain States, the condition is most prevalent in Oklahoma, Tennessee, and North and South Carolina.

About one week after being bitten by the tick, the individual manifests a discrete, macular rash that blanches with pressure. Typically, the rash begins on the wrists and then spreads to the rest of the body. However, in about 15% of the cases no rash appears. Treatment is antibiotic medication. This is a serious infection. When untreated, the mortality rate is approximately 20%.

Autoimmune and connective tissue disorders

Lupus erythematosus (ICD: 695.4)

A chronic and recurrent disorder primarily affecting the skin and characterized by sharply circumscribed macules and plaques displaying erythema, follicular plugging, scales, telangiectasia, and atrophy. (Merck Manual, p. 430)

- Systemic lupus erythematosus or SLE is a chronic autoimmune inflammatory condition that affects many body systems, including the skin. Ninety percent of the cases occur in women, primarily in the 30-50 year age range. Skin manifestations include a malar or 'butterfly' rash on the upper face. With discoid lupus, when heavily scaled lesions on the body are removed, the underlying skin and hair follicle may present a 'carpet tack' appearance. Fever, photosensitivity, polyarthritis, and oral ulcers are common. Medical treatment is non-steroidal or steroid medication and protection from sunlight. Nutritional and lifestyle changes, such as management of allergies and correction of a 'leaky gut' syndrome provide many of these women symptom relief without taking the drugs.

Scleroderma (ICD: 710.1)

A chronic disease of unknown cause, characterized by diffuse fibrosis; degenerative changes; and vascular abnormalities in the skin (scleroderma), articular structures, and internal organs (especially the esophagus, GI tract, lung, heart, and kidney). (Merck Manual, p. 431)

- The word scleroderma literally means thickened or 'hard skin'. As with SLE, scleroderma is a connective tissue disorder that occurs primarily in women. Her face appears tight with thin lips and an apparent inability to show facial expressions. Many of these women manifest the CREST syndrome:

  Calcinosis cutis – calcium deposits in the skin that create firm subcutaneous nodules

  Raynaud's phenomenon – spasm of digital arteries which creates cold discolored fingers

  Esophageal dysfunction – tissue hardening may create lower esophageal scarring and stricture

Sclerodactyly – skin tightening can create tapering fingers
with tight, shiny skin

Telangiectasia – dilated blood vessels, especially on the
face, trunk, and hands

According to the Merck Manual, "*No drug can stop the progression of scleroderma.*" Nutritional and lifestyle changes are a much safer alternative to drug therapy of the patient's symptoms.

Dermatomyositis (ICD: 710.3)

Systemic connective tissue diseases characterized by inflammatory and degenerative changes in the muscles (polymyositis) and frequently also in the skin (dermatomyositis), leading to symmetric weakness and some muscle atrophy, principally of the limb girdles. (Merck Manual, p. 434)

- Dermatomyositis is essentially the skin manifestation of polymyositis. The lesions include a reddish purple rash (heliotrope) and edema around the eyelids, which may resemble the lupus 'butterfly' rash. These lesions may spread to the scalp, upper chest, and arms. If the individual manifests flat-topped violaceous papules on the knuckles, these are referred to as Gottron's papules. When polymyositis manifests, the individual may present with tenderness, weakness, and atrophy of the proximal upper and lower extremity muscles. As with any suspected muscle disease, serum CPK should be evaluated. Unfortunately, individuals with polymyositis are much more likely to have an associated malignancy of the breast, lung, ovary, or gastrointestinal system. Symptomatic management of polymyositis includes prednisone and methotrexate. Obviously, when an associated malignancy is found this requires comprehensive evaluation and treatment.

Neurofibromatosis (ICD: 237.71)

Autosomal dominant disorders designated type 1 (peripheral neurofibromatosis, von Recklinghausen's disease) and the rarer type 2 (central neurofibromatosis), which is characterized by bilateral acoustic neuromas. (Merck Manual, p. 1496)

- Neurofibromatosis, sometimes called von Recklinghausen's disease, is an inherited autosomal dominant condition that affects ectodermal tissue. The condition may be mild, manifesting only freckling and café au lait macules. When freckling occurs in the axilla or groin area, this is referred to as Crowe's sign. Examination of the iris may display Lisch nodules, pigmented spots that are melanocytic hamartomas. At times the condition becomes extremely disfiguring with pedunculated tumors and skeletal abnormalities, such as with 'the Elephant man'.

Treatment of this genetic condition is cosmetic: surgical removal of large tumors.

Erythema multiforme (ICD: 695.1)

An inflammatory eruption characterized by symmetric erythematous, edematous, or bullous lesions of the skin or mucous membranes. (<u>Merck Manual</u>, p. 824)

- Erythema multiforme is a relatively common hypersensitivity skin reaction. Many factors, such as infection, drugs, contact allergens, or autoimmune connective tissue disorders can initiate the lesions. A prodrome of fever, malaise, and itching or burning may precede eruption of the lesions. The lesions, typically on the hands or face, present as red to purple macules and papules with an iris or target pattern. A more advanced form of this condition is Stevens-Johnson syndrome, also called erythema multiforme major. Erythema multiforme is a self-limiting condition and usually resolves in one month without treatment. When an underlying infection is present, this must be treated appropriately.

Erythema nodosum (ICD: 695.2)

An inflammatory disease of the deep dermis and subcutaneous fat (panniculitis) characterized by tender red nodules, predominantly in the pretibial region but occasionally involving the arms or other areas. (<u>Merck Manual</u>, p. 825)

- Erythema nodosum is a hypersensitivity skin reaction to a variety of infections or allergens. The lesions manifest primarily on the limb extensor surfaces, especially the shins. Typically there is a prodrome of fever, malaise, and arthralgia for several weeks prior to the lesions appearing. The name erythema nodosum describes the lesions: they display a red, bruiselike appearance, but have a nodular consistency upon palpation. Again the lesions are self-limiting. However, an underlying infection may require treatment.

Hypersensitivity vasculitis (ICD: 287.0)

Inflammation of blood vessels, which is often segmental, may be generalized or localized and constitutes the basic pathogenetic process of various rheumatic diseases and syndromes. (<u>Merck Manual</u>, p. 437)

- Hypersensitivity vasculitis is inflammation and fibrosis of the postcapillary venules. The reaction may be triggered by drugs, infection, or occur with connective tissue diseases, such as RA, SLE, or Sjögren's syndrome. The lesions manifest as 'palpable purpura' on the legs, especially the shins. The lesions usually heal within one month without treatment, however the underlying cause must be treated appropriately.

- Other vasculitis syndromes include Kawasaki's disease, an acute multisystem vasculitis affecting primarily infants and children. Children with Kawasaki's disease typically manifest conjunctivitis, oral erythema, cervical lymphadenopathy, and cardiac abnormalities, in addition to desquamation on the hands and feet.
- Wegener's granulomatosis is a severe form of systemic vasculitis that may manifest skin lesions, in addition to lung and kidney pathology.
- Obstruction to arterial inflow or venous outflow in the skin may create a bluish or cyanotic discoloration in a netlike pattern, referred to as livedo reticularis.

Photosensitivity and pigmentary disorders

Phototoxic reaction (sunburn) (ICD: 692.71) (Merck Manual, p. 826)

- Sunburn is the inflammatory skin response to excessive exposure to ultraviolet radiation from the sun or an artificial light source. Sunburn manifests as erythema, edema, vesicles, and bullae. The tendency to sunburn is related to an individual's skin phototype (SPT). The paler the skin, the greater the risk:

SPT	Skin color	Response to sunlight
I	pale white	does not tan, burns easily
II	white	tans with difficulty, burns easily
III	white	tans after initial sunburn
IV	light brown	tans easily
V	brown	tans easily
VI	black	becomes darker

Repeated episodes of sunburn damage causes photoaging, or dermatoheliosis.

Photoallergic reaction (ICD: 692.72) (Merck Manual, p. 828)

- When an individual is taking medication, such as an antibiotic, this drug can produce a phototoxic byproduct when exposed to UVA sunlight. This photoproduct is what causes an eczematous dermatitis, similar to sunburn.

Hyperpigmentation (ICD: 709.00)

Abnormally increased pigmentation. (Merck Manual, p. 836)

- Café au lait spots are light brown macules, such as seen with neurofibromatosis.
- Solar lentigo are hyperpigmented macules caused by melanocyte hyperplasia. They typically occur during middle age in sun exposed

areas, such as the neck and back of the hands. The lay term for lentigo is 'liver spot'.

- Melasma manifests as facial hyperpigmentation, often in a malar pattern. Pregnancy is the most common cause of melasma, which is why it is sometimes referred to as the 'mask of pregnancy'. However, it can also occur in women who taking birth control pills. Typically, the lesion slowly fades after pregnancy or stopping birth control medication.

Hypopigmentation (ICD: 709.00)

A congenital or acquired decrease in melanin production. (<u>Merck Manual</u>, p. 835)

- Vitiligo is an inherited condition affecting approximately 1% of the population. The absence of melanocytes manifest as areas of skin depigmentation. Common sites include the hands, face, body folds, and genitalia. The lesions may manifest according to Koebner's phenomenon, at sites of previous trauma. Medical treatment may include repigmentation of vitiligo spots with photochemotherapy, or depigmentation of normal surrounding skin to achieve a uniform skin color.

- Albinism is a comparatively rare (1 in 20,000) genetic defect that impairs melanin synthesis. The individual has a normal amount of melanocytes, but the lack of melanin pigment produces white skin, yellow white hair, and the iris manifests an almost translucent pink eye color. Albinos must limit sun exposure, as they are at greatly increased risk of sunburn and skin cancer.

Benign skin tumors

Nevi (ICD: 631)

Circumscribed pigmented macules, papules, or nodules composed of clusters of melanocytes or nevus cells. (<u>Merck Manual</u>, p. 838)

- A nevus, more commonly know as a mole, is a benign skin tumor comprised of melanocytes. Nevi are very common, often present at birth. However, when nevi appear after age 30 it is important that they are examined, as about 50% of malignant melanoma develops from the melanocytes present in nevi.

Seborrheic keratosis (ICD: 702.19)

Pigmented superficial epithelial lesions that are usually warty but may occur as smooth papules. (<u>Merck Manual</u>, p. 841)

- Seborrheic keratosis is a benign epidermal lesion very common in later life. The lesion presents as a flat or slightly elevated accumulation of cells with a 'stuck on' appearance. The color is light brown to black with a 'greasy' appearance. Seborrheic keratosis does not require treatment, but may be removed for cosmetic purposes.

Skin tags (ICD: 757.39)

Common soft, small, flesh-colored or hyperpigmented pedunculated lesions, usually multiple and occurring mainly on the neck, axilla, and groin. (Merck Manual, p. 840)

- Skin tags, also referred to as acrochordons, are small flesh colored pedunculated papules. They are common, especially after age 30, and manifest primarily in the axilla and neck. Skin tags do not require treatment, but are often removed for cosmetic reasons. One treatment is to tie a fine thread tightly around the base of the polyp. This ligature cuts off the blood supply and the skin tag will atrophy and fall off.

Lipoma (ICD: 214.9)

Soft, movable, subcutaneous nodules with normal overlying skin. (Merck Manual, p. 840)

- A lipoma is a subcutaneous nodular accumulation of fat cells. It palpates with a rubbery, movable consistency. Lipomas are common and benign, requiring no treatment. When the nodule occurs in a bothersome location, such as the belt line or bra strap line, a minor surgery excision will provide relief.

Keloid (ICD: 706.1)

A smooth overgrowth of fibroblastic tissue that arises in an area of injury or, occasionally, spontaneously. (Merck Manual, p. 842)

- A keloid is a fibrotic overgrowth of scar tissue. Keloids are more common in African Americans and tend to be located in body regions where acne occurs. Surgical excision may not be a viable option, as it tends to initiate further keloid formation. Laser treatment or injection of the scar with corticosteroids has shown some success in helping to soften and flatten the lesion.

Malignant skin tumors

Basal cell carcinoma (ICD: M8090/1)

A superficial, eroding ulcer that derives from and resembles epidermal basal cells. (Merck Manual, p. 842)

- Basal cell carcinoma is the most common skin cancer and is malignant and aggressive. However, because it appears incapable of growing without the basal stroma, it rarely metastasizes. The lesions manifest primarily on the head and neck, especially the nose. It appears as a pink dome shaped papule with telangiectasic vessels on the surface. As the papule enlarges, the center flattens and may ulcerate and bleed, presenting a 'rodent ulcer'. This cancer should be surgically excised as soon as possible. With appropriate care, the cure rate approaches 99%.

Squamous cell carcinoma (ICD: M8070/3)

Cancers that arise from the malpighian cells of the epithelium and that usually occur on sun-exposed areas. (Merck Manual, p. 843)

- Squamous cell carcinoma is the second most common skin cancer, and develops when atypical squamous cell keratinocytes invade the epidermis and grow within the dermis. The lesions occur primarily in sun exposed areas (head, neck, and hands), and are most prevalent in skin phototypes I & II. Squamous cell carcinoma of the lip occurs primarily in smokers. The physical appearance of squamous cell carcinoma is variable. It may present as an irregular red or brown patch that develops a thick scale and friable surface which ulcerates. Alternatively, the tumor may be elevated, soft and moveable, with a red inflamed base. The *in situ* form of squamous cell carcinoma, referred to as Bowen's disease, presents as a solitary red scaling plaque. As with basal cell carcinoma, surgical excision is indicated and has a high cure rate when the cancer has not metastasized to a distant site.

Malignant melanoma (ICD: M8742/3)

A malignant melanocytic tumor arising in a pigmented area: skin, mucous membranes, eyes, and CNS. (Merck Manual, p. 843)

- Malignant melanoma is cancer of pigmented skin cells, the melanocytes. It is the most serious of all skin cancers, accounting for approximately 2% of all cancer deaths. The median age of onset is 53, with lesions manifesting primarily on the back and lower legs. All skin lesions should be evaluated using the ABCD guideline:

    A – Asymmetry (one half does not look like the other half)

    B – Border irregularity (scalloped or pseudopod)

    C – Color is varied (mixtures of black, brown, pink, gray, or white)

    D – Diameter greater than 6 mm (the size of a pencil eraser)

Suspicious skin lesions must be biopsied. Prognosis is based upon Clark's scale:

Level I	–	Confined to the epidermis (*in situ*)
Level II	–	Invasion into the papillary dermis
Level III	–	Invasion filling the papillary dermis

Level IV   –   Invasion of the reticular dermis

Level V   –   Invasion of the subcutaneous fat

The treatment is complete surgical excision of the lesion and the underlying dermis. Level I lesions have a 95% five year survival rate. However, individuals with level V lesions that have metastasized have less than 5% five year survival rate.

Vascular lesions

Spider angioma (ICD:) 448.1

A bright red, faintly pulsatile vascular lesion consisting of a central arteriole with slender projections resembling spider legs. (Merck Manual, p. 841)

- Spider angioma is a common benign condition that occurs in 10-15% of adults, usually women. Because the lesions occur most commonly in pregnant women, spider angioma are thought to be related to excess estrogen. The lesion presents as a central red papule with multiple telangiectasic capillaries radiating from the center. The condition usually resolves without treatment. However, if the individual desires for cosmetic reasons, it can be removed with laser treatment.

Venous lake (ICD: 448.9)

- A venous lake is essentially a capillary dilation, similar in appearance to a varicose vein. It appears as a dark blue or purple papule, most often on the lip or oral mucosa. The lesions do not resolve, however they can be removed for cosmetic reasons by laser or electrocautery.

Port wine stain (ICD: 757.32)

A flat pink, red, or purplish lesion present at birth. (Merck Manual, p. 840)

- A port wine stain is a 'birthmark', a flat, irregular, red patch, often found on the face. They do not disappear with the passage of time. They do not require treatment, but can be treated by laser for cosmetic reasons.

Hemangioma (ICD: 757.32)

A raised bright red vascular lesion consisting of proliferations of endothelial cells. (Merck Manual, p. 840)

- Hemangioma is a benign vascular tumor. They appear as a red to purple dome shaped nodule. Strawberry hemangioma are present at birth, often on the face, and usually disappear in early childhood. Cherry angioma, sometimes called senile hemangioma, are small red spots found on the trunk of many elderly adults. These spots do not resolve spontaneously. However, they can be removed for cosmetic reasons.

Hair disorders

Alopecia (ICD: 704.00)

Partial or complete loss of hair. (Merck Manual, p. 814)

- Alopecia is loss of hair. Androgenic alopecia, or male pattern baldness, is very common. By age 50 one-half of all males show some degree of hair loss. The most common pattern is M-shaped, where the hair recedes on the front and vertex of the head. No treatment is required for common baldness. However, the medication Minoxidil (Rogaine) does appear to stimulate hair regrowth. Alopecia areata is a patchy loss of hair in a circumscribed area. The cause is speculative and the hair usually regrows spontaneously in 1 to 3 months.

Hirsutism (ICD: 704.1)

Excessive hair growth. (Merck Manual, p. 814)

- Hirsutism is excessive growth of facial or body hair. When a woman has excessive production of androgenic hormones, this can stimulate the abnormal development of chest hair or a beard. While excessive body hair is not a serious condition, the underlying cause may be. Conditions such as an ovarian or adrenal tumor must be investigated. Hypertrichosis refers to excessive growth of hair in areas that are not androgen dependent.

Nail disorders

Nails are hard plates of keratin at the tips of the fingers and toes. In animals, the nails are claws that can be used as a weapon. In humans, fingernails aid in being able to pick up small objects. The nail plate is normally slightly translucent and shows a pink color from the underlying nail bed which is highly vascular. The proximal nail bed is the matrix where the nail is formed and grows out. The lanula is the white semilunar area of the nail plate overlying the matrix. The proximal nail fold is the cuticle that protects the matrix. The hyponychium is the area underneath the distal nail plate where the skin seals off the end of the nail bed. The fingernails and nailbeds display changes with a variety of infections and systemic illnesses:

Paronychia (ICD: 681.9)

Acute or chronic infection of the periungual tissues. (Merck Manual, p. 800)

- Paronychia is an infection of the nail fold near the cuticle, usually with *Staphlococcus aureus*. An ingrown toenail, often caused by improper nail trimming, is an example of paronychia.

Felon (ICD: 681.01)

*Infection of the pulp space of a phalanx. (*Merck Manual*, p. 495)*

- A felon is an infection of the pulp on the palmar surface of the finger pad. Because of the fibrous septa within the finger pad, these infections may form an abscess requiring incision and drainage.

Onychomycosis (ICD: 110.1) (Merck Manual, p. 803)

- Onychomycosis, or tinea unguium, is a fungal infection of the nail. It is very common, occuring to some degree in most elderly people. Nails with fungal infection usually have a yellow brown crumbling appearance.

Psoriatic nails (ICD: 696.1) (Merck Manual, p. 817)

- Psoriasis is a systemic condition, and up to 50% of psoriasis sufferers manifest psoriatic nail lesions. Onycholysis is separation of the nail from the underlying nail bed. In addition to manifesting onycholysis, psoriatic nails appear pitted with an 'oil staining' appearance of the nail and adjacent skin.

Digital clubbing (ICD: 781.5)

*Enlargement of the terminal digital phalanges with loss of the nail bed angle. (*Merck Manual*, p. 520)*

- When viewed from the side, the angle formed where the nail joins the cuticle is approximately 160 degrees. When an individual is hypoxic, such as with chronic heart or lung disease, the base of the nail becomes edematous and this angle increases to greater than 180 degrees. The finger pads also appear enlarged and swollen, and the nail manifests a downward curve toward the distal edge.

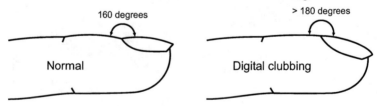

Longitudinal ridging (ICD: 703.9)

- Longitudinal ridging, parallel to the long axis of the finger, is a relatively common finding in the elderly, considered to be a normal variant. However, many nutritional doctors consider longitudinal ridging to represent a subclinical deficiency of hydrochloric acid, calcium, or zinc. Occasionally longitudinal brown streaks are seen under the nails. These streaks, caused by capillary bleeding under the nail, are referred to as 'splinter hemorrhages' and are classically associated with subacute bacterial endocarditis.

Beau's lines (transverse ridging) (ICD: 703.8)

- Beau's lines are transverse ridging or grooves parallel to the end of the nail. As the nail grows out from the matrix, illness or infection can impair nail growth which manifests as a transverse ridge. Typically Beau's lines affect multiple nails. If just one nail is affected, trauma to the matrix is a more likely cause, such as when the individual repetitively picks at the cuticle causing 'habit-tic dystrophy'.

Terry's nails (ICD: 703.9)

- The proximal white portion of the nail plate, the lanula, is normally narrow. When a patient has hypoalbuminemia, such as with liver failure, the nail bed becomes edematous, thus enlarging the lanula. This enlargement, leaving just a narrow band of pink at the distal nail, is referred to as Terry's nails.

Lindsay's nails (ICD: 703.9)

- Lindsay's nails appear similar to Terry's nails. They are also known as 'half-and-half' nails because the proximal half of the nail is white and the distal half is pink. Lindsay's nails are classically associated with uremia and chronic renal failure.

Koilonychia (ICD: 703.8) (Merck Manual, p. 858)

- Koilonychia is when the nail becomes thin and curves upward in a spoon-like fashion. This condition is classically associated iron deficiency anemia.

Study Guide Objectives

o Know the structure and function of the layers of skin: dermis, epidermis, stratum germinativum, stratum corneum.
o Where is glabrous skin located?
o Know which skin lesions are primary, arising from previously healthy skin, or secondary resulting from a change in the primary lesion.
o For each of the primary, secondary, and vascular skin lesions know the definitions and the examples of each.
o Know the pattern of skin lesions and the examples of each.
o Know the difference between open and closed comedones.
o Know the differences betweek acne vulgaris vs. rosacea.
o Rhinophyma is associated with which skin condition?

- A 'double comedone' lesion is characteristic of what skin condition?
- Atopic dermatitis is also known as _____.
- What does the term atopic refer to?
- The technical term for hives is _____.
- Which skin condition manifests scaling with a greasy consistency?
- Which skin condition causes 'cradle cap'?
- Which skin condition causes dandruff?
- Which skin condition is characterized by a 'herald patch'?
- Which skin condition is characterized by a Wickham's striae?
- Which of the bullous skin conditions is serious and can be fatal if untreated?
- Which skin condition is characterized by honey yellow crusted vesicles on a child's face?
- A diffuse infection of the dermis and subcutaneous tissue, characterized by edema, erythema, and pain is referred to as _____.
- Which skin condition is also known as St. Anthony's fire?
- Pastia's lines are associated with which skin condition?
- Which skin condition manifests a bright red tongue with prominent papillae, referred to as a 'strawberry tongue'?
- Which condition is caused by the *Treponema pallidum* organism?
- Condyloma lata are moist pink lesions associated with which condition?
- Which sexually transmitted condition is characterized by flesh colored papules that are centrally umbilicated?
- Which sexually transmitted condition is caused by the same virus that is implicated in cervical cancer?
- Genital warts are associated with which sexually transmitted infection?
- Which skin condition is caused by the human papilloma virus?
- Herpes genitalis is caused by the _____ virus.
- Which infection may manifest as shingles in later life?
- Which condition manifests Koplik's spots?
- If a pregnant woman becomes infected with _____ during her first trimester, her child is at risk for birth defects.
- Which skin condition is caused by the *Pityrosporum orbiculare* organism?
- Know the names for tinea infection of various body regions, eg. body, scalp, beard, hands, nails, etc.
- 'Ringworm' is the common name for the lesions seen with a _____ infection.
- The sarcoptes mite causes _____.
- _____ is caused by infestation with lice.
- Which skin condition is caused by a nematode infestation.
- Which skin condition is caused the *Borrelia burgorferi* spirochete.
- Which skin conditions manifest a malar rash?
- Which skin condition presents a 'carpet tack' appearance when the lesions are removed?

- o Which skin condition manifests the CREST syndrome?
- o Know the components of the CREST syndrome.
- o What is a heliotrope and what condition is it associated with?
- o What are Gottron's papules and what condition are they associated with?
- o What lab test is indicated in the evaluation of dermatomyositis?
- o Von Recklinghausen's disease is another name for which skin condition?
- o What is Crowe's sign and what condition is it associated with?
- o What are Lisch nodules and what condition are they associated with?
- o John Merrick, more commonly known as 'the Elephant man', probably suffered from which skin condition?
- o Stevens-Johnson syndrome is a severe form of which skin condition?
- o Which skin condition manifests 'palpable purpura'?
- o Kawasaki's disease is a form of which skin condition?
- o What is livedo reticularis?
- o Which skin phototypes are at greatest risk of sunburn?
- o Café au lait spots are associated with which skin condition?
- o Lentigo is the technical term for what is commonly referred to as

   _____.
- o What is melasma and what condition is it associated with?
- o Which skin condition is referred to as the 'mask of pregnancy'?
- o Approximately 50% of malignant melanoma develops from

   _____.
- o Which skin condition presents with an accumulation of cells having greasy 'stuck on' appearance?
- o Who is most likely to get keloids and in what locations?
- o What is the most common skin cancer?
- o Which skin cancer appears as a pink dome shaped papule with telangiectasic vessels on the surface?
- o Which skin cancer manifests a 'rodent ulcer'?
- o Bowen's disease is the *in situ* form of which skin cancer?
- o Which is the most serious form of skin cancer?
- o Know the ABCD guidelines for evaluating suspicious skin lesions.
- o Which grade of malignant melanoma on Clark's scale is most serious, having the poorest survival rate?
- o Know the definition of hirsuitism and hypertrichosis.
- o Know the structure and function of the tissues that form and surround the nail.
- o Know the definition and significance of:
  - o paronychia
  - o felon
  - o onychmycosis
  - o psoriatic nails
  - o onycholysis
  - o digital clubbing
  - o longitudinal ridging
  - o Beau's lines

- Terry's nails
- Lindsay's nails
- Koilonychia

5 – Head & Neck

Anatomy & Physiology

Knowledge of anatomy is essential in Diagnosis. When charting or conversing with other health professionals, we must describe the abnormalities in relation to known anatomical landmarks. Physiology helps us to understand the *mechanism* of the abnormalities we find. When you know <u>why</u> an abnormal pattern is present, you can often form a mental picture of the condition. This is always preferable to memorization of facts.

The regions of the head usually take the name of the underlying bone. The cranial vault is comprised of the frontal, parietal, sphenoid, temporal and occipital bones. The midline anterior and posterior fontanels and the bilateral sphenoid and mastoid fontanels are membranous areas where the cranial bones meet. While it is commonly taught that the cranial sutures fuse in adulthood, several chiropractic and osteopathic techniques obtain excellent results from adjustment of these supposedly immovable cranial bones. The nasal, zygomatic, ethmoid, lacrimal, maxillary, and mandible bones comprise the facial bones. The air sinuses located within the frontal and zygomatic bones serve to lighten the skull, and also introduce a resonant tone to spoken voice sounds.

Overlying the facial bones are many muscles, innervated mostly by cranial nerve VII, with the jaw muscles innervated by cranial nerve V. Sensation to the face is via cranial nerve V. The temporal artery is palpable just anterior to the ear. The salivary glands are located near the jaw, producing starch digesting enzymes, as well as saliva to moisten the food:

- The parotid glands lie over the mandible, anterior to the ear.
- The submandibular glands are beneath the mandible, anterior to the angle of the jaw.
- The sublingual glands, not palpable from the exterior, are located in the floor of the mouth.

A major landmark of the neck is the sternocleidomastoid (SCM) muscle which originates from the medial clavicle and inserts at the mastoid process behind the ear. The SCM muscle divides the neck into anterior and posterior triangles. The anterior triangle contains the trachea, thyroid gland and the carotid arteries. The external jugular vein is visualized primarily in the posterior triangle.

The thyroid cartilage is a shield shaped structure that produces the prominent 'Adam's apple', usually more noticeable in males. The lobes of the highly vascular thyroid gland lie inferior and lateral to the thyroid cartilage, with a narrow isthmus connecting the two lobes. Goiter, a visually and palpably enlarged thyroid gland, is seen with hyperthyroidism.

The eyes, ears, nose, and throat provide many avenues for bacteria to enter the body. Multiple chains of lymph nodes and ducts drain the head and neck to help protect against these foreign invaders. Ten pairs of nodes may be palpable within the head and neck:

- Occipital - at the base of the skull
- Postauricular - behind the ear
- Preauricular - in front of the ear
- Tonsillar (aka retropharyngeal or jugulodigastric) - at the angle of the jaw
- Submandibular - under the jaw on the side
- Submental - under the jaw in the midline
- Superficial (anterior) cervical - in anterior triangle and over the SCM muscle
- Posterior cervical - behind the SCM muscle in the posterior triangle
- Deep cervical - deep under the SCM muscle (often not palpable)
- Supraclavicular - just above and behind the clavicle

History

Do you experience unusually frequent or severe headaches?

- Factors relating to location, quality, severity, and chronology are key to diagnosing headaches.
- Associated symptoms: nausea, vomiting, visual changes, hypertension, fever.
- Medications: Birth control pills (BCP), Alcohol (EtOH), over the counter (OTC) nonsteroidal antiinflammatory drugs (NSAID).
- Triggering foods or environmental substances: A double blind clinical trial found that 93% of children with severe frequent migraine headaches showed significant reduction of symptoms when their allergic foods were removed (Lancet, 1983 Oct 15;2(8355):865-9).
- Family history: Migraine's are often familial.

Have you experienced any recent injury to your head?

- Onset: You must detail the circumstances of the injury. Did you fall? What hit your head? Did you experience loss of consciousness (LOC)? How long were you unconscious? Which came first, the fall or LOC? Loss of consciousness *before* the fall may have been caused by a cardiovascular event.
- Associated symptoms: headache, nausea, vomiting, visual changes, numbness, tingling, weakness, watery discharge from nose or ear, dizziness, blackout, seizure, history of heart trouble or epilepsy.

Do you have a painful or stiff neck?

- Onset: Sudden or gradual onset? Fever? Acute onset of a stiff painful neck with a fever suggests meningeal irritation. If you suspect meningitis, what orthopedic tests should you perform?
- Associated symptoms: numbness, tingling, or weakness in the shoulders, arms, or hands, limited range of motion, fever.

Do you have any lumps or swelling in the neck?

- Onset: How long have you had it? Has it changed in size?
- Associated symptoms: Difficulty swallowing? Do you smoke? A persistent neck lump is suspicious for cancer until proven otherwise.
- Neck swelling with associated tremor or tachycardia suggests hyperthyroid goiter.

Examination

Inspect and palpate the face and skull

- A skull with 'normal' size and shape is described as normocephalic. Microcephaly refers to an unusually small, and macrocephaly refers to an unusually large head.
- Note any scars, lumps, rashes, hair loss, or other lesions. Palpate hair texture.
- Palpate the skull for areas of tenderness or deformity. A temporal artery that is tender and manifests a hard consistency upon palpation suggests temporal arteritis. When an arterial abnormality is suspected, you should auscultate for a bruit. A bruit is a soft low pitched whooshing sound created by blood moving through a narrowed artery. It is a low pitched pulsatile sound that is best heard with the bell of the stethoscope.
- Palpate the temporomandibular joint (TMJ). Place the tips of your index fingers directly in front of the tragus of each ear. Ask the patient to slowly open and close their mouth. Observe for symmetry of jaw tracking, while you also palpate for clicking or crepitus. Jaw range of motion can be assessed by asking the patient to place two knuckles between their front teeth.
- Inspect the face for asymmetry, involuntary movements, or edema. Many conditions present with abnormal facial appearance or facies. Marked asymmetry of facial muscles suggests nerve damage, either from Bell's palsy or stroke.

Inspect and palpate the neck

- Inspect the neck for asymmetry, scars, or other lesions. Torticollis or "twisted neck" appears as a laterally flexed and rotated neck. Anterior head carriage is a frequently seen muscular imbalance. Prominent jugular venous pulsations may occur with congestive heart failure (CHF).

- While neck range of motion (ROM) testing is a part of every chiropractic workup, it is also a part of the head and neck 'physical' examination.
- Palpate the neck to detect areas of tenderness, deformity, or masses. The posterior neck muscles should be supple, symmetrical and free of spasm or trigger points.
- Place your thumbs or index fingers alongside trachea just above suprasternal notch to verify that the trachea is midline. The trachea may be *pushed* toward the healthy side by tumor or pneumothorax. The trachea may be *pulled* toward the diseased side by pleural adhesions or a large atelectasis. Tracheal tugging, or a rhythmic downward pull in time with the heartbeat, suggests an aortic aneurysm.
- The thyroid gland may be palpated from either the front or from behind. Palpate gently and avoid any movements that might elicit a choking sensation from your patient. Relax the SCM muscle by having the patient laterally flex the head toward the side being palpated. Use the fingers of one hand to lightly push trachea laterally. With the thumb and fingers of other hand try to 'trap' the lateral lobe of the thyroid gland between your fingers as the patient swallows. Repeat this procedure for the opposite lobe of thyroid gland. If thyroid enlargement is noted, auscultate for vascular bruits using the bell of your stethoscope.
- From either the front or behind the patient, palpate all ten pairs of lymph nodes. Use a gentle circular motion underneath the pads of your fingertips to compress the tissue against the underlying muscle. The deep cervical lymph nodes are difficult to palpate. With the head tipped toward the side being examined, use the fingers to gently palpate underneath the SCM muscle.
- Neck lymph nodes are not normally palpable. However, a palpable lymph node is still normal provided it is: small (< 1 cm), moveable, soft, and nontender. Abnormal nodes may be: enlarged, fixed, hard, and painful. During your palpation of the neck lymph nodes you will also palpate the submandibular salivary gland underneath the jaw. Parotid gland tissue, overlying the angle of the jaw, is usually too amorphous to be palpable, unless the individual has mumps. The sublingual salivary gland can only be palpated underneath the tongue with a gloved finger.
- While axillary lymph nodes are normally examined during the breast examination, if a breast examination is not a part of your routine physical examination (PE), it is advisable to go ahead and screen the infraclavicular and axillary lymph nodes at this time.
- Complete examination of the head and neck will also include checking facial skin sensation (CN V), strength of jaw muscles (CN V), and facial movements (CN VII).

Sample Documentation

The skull was symmetrical and normocephalic. No lumps, lesions or tenderness were noted. The hair was of normal texture. The temporal arteries were palpable bilaterally, but free of tenderness. The facial features were symmetrical. No drooping or facial weakness was noted. The sinuses were not tender to palpation or percussion. The jaw muscles were strong. TMJ motion was smooth and free of clicking or crepitus. The neck was supple with full range of motion. The trachea was midline. The lateral lobes of the thyroid were palpable but not enlarged. Head and neck regional lymph nodes were not palpable. No jugular venous pulsations were visible, and upon auscultation the carotid arteries were free of bruits.

Abnormal Findings

Abnormal facial appearance (facies) associated with a condition or chronic illness:

Giantism and Acromegaly (ICD: 253.0)

Syndromes of excessive secretion of GH (hypersomatotropism) nearly always due to a pituitary adenoma of the somatotrophs. (Merck Manual, p. 74)

- Acromegaly results from an excessive production of growth hormone (GH). The condition usually begins in middle age. The word acromegaly literally translates as 'extremity enlargement'. GH stimulation results in abnormal enlargement of the hands, feet, and facial bones, especially the brow, jaw, and nose.
- Much less commonly, the GH stimulation begins in childhood. When bone growth occurs prior to closure of the epiphyses, pituitary giantism or height of 7-8 feet may result.
- In addition to bone and soft tissue overgrowth in the face, which causes prominence of the brow, jaw, nose, ears, and lips, the skin is coarse and thickened. In females hypertrichosis may manifest. The voice may become deeper due to enlargement of the vocal cords. As various tissues enlarge, nerve compression may result in peripheral neuropathies. Acromegaly places the individual at increased risk of diabetes, hypertension, and heart disease.
- In over 90% of the cases the excessive production of growth hormone is caused by a benign pituitary adenoma. In addition to growth hormone production, the tumor can cause headaches and visual disturbances (bitemporal hemianopia). *EYE CHANGES*
- The tumor is diagnosed via blood analysis of GH, as well as CT or MRI imaging of the tumor.
- Treatment consists of surgical removal of the tumor, radiation therapy, or pharmaceuticals which suppress GH production.

Hyperthyroidism (ICD: 242.9)

A clinical condition encompassing several specific diseases, characterized by hypermetabolism and elevated serum levels of free thyroid hormones. (Merck Manual, p. 86)

- While there are other causes of hyperthyroidism, such as thyroid cancer and inflammatory thyroiditis, about 85% of hyperthyroidism is caused by Grave's disease.
- Grave's disease is essentially an autoimmune disorder in which the body produces antibodies which bind to TSH receptors. This causes decreased TSH production, which in turn triggers the thyroid gland to produce excess thyroxine (T4) and triiodothyronine (T3).
- The condition is relatively common, affecting about 1% of the population, and is much more common in women than men (5:1). Symptoms usually manifest in early adulthood, and the initial episode may occur after a physical or psychic shock. The condition appears to have a genetic predisposition.
- The cardinal signs of Graves disease are: thyroid enlargement (goiter), exophthalmos, tachycardia, and tremors. Additional symptoms may include nervousness, heat intolerance, moist skin, diarrhea, fatigue, and weight loss. In women, amenorrhea may manifest as a consequence of excess thyroid hormone.
- Upon examination, the thyroid gland is palpably enlarged. When this is felt, you should auscultate for the presence of bruits of the thyroid vasculature. The forward displacement of the eyeballs results in eyelid retraction or 'lid lag' where the upper eyelid is above the limbus of the iris and the white sclera is visible. The term 'lid lag' may initially suggest pathology of the eyelid muscles, but this is not the case. Rather as was originally described by von Graefe, "...as the cornea looks down, the upper eyelid does not follow."
- Laboratory evaluation should include a thyroid panel, which will typically disclose elevated T3, T4, & FTI, and decreased TSH. When tremor is present, hyperrreflexia may be evident. In the presence of tachycardia, an ECG is prudent to rule out intrinsic cardiac pathology.
- Medical treatment may involve antithyroid medication, or radioiodine therapy. If the patient is not responsive to this therapy, a subtotal thyroidectomy may be performed.
- A 'thyroid storm', while a rare consequence of hyperthyroidism, can lead to potentially fatal cardiac complications.
- Natural therapeutic management of hyperthyroidism is geared toward reduction of autoimmune tendencies.

Hypothyroidism (ICD: 244) – MORE COMMON

The characteristic clinical response to thyroid hormone deficiency in the adult. (Merck Manual, p. 93)

- Approximately 95% of hypothyroidism is 'primary', caused by deficient production of thyroid hormone. Less commonly, the condition is 'secondary' to inadequate stimulation by the pituitary gland.
- In countries with poor nutritional resources, iodine deficiency is a common cause of hypothyroidism. In the United States, Hashimoto's autoimmune thyroiditis is the most common cause. Iatrogenic hypothyroidism is a common sequela of surgical or radiation treatment for Grave's hyperthyroidism.
- Hashimoto's thyroiditis is more common in women than men (8:1), and is most common after age 40. It is estimated that 3-7% of the population have clinical and subclinical hypothyroidism. As with hyperthyroidsim, it is important to inquire about a family history of thyroid problems.
- The autoimmune pathology involves lymphocytic infiltration of thyroid glandular tissue with consequent loss of function. This same autoimmune pathology may also occur in adrenal and pancreatic tissue, resulting in other insufficiency conditions such as Addison's disease, and diabetes mellitus.
- Congenital hypothyroidism causes the diminished physical and mental development referred to as cretinism. In its extreme form, **TQ** acquired adult hypothyroidism manifests as myxedema.
- Myxedema takes its name from the non-pitting pseudoedema caused by infiltration of tissues with the mucopolysaccharide, hyaluronic acid. This tissue infiltration causes puffiness of the face, especially around the eyes (periorbital edema). The infiltration also affects the tongue and mucous membranes of the mouth, nose, and throat. *EARLY SIGNS*
- Early hypothyroidism may present with depression, weakness, and fatigue. The woman may find that she seems to gain weight, regardless of how little she eats. The lowered basal metabolic rate produces a decreased body temperature and she continually feels cold. Decreased thyroid function may cause prolonged and heavy menstrual bleeding. *ALSO HEAVY BLEEDING, HAIR FALLS OUT*
- As the condition becomes more pronounced, the skin is typically coarse and dry and may have a yellow hue. The hair may also become coarse and dry and falls out, especially at the lateral margins of the eyebrows. The voice becomes husky, and the speech may be slow. When the condition is prolonged, mental function is impaired. *MENTAL FUNCTION*
- Upon examination, a nontender enlargement of the thyroid (goiter) may be present. The facial expression is dull and periorbital puffiness is common. The tissue infiltration can cause cardiac enlargement, which may present with bradycardia and diastolic hypertension. Bilaterally decreased achilles tendon reflexes may be an early sign of low thyroid function.
- The individual usually feels cold due to the decreased basal metabolic rate (BMR). Daily measurement of the basal body temperature is an excellent method to assess thyroid function. If your morning body

temperature is consistently below 97.2° F, suspect low thyroid function.

- Lab testing should include a thyroid panel, which will show decreased T3 & T4. With primary thyroid dysfunction TSH will be elevated. However, when hypothyroidism is due to secondary pituitary dysfunction, the TSH is low. Additional lab testing should include a CBC to assess anemia, and a chem screen to assess cardiac function. The serum cholesterol is generally high, and decreases with treatment.

- Medical management involves treatment with synthetic thyroxine (Synthroid), or desiccated glandular preparations (Armour thyroid).

- Many natural physicians use nutritional supplements that also include glandular tissue extracts, as well as iodine and tyrosine, essential thyroid nutrients.

- An excellent online summary of the clinical management of hypothyroidism is found on Medscape:
  http://primarycare.medscape.com/Medscape/endocrinology/Clinical
  Mgmt/CM.v02/pnt-CM.v02.html

The following is a summary of the different manifestation of thyroid disorders: KNOW FOR TEST   METABOLIC RATE IS SLOW
                          FAST

Increased thyroid function	Decreased thyroid function
weight loss	weight gain
prefers cool temperature	prefers warm temperature
easily irritated	lethargic
increased bowel frequency	constipation
fine hair texture	coarse hair texture
moist skin	dry skin
exophthalmos	periorbital puffiness
possible neck swelling from goiter	no neck swelling
possible amenorrhea	possible hypermenorrhea

METABOLIC RATE→ (handwritten note beside table)
IN OVERTIME
BULDING EYES→ exophthalmos
EYE BAGS periorbital puffiness
PERIOD LOSS   HEAVY BLEEDING

Addison's Disease (Primary or Chronic Adrenocortical Insufficiency) (ICD: 255.4)   TAN   JFK HAD THIS DISEASE

An insidious, usually progressive disease resulting from adrenocortical hypofunction. (Merck Manual, p. 101)

- Addison's disease is a rare condition (4 in 100,000) that can occur at any age and affects both sexes equally. While infections such as TB may cause adrenal hypofunction, the majority of the time (80%) an autoimmune destruction of adrenal tissue is the cause.

- Located above each kidney, the adrenal glands secrete several hormones. Cortisol helps with the regulation of blood sugar and immune function. Aldosterone regulates the level of sodium and potassium in the blood, and thus affects blood pressure. A deficiency of both of these hormones accounts for the symptoms seen with Addison's disease.

- Weakness, fatigue, anorexia and weight loss are the predominant symptoms. Abdominal pain, nausea, and diarrhea are also common. Skin hyperpigmentation may result in a 'tan' appearance (even on areas of skin not exposed to the sun), especially over skin creases or pressure points. A bluish black discoloration of mucous membranes may be visible. Paradoxically, areas of vitiligo may also occur.

- Upon examination, the individual may present as very thin and gaunt looking, with what appears initially to be a good tan. When you suspect Addison's disease, assess orthostatic hypotension. If the systolic blood pressure drops more than 20 mm Hg when moving from the supine to standing, this is a positive Ragland's test, which may indicate adrenal insufficiency.

- Laboratory evaluation should include a chem panel. Low sodium with high potassium is typical of Addison's disease, with a sodium:potassium ratio of < 30:1. Hypoglycemia often goes hand in hand with decreased adrenal function. Decreased kidney function will lead to elevated BUN. Decreased serum or salivary cortisol may be measured directly. ACTH should also be measured. When adrenal hypofunction is primary, ACTH will be elevated. If adrenal hypofunction is 'secondary' to pituitary failure, ACTH will be low. The CBC may show a decreased white blood count, most of which is from neutropenia, producing a relative rather than absolute lymphocytosis.

- A KUB film or abdominal CT may show adrenal calcification.

- Medical management involves exogenously supplied cortisone, which can effect remarkable changes. John Kennedy is probably the most famous person to have had Addison's disease. Pictures taken of him before and after corticosteroid treatment show a dramatic change in his appearance.

- An individual with known Addison's disease should be advised to wear a medic alert bracelet, as an acute adrenal crisis is a medical emergency that can be fatal if not treated promptly.

- While overt Addison's disease is rare, applied kinesiology practitioners frequently find subclinical adrenal hypofunction in their patients. These individuals may do well most of the time, but when placed under stress, which exhausts their limited adrenal function, their symptoms become much worse. Dietary, nutritional, and structural adjustments may produce substantial benefit for these individuals. Inasmuch as this is primarily an autoimmune disorder, management of allergies is crucial.

Cushing's Syndrome (ICD: 255.0) OPPOSITE OF ADDISON'S

A constellation of clinical abnormalities due to chronic exposure to excesses of cortisol (the major adrenocorticoid) or related corticosteroids. (Merck Manual, p. 106)

61

CENTRAL OR TRUNKAL OBESITY

- Cushing's syndrome is a comparatively rare condition that is sometimes referred to as 'hypercortisolism'. While the condition may be 'endogenous', the result of an ACTH secreting pituitary tumor or a local adrenal tumor, more commonly the condition is 'exogenous', the result of long term medical treatment with corticosteroid drugs. Iatrogenic Cushing's syndrome may develop as a consequence of prednisone treatment for conditions such as rheumatoid arthritis.
- One of the functions of cortisol is to control the fluid balance within the body. As such, excess cortisol causes fluid retention that manifests as a rounded 'moon' facies. In females, virilism, with hypertrichosis and temporal balding may occur. Truncal obesity may result in a 'buffalo hump' in the cervicodorsal region. The skin may be thin and reddened. Abdominal striae may be present. Overall the patient may present with central obesity and thin extremities.
- Physical examination will present the physical appearance already described. Additionally, fluid retention may also manifest as hypertension. When the condition is long standing, muscle weakness and osteoporosis will be evident.
- Laboratory workup involves measurement of serum cortisol and ACTH. Measurement of the amount of cortisol excreted in a 24 hour urine sample is also helpful. The chem panel will likely show increased glucose and decreased potassium. Sodium may be normal or slightly elevated. The CBC may show polycythemia, neutrophilia, and lymphocytopenia. A routine UA may disclose glycosuria. A dexamethasone suppression test is used distinguish pituitary from non-pituitary causes of Cushing's syndrome.
- Medical management of Cushing's syndrome is directed toward the cause. If a pituitary tumor is present, surgery or radiation therapy will likely be performed. If an adrenalectomy was performed, it is probable that the individual will now require corticosteroid replacement therapy for the remainder of their life.
- When Cushing's syndrome is secondary to exogenously supplied corticosteroids, the dosage of the drug must be adjusted downward to a level that is just sufficient to control the symptoms of the condition the drug is being used to treat.
- Dietary changes and nutritional supplements are often very effective in chronic autoimmune conditions that cortisone is used to treat. As such, natural therapeutics may benefit many cases of iatrogenically induced Cushing's syndrome.

Parkinson's Disease (ICD: 332.0) MICHEAL J. FOX

An idiopathic, slowly progressive, degenerative CNS disorder characterized by slow and decreased movement, muscular rigidity, resting tremor, and postural instability. (Merck Manual, p. 1466)

- Parkinson's is referred to as 'shaking palsy'. Overall, it presents with the triad of rigidity, tremor, and a flexion posture. For reasons that are not clear, the substantia nigra region of the brain fails to produce sufficient quantity of the neurotransmitter dopamine. This deficiency results in impairment of muscle tension and movement.

- The condition typically manifests at about age 55-60, however it can manifest at a younger age such as with the actor Michael J. Fox. Parkinson's is the fourth most common neurodegenerative disease and affects about 1% of those over 65 years of age.
- The facial rigidity causes the 'Parkisonian mask', a face that is flat and expressionless. The patient may have difficulty closing the mouth and may drool. The facial skin is often greasy. With flexion of the neck, they peer upward in order to see forward.
- The bradykinesia of Parkinson's is readily apparent by watching the eyes blink. Most people will normally blink their eyes about 20-30 times a minute. An individual with Parkinson's disease will blink more slowly, in severe cases only 5-6 times a minute. BLINK SLOWLY
- The tremor affects the fingers and hands most severely, causing a 'pill rolling' movement of the thumb and fingers. The resting tremor may diminish with voluntary movement and sleep. SHAKING
- The muscular rigidity and forward flexion of the trunk may cause a shuffling gait. Over one hundred years ago Parkinson wrote, "*He is irresistibly impelled to take much quicker and shorter steps, and thereby to adopt unwillingly a running pace.*"
- The symptoms appear gradually, and with time the condition becomes a chronic and progressively worse. There is no cure for this condition, but pharmacological agents such as Sinemet may lessen the tremors. Eventually the patient may succumb to conditions such as pneumonia, stroke, or death from complications from a fall.
- While Parkinson's disease is usually diagnosed from signs and symptoms, there are cellular changes that cause the neurological manifestations. Specifically, the presence of eosinophilic granular inclusions in the neurons of the substantia nigra, locus ceruleus, and brain stem are referred to as Lewy bodies.
- A good online summary is found on Postgraduate Medicine, July 1999. ATTENTION TREMOR - ONLY WHEN MOVING
RESTING TREMOR - WHEN RESTING

Bell's Palsy (ICD: 351.0)

Unilateral facial paralysis of sudden onset and unknown cause. (Merck Manual, p. 1461)

- Bell's palsy is unilateral facial paralysis of sudden onset. While the cause is unknown, we suspect it is viral, sometimes occurring after exposure to cold. One theory suggests compression of an inflamed facial nerve as it passes through the temporal bone.
- This condition must be distinguished from a cerebrovascular accident. Bell's palsy affects the entire half of the face, both the upper and lower facial muscles. In contrast, with a stroke, the frontalis and orbicularis oculi muscles are less affected.

- In addition to facial weakness, the individual may experience pain behind the ears and have a history of a recent upper respiratory infection (URI). With an inability to adequately close the affected eye, there may be excessive tearing.
- Medical management involves oral corticosteroids and eye lubricants, such as *Tears Naturale*.
- Many chiropractors have found that electrical stimulation of the facial nerve can produce dramatic recovery. Early intervention can lessen the severity of the impairment. Because this condition can recur, every new patient with Bell's palsy in their history should be counseled to come in for treatment as soon as possible after the onset of symptoms.

Ischemic Stroke (ICD: 436)

Stroke in evolution (evolving stroke): An enlarging brain infarct manifested by neurologic deficits that worsen over 24 to 48 h.
Completed stroke: Brain infarct manifested by neurologic deficits that signify stable injury. (Merck Manual, p. 1421)

- Stroke is the third leading cause of death the US. Each year more than 500,000 Americans have a stroke, and 145,000 die from stroke-related illness. For those who survive their stroke, many experience disability and impairment of their daily activities, some requiring years of long term nursing care. When both the cost of treatment and the loss of job productivity are considered, strokes cost $43 billion each year in the US.
- A stroke or cerebrovascular accident (CVA) results in paralysis of the lower facial muscles. Bilateral cerebral innervation of the upper facial muscles maintains the ability to wrinkle the forehead and close the eyes. These motions <u>are</u> impaired with Bell's Palsy. There will also be numbness of the face which is unlikely to manifest with Bell's Palsy.
- In addition to numbness and weakness of the face, there will likely be paralysis of the arm and leg on the same side. Other symptoms may include:
    o Sudden confusion, trouble speaking or understanding
    o Sudden trouble seeing in one or both eyes
    o Sudden trouble walking, dizziness, loss of balance or coordination
    o Sudden severe headache with no known cause
- Strokes originate from a blockage of blood flow from one of three causes:
    o Thrombosis - formation of a blood clot within a brain artery, most likely from atherosclerotic narrowing.
    o Embolic - lodging of a blood clot in the brain that has formed elsewhere in the body, such as from the heart. If the onset of symptoms is sudden and maximal within a few minutes, the cause is more likely from an embolism.

- o Hemorrhagic - bleeding within the brain, such as from a ruptured aneurysm.
- o If treated within a few hours with clot busting drugs (streptokinase and t-PA), recovery can be dramatic.
- Prevention of known risk factors is key:
  - o smoking
  - o high blood pressure
  - o high cholesterol and triglycerides
  - o obesity
  - o diabetes
  - o heavy alcohol use

Down's Syndrome (ICD: 758.0)

A chromosomal disorder usually resulting in mental retardation, a characteristic facies, and many other typical features, including microcephaly and short stature. (Merck Manual, p. 2233)

- Down's syndrome or trisomy-21, is a genetic defect caused by an extra chromosome. The incidence is about one in 700 live births, 50% born to mothers over 35. The condition is suspected at birth when the infant has characteristic facial features, is placid (does not cry), and the muscles are hypotonic.
- Physical and mental development is retarded. The slanted eyes, flat nasal bridge, and epicanthal folds give a mongoloid appearance. The nose is small and flat. There may be ear dysplasia and the ears may be low set. The mouth is often held open by a thick protruding tongue. The hands may have a single palmar crease (simian crease). The fingers are short and the 5th finger may have only two phalanges. There may be a wide gap between the 1st and 2nd toes.
- Dislocation of the atlas has been reported, due to a congenital anomaly of the transverse portion of the cruciate ligament.
- While these children can live long and relatively productive lives, the aging process appears to be accelerated and life expectancy is decreased due to increased susceptibility to leukemia and heart disease.

Fetal Alcohol Syndrome (ICD: 760.71) (Merck Manual, p. 2158)

- The developing fetus is exquisitely sensitive to the health of the mother and substances in her blood circulation. For this reason, women who might be pregnant should exercise caution with taking drugs, even OTC medicine. Many people do not appreciate that alcohol is a drug, which can adversely affect the developing fetus.
- In the US, the incidence of fetal alcohol syndrome (FAS) is 1-2 per 1,000 live births. If the alcohol abuse is early in the pregnancy, the damage may cause miscarriage. As such, the true incidence is probably higher. An estimated 30-50% of women who drink heavily during their pregnancy will deliver children with fetal alcohol syndrome. It is probable that mothers who are light to moderate

drinkers during their pregnancy are also damaging the fetus, although to a less obvious extent.

- The child of a mother with excessive alcohol intake during pregnancy appears similar to a Down's syndrome child. The eyes are wide spread with inner epicanthal folds. The nose is short and the philtrum, the midline groove above the upper lip, is poorly formed. The upper lip may be thin.
- As this child grows older, mental and behavioral impairment may manifest. The child may be slow to develop language skills. The child may be impulsive and 'hyperactive'. These children seem unable to 'learn from their mistakes', and exhibit signs of mental retardation.
- Once the damage is done, there is no known treatment. Prevention, is the key. Any woman of child bearing age who might become pregnant should be very cautious about drinking alcohol or taking drugs. Damage to the fetus can occur before she misses her period and discovers she is pregnant.

Hydrocephalus (ICD: 742.3) (Merck Manual, p. 2223)

- Hydrocephalus literally means 'water on the brain'. Cerebrospinal fluid or CSF is constantly produced by the choroid plexus in the ventricles of the brain. This fluid bathes the brain and spinal cord. When there is a restriction of CSF flow this can cause enlargement of the brain.
- If the enlargement occurs during fetal development, the head may become too large for a vaginal delivery and a cesarean section may be required. If the enlargement begins after birth, the head will become larger than normal. This progressive enlargement of the head produces dilated scalp veins. The face appears small in comparison to the enlarged cranium.
- One of the causes of hydrocephalus is meningomyelocele. Like spina bifida, taking extra folic acid can help prevent this condition. As such, all women of childbearing age should be taking nutritional supplementation that includes folic acid.
- With early diagnosis, a surgical shunt can reduce the pressure, offers the child the best chance of normal development.

Allergic Facies (ICD: 995.3)

Atopic Dermatitis: Chronic, pruritic, superficial inflammation of the skin, frequently associated with a personal or family history of allergic disorders (eg, hay fever, asthma). (Merck Manual, p. 788)

- About 65% atopic dermatitis sufferers begin to manifest this condition in infancy. It may begin as a rash on the cheeks which spreads to the rest of the face. Severe itching may cause the child to scratch until bleeding develops.
- Food and environmental allergies can cause facial features such as 'allergic shiners', dark, puffy shadows below the eyes, or an 'allergic

salute', a transverse ridge above the tip of the nose, caused by the child using the back of the hand to wipe their nose.

- While some physicians consider milk allergy to be controversial, many of these children improve dramatically when milk products are removed from their diet. Calcium fortified milk substitutes are much less allergenic for these children.

Headache

- Headaches account for 80 million doctor appointments in the US each year.
- Collectively headaches account for 157 million lost workdays each year.
- Over 45 million Americans experience recurring headaches.
- It is estimated that 50 million <u>pounds</u> of aspirin are taken each year for headache relief.

While there are over one dozen known types of headache, the vast majority of headaches are either muscle contraction tension headaches (vertebrogenic headache is often considered a type of tension headache), or vascular migraine headaches. History is where the diagnosis is usually made. You will learn more detail on headache diagnosis in your clinical neurology training, but the following is a brief summary of three of the more common types of headache.

Muscular Tension Headache (ICD: 307.81)

Headache that lasts 30 min to 7 days and is non pulsating, mild to moderate in severity, bilateral, not aggravated by exertion, and not associated with nausea, vomiting, or sensitivity to light, sound, or smell. (<u>Merck Manual</u>, p. 1378)

- Bilateral, may begin in sub-occipital region.
- Generalized ache or feels like a constricting band around the head.
- No pre-headache prodrome.
- Affects both sexes equally.
- No associated symptoms.

Vascular Migraine Headache (ICD: 346.9)

Headache that lasts 4 to 72 h, is throbbing, is moderate to severe in intensity, is unilateral, becomes worse with exertion, and is associated with nausea, vomiting, or sensitivity to light, sound, or smell. (<u>Merck Manual</u>, p. 1376)

- Unilateral, may begin around the eye or temple.
- Throbbing or pounding quality.
- May experience prodromal visual changes, such as blind spots or flashing lights. The presence of prodromal symptoms during the 30 minutes prior to the onset of the headache is what characterizes 'classic' vs. 'common' migraine headaches.

- 75% of migraine sufferers are women; there is probably a familial tendency toward migraine.
- May experience associated symptoms of nausea, vomiting, numbness, visual disturbances.

Cluster Headache (ICD: 346.2)

Headache that lasts 15 to 180 min, is severe, is unilateral, is located periorbitally and/or temporally, occurs up to 8 times per day, and is associated with at least one of the following: tearing, red eye, stuffy nose, facial sweating, ptosis, or miosis. (Merck Manual, p. 1377)

- Cluster headaches share some similarities with migraine headache, as well as some important differences:
  - o As indicated by the name, the attacks occur in a cluster of episodes followed by pain free periods of weeks to years.
  - o The attacks are more frequent in the spring and fall, in contrast to migraine which has no seasonal predilection.
  - o Approximately 90% of cluster headache sufferers are male, vs. approximately 70% of migraine sufferers are female.
  - o Cluster headache shows no familial tendency, as does migraine headache.
  - o Cluster headache does not have a visual prodrome, or nausea and vomiting.
  - o Instead, cluster headache is frequently associated with tearing of the eye, nasal congestion, and possibly ptosis and miosis.
  - o While the quality of cluster headache <u>may</u> be described as 'throbbing', more typically it is described as sharp and stabbing, or 'boring'.

Other less common causes of headache include meningitis, sinusitis, hypertension, temporal arteritis, brain tumor, or subdural hematoma. The consequences of missing the diagnosis of these more serious causes of headache can be devastating to your patient's well being, as well as your professional career. As such, with headache you must always investigate:

- Was there trauma?
- Is the condition acute or chronic?
- Are the headaches unrelenting, getting progressively worse?
- Is there nuchal rigidity?
- Is there a fever?
- What is the blood pressure?
- Is there tenderness of the superficial temporal artery?
- Is there papilledema?
- Do the sinuses transilluminate?

An excellent online book on diagnosing and managing headaches is found on Medscape:

http://www.medscape.com/PCI/headaches/public/headaches-about.html

Study Guide Objectives

o   Know the anatomical structures and landmarks of the head and neck.
o   Know the locations of the skull fontanelles.
o   Know which bones form the cranial vault.
o   Know which bones form the facial bones.
o   Know the cranial nerve innervation supplying sensation and motor function to the face.
o   Know the names and locations of the neck lymph nodes.
o   Know the names and locations of the salivary glands.
o   Know the pertinent history questions for head and neck conditions.
o   What are bruits and how they are detected?
o   Know the four conditions that cause tracheal deviation and which way they push or pull the trachea.
o   Know the cause of 'tracheal tugging'.
o   Know what constitutes normal and abnormal lymph nodes.
o   Know the signs and symptoms associated with the various head and neck conditions discussed.
o   Know which hormones are involved in either excess or deficiency for the head and neck conditions discussed.
o   Know the distinguishing characteristics between hypothyroidism vs. hyperthyroidism.
o   Know the differences between how hypo vs. hyper adrenal function manifests.
o   Know the triad that manifests with Parkinson's disease.
o   Know how Bell's palsy manifests different from a stroke (CVA).
o   Know which head and neck conditions cause skull enlargement.
o   Know the distinguishing characteristics for the various types of headaches.
o   Know the factor that distinguishes common vs. classical migraine headache.
o   Know the differences between migraine vs. cluster headache.
o   Know the danger signals for the less common causes of headache.

6 – Eyes

Anatomy & Physiology

The eyes, one of our most important sensory organs, help us to perceive our environment. Because they are so important, they are well protected within the bony orbit. The upper and lower eyelids provide further protection from injury. The eyelashes are extensions of the eyelids to help shield the eyes from dust. The canthus is where the upper and lower eyelids meet. The caruncle, a fleshy mass located at the medial canthus, contains sebaceous glands which help to lubricate the eye. The tarsal plates provide rigidity to the shape of the eyelid. Located within the tarsal plates, the meibomian glands provide additional sebaceous lubrication.

The front surface of the eyeball is covered by a thin membrane, the bulbar conjunctiva. This membrane merges with the cornea at the outer portion of the iris. Continuous with the bulbar conjunctiva is the palpebral conjunctiva, which lines the inner surface of the eyelids. The lacrimal gland located at the upper outer portion of the orbit secretes tears. The tears wash across the eye and drain into the puncta, the lacrimal sac, and eventually drain into the inferior meatus of the nose.

Six extraocular muscles innervated by cranial nerves III, IV, and VI provide for motion of the eyeballs. The actions of these muscles are coordinated to provide for parallel, conjugate movement of the eyes.

The eyeball itself is comprised of three layers:

- Sclera - The sclera is the tough white outer layer of the eye which provides support to the inner structures. It is continuous with the anterior cornea. The cornea is very pain sensitive and CN V afferent sensation is responsible for the corneal reflex.
- Choroid - The choroid is a vascular middle layer which provides fluid and nutrition to the inner eye. It is continuous anteriorly with the ciliary body and iris. The ciliary body is a muscle that helps to vary the shape of the flexible lens of the eye. The center of the iris is the pupil. When the iris contracts this decreases the amount of light entering the eye to help with near vision (accommodation). The iris dilates when light is low and to increase the amount of light entering the eye for far vision. Pupillary constriction is controlled by CN III. The choroid layer also has dark pigmentation to ensure that only light from the pupil enters the eye.
- Retina - The nerve fibers that originate visual impulses lie on the retina, the innermost layer. Light striking the rods and cones convert light impulses into neural impulses. The optic nerve and retinal blood vessels enter the eyeball at the optic disc. Since the optic disc is devoid of rods and cones, it produces a 'blind spot' on the visual field.

The arteries and veins usually pass as a pair to each quadrant of the posterior retina. The veins are visualized as darker red and thicker than the arteries. The arteries are more of an orange red color with a thin 'arterial light reflex' when seen via ophthalmoscopy. The retinal background is fairly uniform in color, provided it is free of pathology. The macula contains the fovea centralis where sharper central vision is perceived. The cones, which are responsible for color vision, are most concentrated at the fovea centralis. The macula is visualized approximately two optic disc diameters from the disc, toward the temporal side of the fundus. The macula may be slightly darker, or it may appear quite similar to the rest of the retinal background, except for the lack of blood vessels at the macula.

The images generated at the retina are transmitted via the optic nerve to the visual cortex. These fibers decussate or branch at the optic chiasm near the pituitary gland. Defects in the visual field may provide the clues needed to determine the location of the nerve interruption.

History

Do you have any blurred vision or difficulty seeing?

- Ask about frequency, duration, possible cause, etc. Both eyes? Progressive? Is the visual loss central or peripheral?
    - o Floaters - not bilateral, associated with aging and myopia, but not clinically significant.
    - o Halos around lights - acute angle glaucoma.
    - o Double vision or history of crossed eye - strabismus (inward or outward turn of the eye).
    - o Scotoma or central blind spot - glaucoma, optic nerve disorders.
    - o Night blindness - optic atrophy, glaucoma, vitamin A deficiency.

Do you experience eye pain?

- Sudden onset of eye pain or visual changes should be referred immediately.

Do you experience redness, swelling, or discharge from your eyes?

- Possible infection or inflammation of conjunctiva, iris, eyelids, etc.
- What color is the discharge? Allergies and irritants produce excessive tearing. Thick yellow discharge suggests infection.

Do you have a history of eye problems?

- Do you wear eyeglasses or contact lenses? At what age did you begin wearing them? When was your last eye examination?
- Have you ever been tested for glaucoma? Do you have any family members with glaucoma?

What medicines are you currently taking?

- Increased intraocular pressure and cataracts are side effects of prednisone.
- Are you self treating with any eye medications?

How is your general health?

- Uncontrolled diabetes and hypertension will eventually result in eye problems.

Examination

Visual Acuity

Eye examination begins with testing of visual acuity using the Snellen eye chart. The individual stands twenty feet away from the chart, covers one eye and reads aloud the lowest line they can see clearly. Normal visual acuity is 20/20. The numerator refers to the distance the individual stands from the chart, and always remains 20. Only the denominator changes, and represents the distance at which a 'normal' eye would have been able to read the chart. For example, a person with better than normal vision might be able to read the smaller 20/10 line, which is interpreted as meaning they can read at 20 feet, what a normal eye could have read at 10 feet. Or an individual with much poorer 20/200 vision can read at 20 feet, what a normal eye could have read at 200 feet. The values obtained are recorded as OS (left eye), OD (right eye), and OU (both eyes). If the patient wears corrective lenses, visual acuity is usually tested with them on.

The handheld Rosenbaum and Jaeger eye charts are for testing near vision, not far vision. Many doctors screen near vision with the ability to read newsprint at 12-14 inches. When the individual has difficulty with either near or far vision, send them to an eye doctor. Color vision is not routinely tested. Color blindness is usually the result of a sex linked genetic defect, affecting only males.

Visual Fields

After visual acuity, we test the visual fields. Stand two to three feet in front of the patient and have them look straight at you. Position your fingers behind the patient and slowly bring one hand forward as you wiggle your fingers. Have your patient point to the side where they see your fingers. Many doctors test both eyes at once, however you should be aware that this method does not test the nasal visual field. Since most visual defects involve the temporal fields, this quick screen usually suffices. The more thorough method is to have the patient cover one eye, you cover your opposite eye, and then bring your wiggling fingers from the outside toward the eyes. If your patient's and your own visual fields are normal, both of you should see the fingers at about the same time.

73

Approximate normal ranges for peripheral field of vision are: temporal 90 degrees, inferior 70 degrees, nasal 60 degrees, superior 50 degrees.

Extraocular Muscle Function

We next observe the position and alignment of the eyes and test the function of the extraocular muscles. Shine a light toward both eyes. This produces a reflection or corneal light 'reflex' on each eye (Hirschberg test). This reflection should be seen at the same position for each eye, e.g. 12 o'clock. If one eye is turned out (exotropia), or turned in (esotropia), the light reflex will be asymmetrical. If this occurs, perform the cover-uncover test. Have your patient stare straight ahead at you. As you cover one eye with a card, note if the uncovered eye shifts focus. Next remove the card and note if that eye jumps to reestablish fixation. Either of these indicates amblyopia, or a 'lazy eye'.

The diagnostic positions test assesses the 'cardinal fields of gaze' (not to be confused with visual fields). Hold your finger or an object about one foot in front of your patient's eyes. Using either an 'H in space' or six diagonal movements, assess the parallel tracking of both eyes. Take the object out far enough to test for 'end point' nystagmus. Nystagmus is a rhythmic oscillation of eye motion. End point nystagmus usually has a fast component in the direction of gaze followed by a slow return toward the midline. A few beats of end point nystagmus at the extreme lateral gaze is acceptable. When this is seen, hold your finger in that position, to wait for the oscillations to abate. If the nystagmus remains, this is abnormal, and may indicate a neurological problem, such as multiple sclerosis (MS). Typically pathological nystagmus is present in the full range of motion, not just at the end point. When the nystagmus has a cerebellar cause, the nystagmus is usually greater when the eyes turned toward the side of cerebellar lesion.

After completion of the 'H in space' or six diagonal movements, bring your finger toward the bridge of the patient's nose to check for convergence. Upon completion of assessing extraocular muscle function, ask your patient if any of these motions caused him to see double, as ocular muscle palsy may manifest as double vision when the muscle weakness is stressed to its endpoint.

External Ocular Structures

Inspect the external eye structures:

- Inspect the eyebrows for thinning of the lateral margins, which may indicate hypothyroid tendencies.
- Inspect the eyelids and lashes for ptosis, eye protrusion, deformities, or asymmetry.
    - Ptosis - indicates oculomotor nerve damage and may be seen with myasthenia gravis and Horner's syndrome.

- o Exophthalmos - Normally the sclera is not visible at the upper iris margin. If the eyeball protrudes forward and the sclera <u>is</u> visible between the lid margin and the iris, this is referred to as 'lid lag', and suggests hyperthyroid tendencies.
  - o Epicanthal folds suggest Down's syndrome.
  - o The eyelashes should not turn in (entropion) or turn out (ectropion).
  - o Various pathologies such as hordeolum (sty) or chalazion are seen at the lid margins.
- Inspect and palpate the lacrimal apparatus.
  - o The lacrimal gland may be palpable as a slight swelling at the outer margin of the upper eyelid.
  - o Gentle pressure underneath the medial canthus should not be painful. Tenderness or regurgitation of fluid from the puncta may indicate blockage of the nasolacrimal duct.
- Inspect the conjunctiva and sclera.
  - o Use your thumbs to gently draw the lower eyelids down. Ask the patient to look up, to each side, and down. This will help you to visualize the sclera and conjunctiva.
  - o Jaundice produces a yellowing of the normally white sclera.
  - o Anemia manifests as a pallor of the normally pink conjunctiva.
  - o Reddening of the sclera is present with conjunctivitis, iritis, and subconjunctival hemorrhage.
  - o A yellowish growth on the medial sclera may represent a pinguecula or pterygium.
  - o Eversion of the upper eyelid is not normally performed unless there is a specific reason, such as searching for a foreign body.
- Inspect the cornea and lens.
  - o Shine a light from the side to illuminate the cornea. Clouding of the lens indicates cataract.

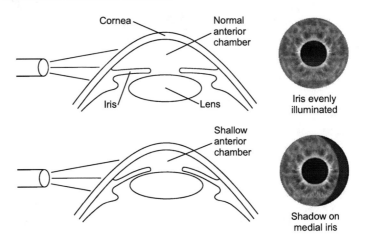

- If an individual has glaucoma, increased intraocular pressure will press the lens and iris of the eye anterior, creating a shallow anterior chamber. Normally when a light is directed from the side, the iris is a uniform color. However, with a shallow anterior chamber, the temporal side closest to the light is illuminated, while a shadow is cast on the medial side furthest from the light. This test is used as a screening examination for possible glaucoma.
- If glaucoma is suspected, the patient should be referred for tonometry readings from an ophthalmologist or optometrist. It is unlikely that glaucoma will be perfectly symmetrical. When palpating over the closed eye, you <u>may</u> be able to palpate increased firmness on that side, and the patient may also experience tenderness upon palpation.
- Observe the size and shape of both pupils. To assess direct and consensual pupillary constriction, bring your penlight to just a few inches away from the pupil at an approximately 45 degrees angle. Do <u>not</u> place the penlight directly in front of the eye, as this can trigger near vision accommodation pupillary constriction. Place the spot of light on each pupil two times: once to view direct pupillary constriction in the same eye, and a second time to assess consensual pupillary constriction in the opposite eye.
- To check for accommodation, hold your finger or an object <u>a few inches</u> from their nose. Have the patient alternate between looking at your finger and a distant object behind you. You should observe pupillary constriction as the patient looks at your finger.
- When the pupil size and shape, direct and consensual pupillary constriction, and accommodation are all normal, it is charted as PERRLA: Pupils Equal, Round, Reactive to Light and Accommodation.
- The corneal blink reflex is often omitted from a routine examination, unless the individual is manifesting signs of cranial nerve abnormality. The test is performed by taking a cotton ball or q-tip and drawing out a wisp of cotton to a point. Lightly touch the wisp to the edge of the iris. Alternatively, if you purchased an insufflator bulb for your otoscope, you can direct a puff of air from the side to the anterior surface of the eye. Corneal sensation is innervated by CN V, which will normally cause a blink response in both eyes, via CN VII.

Ophthalmoscopic Examination

- Ophthalmoscopy is one of the more difficult physical examination skills you must master. While the following guidelines should help, proficiency comes only with practice. You will probably have to perform fundoscopy on at least one hundred people before you start to feel comfortable with this task.

- One of the keys to making the job easier is summed up in one word: *stability*. If you hold the ophthalmoscope firmly braced against your cheek, this helps. If you stabilize your body motion by bracing your weight against the exam table (not the patient), this helps. And finally, if you come in close and lightly brace your hand holding the ophthalmoscope against the patient's cheek, this also helps.

- Since we don't use mydriatic drops to dilate the patient's pupils, you should take steps to facilitate maximum pupil dilation. When possible, dim the room lights. It is a good idea to have a dimmer switch on the lights in your examination room for this purpose. With practice, you will learn the optimum light intensity to use on the ophthalmoscope. Too much light causes pupillary constriction and is uncomfortable to your patient. Too little light does not allow you to properly visualize the retinal structures.

- Use your right hand and right eye to examine the patient's right eye, and your left hand and eye to examine the patient's left eye. If you start at the correct angle you increase the probability that you will easily find the optic disc. To do this, position yourself about 15 degrees lateral from the midline. Have the patient focus their gaze at a point behind you on the wall. If the table is high, you will want to pick a point at about eye level. If the patient is sitting on a low table, and they are looking upward at you, have them fixate on a point on the wall such that you will be coming in at that same angle.

- Position the diopter wheel on 0, and from about 12 inches from the patient shine the light toward their pupil. You should see the 'red reflex', the reflection of your light on the retina. While maintaining your focus on this red spot, come in very close to the patient. The closer you come, the larger the field of view you can see through the pupil. Also, when you come in close enough to lightly rest your hand on their cheek, this provides you with a stability point to pivot on when moving your gaze away from the optic disc to the other retinal structures.

- If the retina is not in focus, with the index finger of your examining hand, change the diopter wheel setting until the focus is sharp. If the patient is nearsighted, you will be rotating the wheel toward the – or red numbers. If the patient is farsighted, use the + numbers. The + diopter numbers may be black, blue, or green depending on your ophthalmoscope.

- Once the retina is in focus, find the optic disc. If necessary, follow a blood vessel toward the disc. Remember, the 'V' formed by a branching blood vessel points toward the disc. At the disc, inspect the following:
  - Color - The disc is normally a creamy yellow orange color, however dark skinned individuals have a darker disc color.

- o Margins - The disc margins should be distinct and even, and the blood vessels should not bend when they cross the disc margin.
  - o Cup to disc ratio - The physiological cup is a slightly brighter color than the rest of the disc, and the diameter of the cup should not be greater than one half the optic disc diameter.
- After inspecting the disc, move outward and inspect all four quadrants of the retina. In each quadrant, you will be inspecting the arteries and veins and the retinal background for hemorrhages and exudates.
- Normally a paired artery and vein pass into each quadrant. The veins are darker red and thicker than the arteries, which usually have an 'arterial light reflex' or thin stripe of light down the middle. With hypertension, the arteries may manifest copper wire, or silver wire defects. Where the arteries and veins cross, inspect carefully for 'AV nicking', also a sign of hypertension.
- In the retinal background between the arteries and veins, you are looking for exudates (the white stuff), and hemorrhages (the red stuff). Hypertension may produce local ischemic infarcts which manifest as 'cotton wool' soft exudates. Hard exudates are the lipid remains of blood vessel leakage, a feature of diabetes. Hemorrhages are seen with both diabetes and hypertension.
- After inspecting the four quadrants, attempt to visualize the macula. Because the fovea centralis is the area of greatest visual acuity, it is also the area most uncomfortable with bright light. This is why we perform this part of the exam last. To see the macula, either shift your focus laterally about two disc diameters, or have your patient briefly stare directly into the light. A normal macula is difficult to visualize, and may appear very similar to the retinal background, except for the absence of blood vessels.

Sample Documentation

Visual acuity with the patient wearing corrective lenses was 20/20 in each eye. Visual fields were full and free of defect. The corneal light reflex was symmetric bilaterally. Extraocular movements were full and intact. No nystagmus, ptosis, or lid lag or was noted. The conjunctiva were pink and no lesions were noted at the lid margins. The sclerae were white, with no hemorrhages noted. The cornea and lenses were clear and free of opacity. The pupils were equal, round, reactive to light and accommodation. The corneal blink reflex was not tested. Ophthalmoscopic examination disclosed a normal red reflex bilaterally. The optic discs were cream colored, with distinct even disc margins. The physiological cup to disc ratio was 1:2. Arteries and veins were of normal color and caliber. No AV nicking was noted. The retinal background was free of hemorrhages or exudates. The maculae were not visualized.

Abnormal Findings

Defects of the Visual Field

- A central blind area indicates macular damage possibly from diabetes or macular degeneration.
- Decreased peripheral vision suggests increased intraocular pressure from glaucoma (small central scotomas may also be an early sign of glaucoma).
- A shadow or diminished vision in one quadrant or half of a visual field may indicate retinal detachment.
- Unilateral blindness suggests a lesion of the globe or optic nerve.
- Bitemporal hemianopia is most commonly caused by a pituitary tumor at the optic chiasm.
- Unilateral nasal hemianopia suggests a lesion at the outer uncrossed fibers of the optic chiasm, possibly from pressure of an internal carotid artery aneurysm.
- Homonymous hemianopia, loss of same half of visual field in both eyes, suggests trauma or a lesion at the occipital lobe.

The following shows how some of the more common visual field defects might appear to the patient:

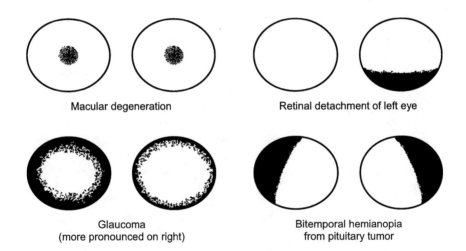

Macular degeneration

Retinal detachment of left eye

Glaucoma
(more pronounced on right)

Bitemporal hemianopia
from pituitary tumor

Abnormalities of Eyelids and Lacrimal Apparatus

Periorbital edema (ICD: 376)

- Periorbital edema is a symptom that may be caused by a variety of conditions, such as renal failure, congestive heart failure, or myxedema. In children, periorbital edema may be due to a *Haemophilus* or *Streptococcus* infection (Merck Manual, p. 2315). Treatment must be directed at the underlying cause.

Orbital Cellulitis (ICD: 376.0)

Inflammation of the orbital tissues caused by infection that extends from the nasal sinuses or teeth, by metastatic spread from infections elsewhere, or by bacteria introduced via orbital trauma. (Merck Manual, p. 706)

- Cellulitis is a bacterial infection beneath the skin. The eye is surrounded by conjunctival membranes. If an infection occurs anterior to these membranes (preseptal), it is referred to as a periorbital cellulitis. An infection posterior to the conjunctival membranes (postseptal), is called orbital cellulitis.
- While orbital infections are not common, they are quite serious because the post conjunctival veins drain into the intracranial area, and meningitis can develop. Prior to the development of antibiotics, the mortality from orbital cellulitis was one in five, and those who did not die may have become blind in that eye.
- As with most infections, a fever may manifest. A CBC will likely show an elevated white count with neutrophilia. When cultured, the infective organism is typically *Staphylococcus, Streptococcus,* or *Haemophilus.*
- Patients with orbital cellulitis require immediate referral for IV antibiotic therapy.

Exophthalmos (Proptosis) (ICD: 376.2)

Protrusion of one or both eyeballs that results from orbital inflammation, edema, tumors, or injuries; cavernous sinus thrombosis; or enlargement of the eyeball (as in congenital glaucoma and unilateral myopia). (Merck Manual, p. 706)

- Exophthalmos, or abnormal protrusion of the eyeball may occur due to a variety of causes. If the condition is bilateral, hyperthyroidism is the most likely cause. If other signs such as tremor and tachycardia are present, this makes the diagnosis of hyperthyroidism more likely. However, also keep in mind that many cases of hyperthyroidism never manifest exophthalmos.
- If the condition is unilateral and pulsatile, an arteriovenous aneurysm of the internal carotid artery is possible. A bruit may be audible with the bell of the stethoscope over the closed eyeball.
- If the condition is non-pulsatile, an infection of the cavernous sinus must be ruled out. This individual will likely have a fever, headache, and may manifest symptoms of a brain infection such as loss of consciousness or cranial nerve palsy. A brain tumor is another possible cause of unilateral non-pulsatile eye protrusion.
- Normally the upper eyelid slightly covers the iris of the eye. If the white sclera is visible between the iris and the upper eyelid, 'lid lag' is present.
- If the eye protrusion is sufficient that the eyelids can no longer cover the eyeball, conjunctival irritation and dryness will result. The patient may report a 'gritty' feeling in the affected eyes, and possibly double

vision. Obviously, all serious eye conditions require prompt medical referral.

Enophthalmos (ICD: 376.5)

- Enophthalmos refers to a backward displacement of the globe in the orbit, or 'sunken eyes'. The cause is usually nutritional wasting (cachexia), or dehydration.

Dacrostenosis (ICD: 375.5)

Stricture of the nasolacrimal duct, often resulting from congenital abnormality or an infection. (<u>Merck Manual</u>, p. 707)

- Dacrostenosis is an obstruction of the nasolacrimal duct. The condition may be either congenital or acquired as the result of an inflammation, deviated septum, or nasal polyps. Trauma that results in fracture of the nasal bones may also cause this condition.
- The condition manifests as epiphoria, chronic overflow of tears past the lid margin due to a blockage of tear drainage. Palpation of the nasolacrimal duct may cause regurgitation of tears from the puncta.
- Conservative treatment involves light fingertip massage of the duct to promote drainage. If the condition does not respond to conservative management, surgical drainage will be required.

Dacrocystitis (ICD: 375.3)

Infection of the lacrimal sac. (<u>Merck Manual</u>, p. 707)

- Dacrocystitis is usually a consequence of dacrostenosis. In addition to epiphoria, the individual may manifest fever and an elevated WBC count, in addition to conjunctivitis and local redness over the lacrimal sac.
- Palpation of the nasolacrimal duct may cause regurgitation of pus from the puncta.
- Conservative management involves hot compresses to promote drainage and healing. If an abscess has formed, incision and drainage and antibiotic therapy will probably be required.

Blepharitis (ICD: 373.0)

Inflammation of the lid margins with redness, thickening, and often the formation of scales and crusts or shallow marginal ulcers. (<u>Merck Manual</u>, p. 708)

- Blepharitis is inflammation of the eyelids. The condition may be either acute or chronic. Acute blepharitis is usually caused by a staphylococcal infection. Chronic blepharitis may be a consequence of seborrheic dermatitis or allergies.
- The condition manifests as persistent redness of the eyelid margins with accumulation of greasy flakes or scales around the base of the eyelashes, usually more noticeable upon awaking in the morning.

- Treatment usually consists of improved eyelid hygiene. It is essential that germs not be transmitted to the eye. As such, it is recommended that the individual not touch their eyes with their fingers. The crusts can be gently removed with a Q-tip soaked in diluted baby shampoo.
- If the condition does not improve with conservative management, an antibiotic such as tetracycline may be required.

Hordeolum (Stye) (ICD: 373.1)

An acute localized pyogenic (usually staphylococcal) infection of one or more of the glands of Zeis or Moll, of the eyelash follicle (external hordeolum), or rarely of the meibomian glands (internal hordeolum, meibomian stye). (Merck Manual, p. 709)

- A hordeolum or sty is an infection of a hair follicle at the lid margin. In about 90-95% of the cases the organism is *Staphylococcus aureus*. The condition usually results from a blockage of Zeis or Moll sebaceous glands.
- Much less common, but more severe when it occurs, an internal hordeolum can result from infection of the meibomian gland. This condition may present similar to a chalazion. However, while the sty is very painful, the chalazion is not.
- Often the sty will come to a head and rupture on its own. If not, it may need to be surgically lanced. If the condition does not respond to conservative measures, oral antibiotics are indicated.

Chalazion (ICD: 373.2)

Chronic granulomatous enlargement of a meibomian gland from occlusion of its duct, often following inflammation of the gland and surrounding tissue. (Merck Manual, p. 710)

- A chalazion is a retention cyst of the meibomian gland. It appears similar to a sty, however the swelling points inward, not to the lid margin, and the contents of the cyst are generally sebaceous, rather than infectious.
- While the condition <u>may</u> have been painful in the early stages, it usually manifests as a chronic painless nodule on the inner eyelid margin.
- About one quarter of chalazia resolve without treatment. Conservative management involves hot compresses, followed by digitally massage the area to break and express the sebaceous nodule. If this does not resolve the condition, surgical removal is necessary.

Entropion (ICD: 374.0) and Ectropion (ICD: 374.1)

Inversion (entropion) and eversion (ectropion) of the eyelid can result from aging or from scar formation. (Merck Manual, p. 710)

- Ectropion is a turning out of the lower eyelid. Entropion is when the eyelid is turned in. The skin of the eye is the thinnest of the body. As such, it tends to sag with aging. Both of these conditions may affect either the upper or lower eyelid, although the lower lid is more commonly affected.

- Both conditions cause excessive tearing (epiphoria) for slightly different reasons. If the lower lid sags sufficiently that it loses contact with the globe, this will disturb the normal drainage flow of tears. The eye will become dry and excessive tearing will result. If the lower eyelid is turned in, rubbing of the eyelashes will irritate the cornea and also cause excessive tearing.
- Conservative care involves lubricating eyedrops to prevent drying of the eye. Surgery (blepharoplasty) may be the only successful long term solution.

Ptosis (ICD: 374.3) (Merck Manual, p. 1454)

- Ptosis is when the upper lid covers all or part of the pupil. The lid should cover part of the iris, but not the pupil. Ptosis may occur with myasthenia gravis, Horner's syndrome, or CN III damage.
- As we age the connective tissue that connects the palpebral muscles to the eyelids may become stretched. This is another possible cause of ptosis. It is not uncommon for patients to develop a 'droopy' upper eyelid following cataract surgery.
- Obviously ptosis may be a symptom of an underlying condition that must be dealt with.

Xanthelasma (ICD: 374.8) (Merck Manual, p. 710)

- Xanthelasma are fatty, yellowish lesions on the upper or lower eyelids. These lesions are benign and not clinically significant. They are most commonly seen with aging.
- It is thought that these deposits are a consequence of lipid metabolism. As such, serum cholesterol and triglycerides should be checked.

Abnormalities of the External Eye, Iris, and Cornea

Acute Conjunctivitis (ICD: 372.0)

An acute conjunctival inflammation, occurring in populations with good hygiene, caused by viruses, bacteria, or allergy. (Merck Manual, p. 711)

- The conjunctiva are clear membranes that protect the eyeball and inner surface of the eyelids. When these membranes become inflamed conjunctivitis, more commonly known as 'pink eye' results. The inflammation may be caused by bacteria, viruses, or environmental causes such as tobacco smoke or chemical burns.
- The condition is quite common, representing about 30% of all eye complaints. If there is a yellow green colored discharge, a bacterial infection from *Staph* or *Strep* is likely.
- Viral and allergic conjunctivitis produce a clear watery discharge with itching. Preauricular lymphadenopathy is common with bacterial and viral conjunctivitis, and uncommon with allergic conjunctivitis.

- Treatment depends upon the cause. Viral and bacterial conjunctivitis are highly contagious, so patients should avoid touching their eyes which can spread the condition to the other eye or to other members of the family.
- Bacterial infection may require a topical antibiotic in the eye. If untreated, bacterial conjunctivitis may progress to more serious conditions such as cellulitis.
- Viral conjunctivitis usually accompanies the common cold, a self limiting condition requiring only supportive care. Allergic conjunctivitis requires elimination of the allergen, such as environmental tobacco smoke.
- An online review article of the causes of 'red eye' is found on: http://content.nejm.org/cgi/content/short/343/5/345

Chronic Conjunctivitis (ICD: 372.1)

A chronic inflammation of the conjunctiva characterized by exacerbations and remissions that occur over months or years. (Merck Manual, p. 715)

- Chronic conjunctivitis may be a consequence of physical conditions which irritate the eye, such as ectropion, entropion, blepharitis, or chronic dacryocystitis. Obviously continued exposure to irritants such as tobacco smoke can cause chronic conjunctivitis.
- Treatment should be directed at the underlying cause.

Trachoma (Granular Conjunctivitis; Egyptian Ophthalmia) (ICD: 076.9)

A chronic conjunctivitis caused by Chlamydia trachomatis and characterized by progressive exacerbations and remissions, with conjunctival follicular hyperplasia, corneal neovascularization, and scarring of the conjunctiva, cornea, and eyelids. (Merck Manual, p. 715)

- While not a common problem in the developed world, trachoma is still a serious health problem in regions where economic and sanitary conditions are poor. Trachoma is one of the oldest documented infectious conditions, first described during the times of the Egyptian pharaohs.
- Chlamydia is an intracellular bacteria that causes scarring of the conjunctiva and cornea. If untreated it eventually causes blindness. Worldwide there are an estimated 146 million cases in need of treatment, and an estimated 15% of blindness worldwide is caused by trachoma.
- Tetracycline ointment in the eye is the usual treatment. If the condition has cause deformity of the eyelid (entropion) surgery will be required.

Scleritis (ICD: 379.0)

A severe, destructive, vision-threatening inflammation involving the deep episclera and sclera. (Merck Manual, p. 717)

- Severe boring eye pain that wakes the individual at night is the most common symptom that causes the patient to seek treatment for this condition. Upon examination, the patch of inflammation on the white sclera may appear a deep blue red or purple color. The individual will also probably experience photophobia or extreme light sensitivity.
- In the majority of cases, the inflammation is a manifestation of an autoimmune inflammatory disorder, such as rheumatoid arthritis, SLE, gout, psoriatic arthritis, or Wegener's granulomatosis.
- The treatment must be directed at the underlying cause. The patient will probably be put on oral corticosteroids, and possibly immunosuppressive drugs, such as cyclosporine.

Uveitis (ICD: 364)

Inflammation of any component of the uveal tract (iris, ciliary body, or choroid). (Merck Manual, p. 725)

- Iritis is inflammation of the iris. Inflammation of the iris and the ciliary body is called iridocyclitis or anterior uveitis. Choroiditis is referred to as posterior uveitis.
- Uveitis may result from a variety of causes such as autoimmune arthritides, bacterial or viral infections, and tuberculosis.
- Symptomatically, the condition presents as eye pain with photophobia. Anterior uveitis is typically more symptomatic than posterior uveitis.
- Upon examination, iritis manifests as a red halo around the iris and cornea. This is different from conjunctivitis, where the redness is seen more at the periphery. Inflammation of the ciliary body can cause both decreased and increased intraocular pressure (IOP). The inflammation may cause decreased aqueous production by the inflamed ciliary body, or intraocular pressure may be elevated as a result of obstructed aqueous outflow.
- Treatment must be directed to the cause. Prompt referral is indicated, as untreated iritis can lead to glaucoma.

Pinguecula (ICD: 372.5)

- Pinguecula are a yellowish thickening of the bulbar conjunctiva. They may be due to prolonged exposure to wind, dust, or other irritants. They occur first at the nasal side, and later at the temporal side of the eye, and are more common with aging. In contrast to the more significant pterygium, pinguecula are harmless.

Pterygium (ICD: 372.4)

- Pterygium are similar in appearance to pinguecula, and may be considered a pinguecula that has progressed beyond the harmless stage. The yellowish thickening has now grown across the cornea, usually from the nasal side, and may interfere with vision if it covers the pupil.

- Pterygium may grow and pull on the cornea sufficiently that they change the refractive properties of the eye, causing astigmatism. When this occurs, or if the pterygium covers the pupil surgical removal is indicated.

Hyphema (ICD: 360.8)

- Hyphema is blood in the anterior chamber of the eye. The usual cause is blunt or penetrating trauma. In the absence of trauma, spontaneous hemorrhage can develop if the individual has a bleeding disorder, such as hemophilia, or as the result of blood thinning medication (coumadin).
- Symptomatically, the individual may present with blurred vision, pain, and photophobia.
- While small amounts of blood may clear without treatment, immediate referral to an ophthalmologist is required, as some cases may have increased intraocular pressure requiring the blood to be evacuated.

Hypopyon (ICD: 360.0)

- Pus in the anterior chamber may be a consequence of untreated iritis. Again immediate referral is indicated.

Cicatricial Pemphigoid (Ocular Cicatricial Pemphigoid; Benign Mucous Membrane Pemphigoid) (ICD: 372.6)

A chronic, bilateral, progressive scarring and shrinkage of the conjunctiva with opacification of the cornea. (Merck Manual, p. 717)

- Pemphigus is a rare autoimmune disorder. The ocular manifestations can cause progressive scarring of the conjunctival membranes, which can eventually result in corneal opacity and blindness. This condition occurs primarily after age 60.
- Medical management of ocular cicatricial pemphigoid involves systemic corticosteroids, although this treatment is usually not curative and only slows the progression of the condition.

Subconjunctival hemorrhage (ICD: 372.7) (Merck Manual, p. 702)

- Subconjunctival hemorrhage is a very alarming condition for the patient. The individual may think they have had a stroke, or may lose sight in their eye. While it is prudent to send your patient to an ophthalmologist for a second opinion, you should endeavor to calm your patient as this condition looks much worse than the actual pathology.
- The sclera of the eye presents with a sudden onset of a distinct, sharply circumscribed bright red area of localized hemorrhage. The adjacent conjunctiva is not inflamed and there is no discharge. The condition is unilateral, not painful, and visual acuity is not affected.
- This blood leakage may have occurred as a result of minor trauma, such as coughing or sneezing. The trauma may have been so minor

that the patient does not recall it. Another common cause of subconjunctival hemorrhage is simply rubbing the eyes with too much force.

- The condition will resolve spontaneously in a few weeks without treatment. However if the condition fails to resolve, or keeps recurring, investigation of a bleeding disorder is indicated.

Superficial Punctate Keratitis (ICD: 370.2)

Scattered, fine punctate loss or damage of epithelium from the corneal surface of one or both eyes. (Merck Manual, p. 718)

- Superficial punctate keratitis presents as multiple small opacities over the cornea. Symptomatically, the individual may experience eye discomfort, as if a foreign body was in the eye, tearing and photophobia. Usually the condition is mild enough that visual acuity is not affected.
- While the cause is not certain, the opacities are thought to be the result of a chronic subclinical viral infection.
- The condition usually resolves without treatment, although the use of artificial tears eyedrops may accelerate resolution. However, recurrence of episodes is common.

Corneal Ulcer (ICD: 370.0)

Local necrosis of corneal tissue due to invasion by bacteria, fungi, viruses, or Acanthamoeba. (Merck Manual, p. 718)

- Corneal ulcers can develop from a variety of causes. One of the more common causes is improper cleaning of contact lenses, which places bacteria and viruses in constant contact with the cornea.
- Symptomatically, the individual will experience tearing, photophobia, and the sensation of a foreign body in the eye. A purulent discharge may develop and if the infection is marked, hypopyon may appear.
- This condition requires immediate referral. Untreated corneal ulcers can lead to the formation of scar tissue, with consequent loss of vision.

Herpes Simplex Keratitis (Herpes Simplex Keratoconjunctivitis) (ICD: 370.4)

Corneal herpes simplex virus infection, with a spectrum of clinical appearances, commonly leading to recurring corneal inflammation, vascularization, scarring, and loss of vision. (Merck Manual, p. 719)

- Herpes simplex is one of the most common of viral infections. The same virus that appears as an oral 'cold sore' can be spread to the eye. The condition may appear initially as small fever blister vesicles on the eyelid margins. This infection can spread to the cornea and cause a characteristic dendrite shaped ulcer.

- While herpes infections are self limiting, ophthalmologic referral is indicated for anti-viral therapy, as these infections can cause permanent scarring of the cornea.

Herpes Zoster Ophthalmicus (Ophthalmic Herpes Zoster, Herpes Zoster Virus Ophthalmicus, Varicella-Zoster Virus Ophthalmicus) (ICD: 053.2)

Varicella-zoster virus infection involving the eye. (Merck Manual, p. 719)

- Herpes zoster is infection with the same virus that causes chicken pox. Once the individual recovered from the initial infection (usually in childhood), the virus remains dormant in the nerve root. As we age, our immune function declines. With this decreased immunity, the virus may become reactivated and recur as shingles.
- We typically associate shingles with a band of vesicles between two ribs. However, in the elderly, herpes zoster ophthalmicus, or shingles of the first division of the trigeminal nerve is a very common initial presentation of shingles.
- The patient may experience severe pain, itching, redness, and fluid filled vesicles on the skin around the eye. If the infection spreads to the orbit, corneal irritation, cataract, or glaucoma can result.
- Medical management with antiviral drugs is indicated to forestall the complications that might cause permanent eye damage.

Keratoconjunctivitis Sicca (Keratitis Sicca) (ICD: 370.4)

A chronic, bilateral desiccation of the conjunctiva and cornea due to inadequate tear volume (aqueous tear-deficient keratoconjunctivitis sicca) or to excessive loss of tears due to accelerated evaporation because of poor tear quality (evaporative keratoconjunctivitis sicca). (Merck Manual, p. 720)

- Keratoconjunctivitis Sicca, sometimes referred to as 'dry eye syndrome' may be associated with the autoimmune condition Sjogren's syndrome.
- Paradoxically, conditions that cause excessive tearing, such as working around smoke can also cause this condition. The steady flow of tears that are constantly produced are 'lubricating' tears' which contain sebaceous secretions to keep the eye from drying out. 'Reflex tearing' is a sudden release of tears when the eye is irritated. If reflex tearing predominates, it will wash away the protective oils and as a result, the eye may become dry.
- The individual may experience burning eye pain, tearing, and photophobia. The Schirmer test measures the ability of the eye to wet a strip of sterile filter paper, thus a measurement of tear production.
- Treatment consists of specialized eyedrops, such as lacrilube, that contain lubricant.

Keratomalacia (Xerotic Keratitis; Xerophthalmia) (ICD: 370.8)

A condition associated with Vitamin A deficiency and protein-calorie malnutrition, characterized by a hazy, dry cornea that becomes denuded. (Merck Manual, p. 722)

- In addition to causing night blindness, a vitamin A deficiency can cause dry eyes (xerophthalmia), dry conjunctiva (xerosis), keratin deposits on the bulbar conjunctiva (Bitot's spots), and a softening of the cornea which may lead to blindness (keratomalacia).

Keratoconus (ICD: 371.6)

A slowly progressive ectasia of the cornea, usually bilateral, beginning between ages 10 and 20. (Merck Manual, p. 722)

- Keratoconus literally means 'cone shaped cornea'. The cornea is normally dome shaped. Because of thinning of anterior surface of the cornea, it protrudes assuming a more cone shaped. The condition is usually bilateral, although not necessarily symmetric.
- While the research is incomplete, keratoconus is probably genetic, and has a higher than expected association with conditions such as Marfan's syndrome and Down's syndrome. The onset is usually during puberty.
- The cornea is responsible for about two thirds of the refractive power of the eye, with the lens contributing only about one third towards focusing the image on the retina. Keratoconus may be detected when the adolescent requires frequent change of their eyeglass prescription, as their vision becomes progressively more near sighted. In some cases, rigid contact lenses offer a better correction. Eventually, if the condition continues to worsen, the individual may require corneal transplantation.
- Patients with keratoconus are advised to avoid rubbing their eyes, as this may make the condition worse.

Corneal Transplantation (Corneal Graft, Penetrating Keratoplasty) (ICD: V42.5)

A surgical procedure to remove the diseased part of the cornea and replace it with a similarly shaped and sized part of a healthy donor cornea. (Merck Manual, p. 722)

- While the cornea usually lasts a lifetime, either through injury, disease, or congenital defect the cornea may become incapable of adequately focusing light onto the retina.
- During the surgery, about two thirds of the old cornea is removed and replaced with a donor cornea. Because the cornea is relatively avascular, corneal transplants have the highest success rates of any transplant surgery.

Arcus senilis (ICD: 379.9)

- This is a grayish white deposit of lipoid material around the limbus of the iris. It has no effect on vision.
- This condition is a 'normal variant' not uncommon in the elderly. While this whitish ring is thought to contain cholesterol, the individual may or may not have elevated serum cholesterol.

Pupil Abnormalities

Anisocoria (ICD: 379.4) (Merck Manual, p. 1454)

- Unequal pupil size may be normal in 5-20% of the population. If both pupils react equally to light and accommodation, this may be of no cause for concern.

Miosis (ICD: 379.4) (Merck Manual, p. 1454)

- Pupils fixed and constricted (< 2 mm). This is seen as a reaction to drugs, such as pilocarpine drops used for treatment of glaucoma.

Mydriasis (ICD: 379.4) (Merck Manual, p. 1454)

- Pupils fixed and dilated (> 6 mm). This occurs with the 'fight or flight' sympathetic response. If the person is unconscious from trauma, fixed and dilated pupils may indicate irreversible brain damage.

Blind eye (ICD: 369.8) (Merck Manual, p. 1454)

- In addition to impaired visual acuity, there will be a lack of direct and consensual pupillary constriction when light is directed into the blind eye.

Oculomotor (CN III) damage (ICD: 951.0) (Merck Manual, p. 1454)

- There will be a dilated pupil that fails to respond to light or accommodation. Ptosis of the upper eyelid and lateral deviation of the eye may be present.

Argyll Robertson pupil (ICD: 379.4) (Merck Manual, p. 1454)

- Small irregular shaped pupils that react to near vision (accommodation), but fail to react to light. It is classically associated with untreated neurosyphillis, however other causes such as polio, multiple sclerosis, syringomyelia, and alcoholism have been reported.

Adie's tonic pupil (ICD: 379.4) (Merck Manual, p. 1454)

- This benign condition results in a unilateral dilated pupil that reacts sluggishly to both light and accommodation. This patient may also have diminished deep tendon reflexes.

Horner's Syndrome (ICD: 337.9)

Variable ptosis, miosis, and anhidrosis developing on the same side of the face after injury to ipsilateral sympathetic fibers in the hypothalamus, brain stem, spinal cord, C-8 to T-2 ventral spinal roots, superior cervical ganglion, internal carotid sheath to the iris, and upper eyelid. (Merck Manual, p. 1455)

- Damage to the eye's sympathetic nerve supply results in a unilateral small pupil. This small pupil will still react normally to light and accommodation. Ptosis, or drooping of the upper eyelid will cause the eye to appear smaller. Less commonly, anhydrosis or a loss of sweating on the same side will occur.
- When Horner's syndrome is seen, a Pancoast tumor should be investigated.

Abnormalities of the Lens and Optic Disc

Cataract (ICD: 366)

Developmental or degenerative opacity of the lens. (Merck Manual, p. 724)

- The lens of the eye is composed of water and protein and should be clear. With aging, the protein can clump together to produce the lens clouding characteristic of cataract. In the early stages, this clouding may be barely visible. However, in time the lens will begin to become opaque. Cataract is the leading cause of blindness. By age 65, about one half of Americans will have a cataract.
- Juvenile cataracts are sometimes the result of diabetes and have a distinctive 'snowflake' pattern.
- The main symptom is a painless loss of vision. Elderly patients may notice this most at night and have difficulty driving at night.
- When you begin ophthalmoscopy, the retina normally appears as a 'red reflex' within the pupil. A small cataract may stand out as a dark shadow on the red reflex. Complete absence of the red reflex suggests a large cataract.
- An additional ophthalmoscopic procedure is to start with a focus on the anterior cornea (+20 diopter). Then, dial down toward a zero diopter until the retina comes into focus. Normally, nothing is 'in focus' until the focal point reaches the back of the eye. If a cloudiness comes into focus during this procedure, this may be a cataract you are visualizing.
- Once the loss of vision begins to prevent or interfere with daily activities, cataract surgery will help the individual return to a more productive lifestyle. During the surgery, the defective lens is removed surgically or by an ultrasound emulsification and suction procedure. An artificial lens is then inserted in its' place.
- Chronic exposure to ultraviolet light is thought to contribute toward cataracts. As such, wearing sunglasses when in direct sunlight is a good preventive measure.

Papilledema (Choked disk) (ICD: 377.0)

Swelling of the optic nerve head due to increased intracranial pressure. (Merck Manual, p. 738)

- Papilledema is sometimes referred to as a 'choked disc'. Increased intracranial pressure causes the optic disc to bulge outward toward the doctor. This pressure may be from a space occupying lesion such as a brain tumor. If trauma has occurred, it is a sign of serious brain injury. Another possible cause is malignant hypertension.
- The underlying condition that is causing the increased intracranial pressure is usually sufficient that the papilledema is almost always bilateral. When the disc bulges out, the physiological cup is difficult to visualize and the margins of the disc are blurred. The blood vessels will curve as they pass over the margin of the elevated disk.
- Papilledema is usually painless and does not cause a significant loss of visual acuity. However, there may be an enlargement of the normal physiological blind spot. Immediate referral is indicated. The underlying cause of the increased intracranial pressure may be life threatening, or sustained pressure may cause optic atrophy and blindness.

Papillitis (Optic Neuritis) (ICD: 377.3)

Inflammation or infarction of that portion of the optic nerve visible ophthalmoscopically. (Merck Manual, p. 739)

- Papillitis may cause a swelling of the optic disc that appears very similar to papilledema. This swelling may be the result of an inflammation such as temporal arteritis, or a demyelinating condition such as MS.
- However, while papilledema is usually bilateral, papillitis is usually unilateral. Another distinguishing characteristic is that while papilledema has minimal effect on vision, the inflammation of optic neuritis does frequently cause blindness and the condition may be painful.

Optic Atrophy (ICD: 377.1)

Atrophy of the optic nerve. (Merck Manual, p. 741)

- Optic atrophy is a sign that manifests with death of optic nerve tissue, resulting in a pale white disc. The retinal vessels may also be smaller and atrophic.
- In some cases, optic atrophy is congenital. Acquired optic atrophy may develop from a variety of causes, such as occlusions of the central retinal vein or artery, glaucoma, or neurological disorders.
- Leber's optic neuropathy is a rare X-linked genetic disorder that affects 20-30 year old males causing progressive optic atrophy and blindness.
- If the atrophy is sufficient that the individual is blind in that eye, both direct and consensual pupillary constriction will be absent when the light is directed into the blind eye.

Glaucoma (ICD: 365)

A group of disorders characterized by progressive damage to the eye at least partly due to intraocular pressure. (Merck Manual, p. 733)

- Glaucoma is the condition of increased intraocular pressure within the eye. The condition may develop as a result of increased production of aqueous humor, inadequate drainage at the canal of Schlemm, or both.
- About 3 million Americans have glaucoma, and worldwide the condition affects 67 million. It is the second most common cause of blindness, and the leading cause of blindness among African-Americans. Many of these individuals are unaware they have the condition, which is why glaucoma is sometimes referred to as the *"sneak thief of sight"*.
- A gradual loss of visual acuity is the first symptom. The individual will notice a blurring of their vision, especially at the peripheral fields.
- When seen through the ophthalmoscope, increased intraocular pressure will create a posterior depression of the optic disc. The physiological cup is prominent and enlarged (cup to disc ratio is greater than 1:2). As contrasted with papilledema, the disc margin is distinct, and the retinal vessels may be displaced nasally as they sink in over the disc margin.
- Increased intraocular pressure can be measured by the eye doctor using puff tonometry.
- Glaucoma is a condition that is 'managed', rather than 'cured'. Medication can decrease aqueous production or facilitate aqueous drainage. As a last resort, laser surgery can enlarge the drainage system. If untreated, glaucoma can eventually progress to optic atrophy and blindness.

Primary Open-Angle Glaucoma (ICD: 365.1)

Glaucoma associated with an open anterior chamber angle. (Merck Manual, p. 733)

- Primary open angle glaucoma is the most common type of glaucoma, accounting for approximately 70-90% of all glaucoma. While the outflow of aqueous humor is restricted, it is not because the anterior chamber angle formed by the iris and cornea is reduced. The condition is typically bilateral and symptoms develop gradually. By the time vision is affected, there may already be permanent damage. Hence the importance of routine screening and early detection.

Angle-Closure Glaucoma (ICD: 365.2)

Glaucoma associated with a closed anterior chamber. (Merck Manual, p. 736)

- Angle closure glaucoma occurs in less than 10% of all glaucoma patients. The outflow of aqueous humor is blocked by a narrow angle where the iris meets the cornea. The condition may be acute or chronic.

- With an acute episode, the rapid increase in intraocular pressure in one eye produces a redness around the iris, and the eye is painful. The pupil may be dilated and react poorly to light. If gentle pressure is applied over the closed eye, the eye will feel more firm than the unaffected eye. Immediate referral is indicated, as optic atrophy and permanent blindness can result within a few hours.

Abnormalities of the Retinal Vessels and Background

Hypertensive Retinopathy (ICD: 362.1)

Retinopathy resulting from high blood pressure. (<u>Merck Manual</u>, p. 729)

- Hypertension causes progressive damage to retinal vessels and the retinal background:
  - o   narrowed retinal arteries
  - o   'copper wire' deformity (widened light reflex)
  - o   'silver wire' deformity (vessel is completely opaque to light)
  - o   A-V nicking
  - o   flame and splinter hemorrhages
  - o   'cotton wool' soft exudates (local ischemic infarcts)
  - o   ischemic papilledema
  - o   perivascular sheathing (perivascular edema may make the arteries appear white and swollen)
  - o   'macular star' hard exudates around the macula

Diabetic Retinopathy (ICD: 362.0)

A variety of pathologic retinal changes characteristic of chronic diabetes mellitus. (<u>Merck Manual</u>, p. 729)

- Diabetic retinopathy affects the veins more than the arteries. Venous stasis results in:
  - o   microaneurysms
  - o   dot & blot hemorrhages
  - o   soft exudates
  - o   hard exudates (lipid remains of vascular leakage)
  - o   neovascularization near the macula is a dangerous complication of diabetes and requires prompt referral if vision is to be preserved.

Central Retinal Artery Occlusion (ICD: 362.3)

Blockage of the central retinal artery, producing painless, sudden, unilateral blindness. (<u>Merck Manual</u>, p. 730)

- A blockage of a main retinal artery by a blood clot can cause sudden loss of vision in one eye. The patient at risk for this condition parallels the risk factors for stroke and heart attack. Central retinal artery occlusion has also been associated with temporal arteritis.

- In some cases, the clot may dislodge, in which case the blindness is temporary. A temporary painless loss of vision in one eye is referred to as amaurosis fugax.
- Occlusion of small arteries causes 'cotton wool' infarcts. When the blood flow to a larger area is blocked, the retina may appear pale and the macula which is normally hard to see appears as a cherry red spot against this pale background.
- Immediate referral is indicated, as the condition may cause permanent blindness.

Central Retinal Vein Occlusion (ICD: 362.3)

Blockage of the central retinal vein, usually occurring in elderly patients. (Merck Manual, p. 731)

- Occlusion of a main retinal vein can also result in painless loss of vision in one eye. The condition occurs primarily in the elderly, probably as a consequence of diabetes or hypertension. The onset of symptoms are slower than with arterial occlusion.
- Obstruction of venous drainage will cause leakage of blood from the capillary bed. This in turn may cause ischemia and 'cotton wool' infarcts. Neovascularization may develop later as an attempt to reestablish normal circulation. Unfortunately, this growth of blood vessels can actually cause further visual loss.

Age-Related Macular Degeneration (Senile Macular Degeneration) (ICD: 362.5)

Atrophy or degeneration of the macula. (Merck Manual, p. 731)

- Age related macular degeneration (AMD) is a very common condition, and is one of the leading causes of visual impairment in the elderly. Vision is lost in the fovea centralis region of the retina. Peripheral vision is spared. For this reason, these individuals are not truly 'blind'. However, daily activities that require central vision, such as reading, watching television, or driving an automobile are severely impaired.
- Approximately 90% of macular degeneration is the atrophic or 'dry' form. Drusen are small yellow spots on the retina that are considered to be a 'normal variant'. Newer research suggests that drusen develop when there is a lack of antioxidants to clear the waste products from the eyes. Drusen are normally small and do not affect vision. However, the retina overlying these spots becomes thin and atrophies when they accumulate. The loss of vision with this 'dry' form of macular degeneration is gradual. There is no known treatment other than nutritional prevention.
- About 10% of macular degeneration is exudative or 'wet' macular degeneration. With this form, neovascularization or new blood vessels develop within the choroid layer. These new vessels can leak fluid or bleed, causing subretinal edema and hemorrhage. This in turn damages the rods and cones in the overlying retina. With the

'wet' form the loss of vision may be sudden and severe. Laser photocoagulation therapy can be used to halt the spread of hemorrhage and vision loss. However, this treatment only prevents a worsening of the condition. It is not capable of restoring vision that has already been lost.

- The American Macular Degeneration Foundation has a website with a printable Amsler grid chart that is used to diagnose the condition: http://www.macular.org/chart.html
- The following Medscape link is a good summary article on macular degeneration: http://www.medscape.com/viewarticle/432579_print

Retinal Detachment (ICD: 361)

Separation of the neural retina from the underlying retinal pigment epithelium. (Merck Manual, p. 731)

- The vitreous is a clear jelly like substance that fills most of the space within the eye. This substance helps to hold the thin retina against the back of the eye. As we age, this vitreous may become more fluid and less jelly like. If the vitreous pulls away from the retina, it can pull the retina with it. Once fluid passes behind the retina, it may continue to detach. Retinal detachment is painless. However, when this occurs the individual may experience a flash of light, or a new 'floater'.
- While retinal detachment can occur at any age, they are most common after age 60. Myopic patients (the globe is elongated in the AP dimension) are at greater risk for retinal detachment.
- Any patient who experiences flashes of light, new 'floaters', or partial loss of one quadrant of the visual field in one eye should have an immediate referral to an ophthalmologist.
- Mild retinal detachments may heal without treatment. Others require laser photocoagulation to 'spot weld' the retina in place.

Retinitis Pigmentosa (ICD: 362.5)

A slowly progressive, bilateral, tapetoretinal degeneration. (Merck Manual, p. 732)

- Retinitis pigmentosa (RP) is a hereditary disorder that affects about one in 3700 people. The condition usually appears between age 10 to 30.
- Pathologically, there is a breakdown of the rods, and to a lesser extent the cones of the retina. Since the rods are needed to see in low light conditions, the individual may first notice that they stumble when moving around objects at night.
- When viewed with an ophthalmoscope, the damaged areas present as dark pigmentation in a bone spicule pattern against the red retinal background.
- Typically vision is lost first at the periphery, thus resulting in 'tunnel vision'. The condition is progressive, although it may take as long as ten years before all vision is lost.

- There is no known treatment for retinitis pigmentosa, although Vitamin A supplementation is thought to slow the progression of the condition.

Refractive Error (ICD: 367) (Merck Manual, p. 741)

- Emmetropia: Normal vision, the cornea and lens focus light correctly on the retina.
- Myopia: Nearsighted, the globe is elongated in the AP dimension resulting in light being focused anterior to the retina.
- Hyperopia: Farsighted, the globe is flattened in the AP dimension resulting in light being focused posterior to the retina.
- Astigmatism: The cornea and lens are not symmetric. This causes light entering the eye to focus in several different points within the eye.

Normal variants

- Scleral crescent: gray white crescent at the optic disc margin.
- Pigmented crescent: black retinal pigment at temporal margin of the optic disc .
- Drusen: Drusen are small yellow dots scattered sporadically on the retina. They are granular deposits that are easily confused with hard exudates. How would you rule out serious disease that causes exudates? Although they may occur coincident with age related macular degeneration, they are usually benign and do not affect vision.
- Myelinated nerve fibers: These present as fine feathery patches that may obscure the disc margin and retinal vessels. They are usually unilateral and are present at birth. While they resemble cotton wool exudates, myelinated nerve fibers are the only white structures with a feathery edge.

General principles of ophthalmoscopy

- Hemorrhages and exudates are never normal.
- Microaneurysms indicate diabetes mellitus until proven otherwise.
- A-V nicking indicates hypertension until proven otherwise.
- Hemorrhages and exudates are not specific for any disease. The eye exam alerts you to the possibility of hypertension or diabetes, but you must follow up with specific tests for those conditions.

Study Guide Objectives

o Know the external and internal anatomical structures of the eye.
o Know the functions of these eye structures.
o Know the cranial nerves involved with specific eye motions, corneal blink reflex, pupillary light reflex, etc.
o What structure provides fluid and nutrition to the eye?
o Which bones form the orbit?
o What anterior eye structure is continuous with the sclera?

- What anterior eye structures are continuous with the choroid?
- What structure produces the 'blind spot' on the visual field?
- Know how to use eye charts and how to document visual acuity.
- Can the Rosenbaum card be used to assess distant vision?
- During visual field testing, which direction provides the greatest field of vision?
- What causes bitemporal hemianopia?
- What is the Hirschberg test?
- Why would you perform the cover-uncover test?
- What is the significance of a few beats of 'end point' nystagmus?
- What is the significance of sustained nystagmus?
- What is the significance of thinning of the lateral margins of the eyebrows?
- What is the significance of epicanthal folds?
- What is the significance of yellow sclera?
- What is meant by PERRLA?
- Know how to test for pupillary light reflex, fixation, and accommodation.
- Know the definition of miosis, mydriasis, anisocoria, Argyll Robertson pupil, Adie's tonic pupil, etc.
- What is strabismus?
- What is scotoma?
- What is amaurosis fugax?
- Which is more serious: pinguecula or pterygium?
- What causes glaucoma?
- Which cranial nerve is involved with herpes zoster ophthalmicus?
- Know the definition of emmetropia, myopia, hyperopia, and astigmatism.
- Which contributes more to refraction of light entering the eye: the cornea or the lens?
- What structure separates the anterior from the posterior chamber of the eye?
- Know the parts and how to use the otoscope/ophthalmoscope diagnostic set.
- Know how to perform the ophthalmoscopic examination of the eye.
- Know what causes the 'red reflex'.
- Know the internal eye structures visible through the ophthalmoscope.
- Know the changes that occur in and around the eye with aging, and causes of decreased visual acuity in an older adult.
- Know the history questions that should be asked for eye conditions.
- Know the signs and symptoms associated with the various eye conditions discussed.
- Know which eye conditions cause visual loss.
- Know which eye conditions cause eye pain.
- Know which eye conditions cause a red eye.
- Know the characteristics of a normal optic disc.
- Know the eye changes pertinent to diabetes vs. hypertensive retinopathy.

- Know the common pathologies responsible for peripheral field defects.
- Know the significance of 'lid lag'.
- Know the significance of a pale optic disc.
- Know the significance of an increased cup to disc ratio.
- Know what causes Argyll Robertson pupil.
- Know the significance of A-V nicking in the retinal background.
- Know the significance of hard and soft exudates in the retinal background.
- Know the significance of hemorrhages in the retinal background.
- Know the significance of papilledema.
- Know the significance of microaneurysms in the retinal background.
- Know the significance of drusen.
- Know the difference between how Horner's syndrome vs. Oculomotor III nerve damage manifests.
- What structures visible on ophthalmoscopy are considered 'normal variants'?

7 – Ears, Nose, & Throat

Anatomy & Physiology

The ear, the body's sensory organ of hearing and equilibrium is divided into three compartments. The external ear begins with the auricle, also called the pinna, which funnels sound into the external auditory canal. This approximately one inch long canal, which terminates at the tympanic membrane, is lined with glands that secrete protective cerumen. When visualized through the otoscope, the tympanic membrane (often charted as TM) appears pearly gray. The circumference of the tympanic membrane is anchored by a fibrous annulus. The eardrum is pulled in slightly by the malleus and is angled inward at the inferior margin. These two factors produce the 'cone of light' at the anterior inferior surface. The umbo, manubrium, and short process of the malleus may be seen through the translucent eardrum. The inferior portion of the drum is taut (pars tensa), while the smaller superior portion is referred to as the pars flaccida.

The middle ear is an air filled chamber within the temporal bone. When intact, the tympanic membrane seals the outer opening. The eustachian canal provides for an air passage between the middle ear and the nasopharynx to equalize pressure on both sides of the eardrum. In adults, this canal angles anteriorly and inferior. In children, this tube is smaller and more horizontal, which allows for easier migration of pathogens to the middle ear. The ossicles (malleus, incus, and stapes) transmit the vibrations created at the tympanic membrane to the oval window of the inner ear.

The inner ear contains the cochlea and semicircular canals. The cochlea is a coiled structure containing the organ of Corti, which has minute hair cells that convert sound vibration into nerve impulses, which are then transmitted to the brain via CN VIII. The semicircular canals contain fluid that shifts with changes of body position, thus helping us to perceive motion and maintain balance.

The nose serves several functions. As the first part of the respiratory tract, the mucous membranes which line the nasal turbinates warm and moisten the inspired air. Hairs located in the vestibule or opening to the nasal cavity also help filter the air we breathe. The external openings of the nose are the nares, separated by the collumella. The sense of smell is mediated by CN I, which has olfactory receptors at the superior nasal cavity. The nasal mucosa is highly vascular, especially at Kiesselbach's plexus of the anterior nasal cavity. As a result nosebleeds often bleed profusely.

The paranasal sinuses are located above and lateral to the nasal cavity. They produce mucous which drains into the nasal cavity. They also serve to lighten the skull and provide resonance to voice sounds. Only the frontal and maxillary sinuses are accessible to examination. The ethmoid and sphenoid sinuses are positioned more midline and deeper within the skull.

The digestive tract begins with the oral cavity. If they have their full complement, adults have 32 permanent teeth to masticate food. Children have 20 temporary or deciduous teeth which erupt at 6 to 24 months, and are replaced by permanent teeth at 6 to 12 years of age. The teeth are firmly anchored in sockets within the maxilla and mandible. The gingiva, or gums protect this connection. The gingiva are continuous with the buccal mucosa, which line the inner surface of the cheeks. The space between the cheeks and teeth is referred to as the vestibule. The roof of the mouth is the hard palate anteriorly, and the soft palate posteriorly. The uvula is an extension of the soft palate that hangs down at the midline. At the floor of the mouth, the tongue is a versatile muscle that moves the food during chewing. The tongue also contains papillae innervated by cranial nerves VII and IX, which mediate the sensation of taste. The inferior midline of the tongue is the frenulum. Wharton's ducts, on either side of the frenulum, are the openings of the submandibular salivary glands. Stenson's ducts, the openings for the parotid gland are located lateral to the posterior tongue, near the upper second molar. When not helping us with chewing, the tongue helps us to modify voice sounds into words. The tonsils are located between the anterior and posterior pillars, which separate the mouth from the oropharynx. The pharyngeal tonsils, or adenoids, are located superior to the hard and soft palate and are not visible on routine examination.

History

Do you have any pain in your ears?

- Was the onset sudden or gradual?
- Have you had any recent trauma?
- Do you swim frequently?
- Have you experienced any recent cold or sore throat symptoms, eg. upper respiratory infection (URI)? Bacterial and viral infections can travel up the eustachian canal to the middle ear. Dental infection can refer pain to the ear.
- Where does it hurt, close to the surface, or deeper?
- Does it hurt if you pull or push on the ear?
- Does your pain change with different head positions?

Do you have a history of ear infections?

- Recurrent ear infections suggest possible allergies, especially to milk products.

Have you noticed any discharge from your ears?

- What is the color?
  - Clear - may be from CSF if trauma was involved.
  - Purulent - infection with otitis externa, or otitis media if drum has perforated.
  - Foul smelling yellow/gray - cholesteatoma
- Was there a relationship between the pain and the discharge? If the pain decreased when the discharge began, this suggests perforation of the eardrum.

Have you had trouble hearing?

- Did the hearing loss occur suddenly or gradually? Some degree of gradual hearing loss with aging is normal (presbycusis). Sudden onset of hearing loss is more ominous and the cause must be determined.
- Have you had trouble with excessive ear wax?

Do you experience ringing in your ears?

- Does your work or recreational activities expose you to loud noises?
- Do you also experience vertigo and nausea? Unilateral tinnitus with these symptoms may suggest Meniere's disease.
- What medications are you taking? Aspirin, some antibiotics (streptomycin, neomycin), and some anti-inflammatory medicines (indomethacin, naproxen) may cause ringing of the ears as an unintended side effect.

Do you experience dizziness or vertigo?

- Do you feel as if the <u>room</u> is spinning (objective vertigo), or as if <u>you</u> are spinning (subjective vertigo)? True vertigo is a sign of neurological or labyrinthine dysfunction. Dizziness that is not true vertigo is more likely a consequence of cardiovascular disease.

Do you have any nasal discharge?

- Is the discharge mucoid or purulent? Mucoid discharge suggests allergic origin. Purulent discharge suggests infection. If you suspect infection, always check for fever. Clear watery discharge with a history of head trauma is an ominous sign of significant cranial injury.

Do you experience frequent colds?

- How often do you have head colds? Most people experience one to two episodes of coryza a year, especially if they are around children. However, frequent repetitive episodes should alert you to the need to support immune function.

Do you have sinus pain or chronic post nasal drip?

- Chronic sinusitis is most likely allergic in origin.

Have you ever experienced trauma to your nose?

- Previous trauma may result in a deviated septum with subsequent obstruction of one of the nares.

Do you experience frequent nosebleeds?

- How often, how much do you bleed, and does it resolve without treatment? Frequent nosebleeds that are not easily controlled should alert you to the possibility of coagulation disorders, such as hemophilia, leukemia, or idiopathic thrombocytopenia (ITP).

Do you have allergies or hay fever?

- Seasonal rhinitis from pollen is common. Year round allergies are more likely caused by dust or pet dander. Allergic load is additive, therefore treatment must also be multi-factorial.
- What OTC remedies do you use? Overuse of antihistamines can irritate the mucosa and result in rebound swelling. Nutritional guidance is essential.

Have you noticed any sores in your mouth?

- The list of mouth lesions is quite large: aphthous ulcers (canker sore), Koplik's spots, leukoplakia, oral candidiasis, glossitis, carcinoma, etc. Chinese and Ayurvedic medicine consider tongue diagnosis much more important than does Western Medicine.

How frequently do you get sore throats?

- Are there known environmental causes, such as exposure to dust or smoke?
- Is there a fever? Do you also have an upper respiratory infection (URI)? Are there white or yellow exudates on the tonsils or pharynx? These signs are highly suggestive of streptococcal infection. A rapid strep test and/or throat culture are indicated.
- Persistent sore throats warrant additional investigation. Is there also splenomegaly or lymphadenopathy? A monospot test for infectious mononucleosis may be in order.

Do you have bleeding gums?

- Pyorrhea or dental caries are the most likely cause. Injury from overly vigorous tooth brushing is another possible cause. If there are other signs of bleeding abnormalities, disorders of coagulation should be investigated. Overt scurvy, while rare, must also be considered.

Do you have any toothache?

- Dental decay should be referred for appropriate dental care. Your nutritional recommendations can go a long way toward helping your patients keep all of their teeth in good health for all of their years.

Do you have any hoarseness or change in voice?

- Acute hoarseness is most likely the result of viral upper respiratory infection, or overuse of the voice.
- Other *'zebra'* causes include diphtheria, carcinoma, or reflux esophagitis.
- If other neurological abnormalities are present, myasthenia gravis or peripheral neuropathy are possible causes.

Do you have difficulty swallowing?

- Dysphagia with heartburn suggests reflux esophagitis.
- Is there difficulty with swallowing both liquids and solids? Difficulty swallowing liquids suggests esophageal spasm or stricture.
- Is there weight loss? Difficulty swallowing solids and weight loss are danger signals for esophageal carcinoma.

Do you smoke?

- Chronic tobacco use (pipe, cigarettes, or smokeless tobacco) is a risk factor for oral cancer, as well as lung cancer.

Examination

Ears

Inspect and palpate the auricles. Ear size is variable and may have no clinical significance. Down's syndrome children usually have small, low set ears. When palpated the auricles should not be tender. When they are, suspect otitis externa. If the mastoid processes are tender, mastoiditis should be investigated.

In order to inspect the tympanic membrane, select the largest speculum which will fit comfortably in the ear canal. For finer control, hold the otoscope as you would a pencil, not like a hammer. Use your right hand when examining the right ear, your left hand for the patient's left ear. Lightly rest the ulnar side of your fingers against the patient's cheek. With this stabilization, if the patient moves, your hand holding the otoscope will also move. This decreases the likelihood of the speculum injuring the patient. For adults, pull the pinna up and back to straighten the ear canal. For a child, pull the pinna down. Tilt the patient's head slightly away from you. Gently introduce the speculum into the ear canal. It is usually best to observe the outside of the speculum at the beginning of insertion. When it is about half way inserted, bring your eye close to the otoscope, and continue to slowly insert the speculum. Once you are able to visualize the tympanic membrane, nothing is gained from further insertion. If your view is blocked by cerumen, or a very narrow canal, just do the best you can and document what you are able to observe. You should never insert the speculum further than is comfortable for your patient.

Note any redness or irritation of the external canal. The tympanic membrane is normally a pearly gray color. Look for the cone of light and other landmarks of the tympanic membrane. If the cone of light is not visible, there may be bulging of the tympanic membrane. If the patient is able to perform a valsalva maneuver, you may be able to observe eardrum mobility. Insufflation involves introducing pressure via a squeeze bulb to the outside of the tympanic membrane. It can only be performed with a special soft speculum that seals the speculum to the ear canal. If you try to seal the ear canal with an ordinary speculum, you will probably hurt your patient.

Ear examination concludes with assessment of hearing. Have your patient close their eyes and block one ear. Rub your thumb and fingers together close to their other ear and ask, "*Can you hear this?*" When they say yes, say "*Tell me when you can no longer hear it.*" As you continue to rub your fingers, take them further away from their ear. When you are about three feet away, if they have not yet said "*now*", stop rubbing your fingers together and wait for them to tell you the finger rubbing has stopped. Repeat the procedure on the opposite ear. If they can hear finger rubbing to 2-3 feet, and it is heard approximately equal in both ears, this is usually considered an adequate screen of hearing.

If the finger friction rub test is abnormal, or if you want to be more thorough, assess hearing using a 256k or 512k tuning fork. The 128k tuning fork is <u>not</u> appropriate to test hearing. It is used to assess the sense of vibration, or to screen for the presence of a fracture.

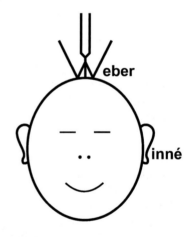

- Weber test: Strike the tuning fork and place it at the midline of the skull. Ask the patient if they hear the sound equally in both ears.
- Rinné test (pronounced RIN-neh): Strike the tuning fork and place it on the mastoid process. Begin timing and ask the patient when they can no longer hear the sound. When they say "*now*", note how many seconds elapsed and place the vibrating tines near their ear and ask them "*can you hear this?*" If they say yes, continue timing until they say the sound disappears again. Normally air conduction is twice as long as bone conduction, after bone conduction has stopped. This is charted as AC > BC or Rinné +. (In orthopedic testing, a positive test result is abnormal, a negative test result is normal. With the Rinné test this pattern is reversed.)
- In practice, you may want to use the following variation of the Rinné test described in the <u>Merck Manual</u> (p. 659):

  "*The stem of a vibrating tuning fork is placed in contact with the mastoid process (for bone conduction); then the tines of the still vibrating fork are held near the pinna (for air conduction), and the patient is asked to indicate which stimulus is louder."*

- Schwabach test: This is not a great test, but it might show up on a board exam. It involves using the tuning fork to compare your patient's bone conduction hearing to your own. We expect the sound to disappear at about the same time for both the doctor and patient.

Nose

Observe the external nares for midline placement of the collumella. A deviated septum may indicate previous nose trauma. If the nares are unequal, have the patient occlude each nostril one at a time and test for unequal air flow. If any external lesions or deformity are noted, palpate for tenderness. The nasal mucosa are very sensitive and easily irritated by inappropriate examination. <u>An ear speculum is the wrong size to use in the nose</u>. A nasal speculum is about 1/4 inch wide and only 1/4 inch deep. This speculum does not irritate the nose, as the much longer ear speculum does. If you do not have the correct speculum, try this: take your thumb or index finger and lift the tip of the nose to increase the size of the nare being examined. Shine your bright light in the opening. You will see more with this method than you will using the wrong size speculum, and your patient will appreciate you not traumatizing their nasal mucosa. Complete examination of the nose would include testing the sense of smell (CN I).

Lightly press on the frontal and maxillary sinuses. The patient will feel pressure, but should not feel pain. If tender, lightly tap the sinus with your finger to test for percussion tenderness. If you suspect sinus inflammation, sinus transillumination is performed by shining a bright light underneath the sinus to check for a fluid level within the sinus. A lack of illumination with sinus pain suggests blocked sinus drainage. A lack of illumination without pain may be the result of sinus agenesis.

Throat

Observe the lips for cracking or cold sores. Board trivia question: What condition causes cherry red lips? Using a tongue blade, inspect the teeth and gums. Dental decay or gingivitis should be referred to a dentist. Observe the dorsum and undersurface of the tongue. Using a tongue blade, push the cheek away from the teeth to inspect the buccal mucosa. Stenson's duct may be visible as a dimple near the upper second molar. Observe the roof of the mouth for conditions such as torus palatinus, or a bruise like macule that is seen with AIDS.

Using the tongue blade to depress the tongue, have the patient say "ahh". The uvula should rise evenly. If it pulls to one side, suspect impairment of CN X. As the patient sticks their tongue out, observe if the tongue deviates to one side. If it does, suspect CN XII impairment.

Inspect the tonsils and posterior pharynx for the presence of inflammation or exudate. Tonsillar enlargement is graded by how far they extend toward the midline. If you are going to treat children in your practice, you may want to have a rapid strep test available in your office, if it is allowed in your state. Regardless of whether you perform the test yourself, or refer the patient out, all questionable cases must be investigated, as untreated streptococcal infection may spread to the heart (endocarditis) or kidneys (acute glomerulonephritis).

Complete examination of the mouth would include testing the gag reflex (CN IX) and the sense of taste (CN VII & IX). During examination of the oral cavity, you may detect the presence of characteristic breath odors. Diabetics often have a sweet fruity breath odor caused by the presence of acetone. An ammonia breath odor may occur with individuals having kidney impairment or in need of bowel detoxification. Obviously dental decay, heavy smoking, and alcohol will also cause breath odors.

Sample Documentation

Upon palpation, the auricles were nontender and free of visible lesion. A small amount of cerumen was visible in the right ear canal. The tympanic membranes were intact, pearly gray in color, with no sign of inflammation. The cone of light and bony landmarks were visualized normally bilaterally. Finger friction rub was heard to three feet bilaterally. Weber's test was heard equally in both ears. Rinné test disclosed AC > BC, and was equal bilaterally.

The nose was symmetric with no skin lesions or deformity. The septum was midline and both nares were patent. Nasal mucosa was pink and moist, with no evidence of polyps or discharge. The sinuses were not tender to palpation or percussion. Transillumination of the sinuses was not performed.

The buccal mucosa and gingiva were pink, moist, and free of lesion. All 32 teeth were present. Multiple mercury amalgam fillings were noted in the posterior molars. The tongue protrudes symmetrically and displays normal papillae. The uvula rises evenly during phonation. The gag reflex was not tested. The tonsils were present, but not enlarged. No inflammation of the posterior pharynx was noted.

Abnormal Findings

Ears

Hearing Loss (ICD: 389)

Deafness can occur from a number of causes, however there are two main categories of hearing loss. It is important that you know representative causes of each type, and how the Weber and Rinné tuning fork tests are used to differentiate between these two types of hearing loss. The following summary shows how each type of hearing loss appears upon examination:

	Weber test	Rinné test	Causes
Normal hearing	Sound heard equally in both ears	AC > BC (Rinné +)	
Conduction hearing loss	Sound lateralizes to the bad ear	AC < BC (Rinné –) or AC = BC (Rinné =)	Impacted Cerumen Perforated TM Otitis Media Otosclerosis
Sensorineural hearing loss	Sound lateralizes to the good ear	AC > BC, but sound is heard for less time in bad ear than in good ear	Congenital Presbycusis Occupational Ototoxic drugs

Conductive hearing loss (Merck Manual, p. 659, 2161)

There are four main causes of conductive hearing loss:

- Impacted cerumen blocks the transmission of sound waves to the tympanic membrane.
- The tympanic membrane is perforated and thus does not move normally when sound strikes the eardrum.
- Otitis media decreases the mobility of the tympanic membrane.
- Otosclerosis of the ear ossicles does not allow normal transmission of motion from the tympanic membrane to the oval window.

Because the normal ear hears room noise that the bad ear does not, the sound of the tuning fork will appear to be heard louder in the bad ear with the Weber test. However, since the conduction of sound via air conduction is blocked, the Rinné will disclose AC < BC or AC = BC.

Sensorineural hearing loss (Merck Manual, p. 659, 2161)

When an individual suffers from sensorineural hearing loss they are 'nerve deaf'. Causes include:

- Congenital – If the mother contracts a rubella infection during the first trimester, the organ of Corti may become irreversibly damaged.
- Presbycusis, the loss of hearing that occurs normally with aging.
- Chronic exposure to loud noise, such as rock musicians, or working around heavy machinery will cause sensorineural deafness.
- Ototoxic drugs – A number of drugs, such as streptomycin and gentamycin are ototoxic. Heather Whitestone was crowned Miss America in 1995. She lost her hearing at 18 months of age following a DPT shot.

With the Weber test, the sound will lateralize to the good ear. Sensorineural hearing loss causes the individual to hear poorly with <u>both</u> air and bone conduction. However, the Rinné test will still show a normal 2:1 ratio of AC > BC. For example in their good ear AC = 60 seconds, BC = 30 seconds; in the bad ear that is nerve deaf AC = 30 seconds, BC = 15 seconds.

Tinnitus (ICD: 388.3)

Perception of sound in the absence of an acoustic stimulus. (<u>Merck Manual</u>, p. 665)

- Tinnitus, or ringing of the ears, is a symptom rather than an anatomical condition. The condition is relatively common, affecting an estimated 30 million Americans.
- Most people experience some ringing in the ears after exposure to loud noises. Other causes include barotrauma, cerumen buildup, Ménière's disease, or as a side effect of ototoxic drugs.
- When there is a correctable cause, treatment is directed to eliminating that cause. Some degree of tinnitus is an expected associated symptom of presbycusis, or age related hearing loss. In fact when tinnitus is present, there is almost always some degree of hearing loss.

Sudden Deafness (ICD: 388.2)

Severe sensorineural hearing loss that usually occurs in only one ear and develops over a period of a few hours or less. (<u>Merck Manual</u>, p. 680)

- A synonym for sensorineural hearing loss is 'nerve deafness'. This is in contrast to a conduction hearing loss, such as caused by a wax obstruction in the ear canal. Some degree of sensorineural hearing loss is a normal consequence of aging. However, in some cases an individual experiences a sudden and severe episode of hearing loss.
- There can be a variety of causes for sudden sensorineural hearing loss (SSHL):
    o Vascular compromise – The blood supply to the cochlea is limited, with no collateral circulation. If this blood supply becomes restricted, essentially a mini-stroke to this blood supply, cochlear function will be compromised.
    o Viral infection – In some cases, the hearing loss is attributed to a recent viral infection, such a measles, mumps, or rubella.
    o Immune – Autoimmune disorders, such as systemic lupus erythematosus, have been known to cause sudden hearing loss.
    o Intracochlear membrane rupture – If the individual sustains trauma, which could include a change in ear pressure with either flying or scuba diving, the delicate membranes within the cochlea may rupture and result in a loss of fluid from the inner ear.

- o Idiopathic – When no cause can be identified, the condition is referred to as idiopathic sudden sensorineural hearing loss (ISSHL). Because of the difficulty in diagnosing sensorineural hearing loss, it is not uncommon for the cause to remain uncertain.
- Symptomatically, the individual may awaken in the morning with a sudden profound hearing loss. Almost always, the condition affects just one ear. Most of these individuals will also experience ringing of the ear, and about one half will also experience vertigo. The condition affects all ages and both sexes equally.
- Clinical evaluation will likely include audiometry, auditory evoked brainstem response testing (ABR), and electronystagmography. An MRI will allow visualization of the inner ear.
- When a cause can be identified, treatment can be directed to that pathophysiology, e.g. clot busting drugs, anti-inflammatory or antiviral medication, etc. However, in many cases, there is no effective treatment. The condition will either recover via the innate healing potential of the body, or it won't. If recovery is going to occur, it usually occurs spontaneously in the first few days or weeks. When the condition persists longer than this, the condition is most likely permanent.

Noise-Induced Hearing Loss (ICD: 388.1) (<u>Merck Manual</u>, p. 680)

- Noise Induced Hearing Loss (NIHL) is one of the most common causes of hearing loss, affecting an estimated 10 million Americans. While some degree of hearing loss is a normal consequence of aging, this process is accelerated by exposure to loud noise.
- Chronic exposure to sound greater than 85 decibels of intensity can result in damage to the cochlea hair cells. A wide variety of occupations routinely involve exposure to loud noises, such as airline pilots, heavy equipment operators, and rock musicians. Even when the exposure is not chronic, a single exposure to a sufficiently loud noise can also result in permanent damage.
- Usually the hearing loss is bilateral and fairly symmetrical. As with many forms of hearing loss, quite often the individual also experiences tinnitus, or a ringing sensation in the ears.
- Prevention is the key. Individuals likely to experience sustained exposure to loud noises should wear ear protection. Once the damage is done, there is no treatment. However, the individual can regain some of the lost function by wearing hearing aids.

Presbycusis (ICD: 389.1)

Sensorineural hearing loss that occurs in people as they age and that may be affected by genetic or acquired factors. (<u>Merck Manual</u>, p. 681)

- As we age, a certain degree of hearing loss is expected. The condition affects about one quarter of individuals in their sixties, and about 40-50% of individuals 75 or older experience presbycusis.

- The causes are multiple. Atherosclerosis and circulatory deficits can affect the health of the sensory hair cells and cause thickening of the basilar membrane of the cochlea. Presbycusis may also represent the manifestation of a lifetime of noise induced hearing loss.
- Typically high frequency hearing is most affected. This is the range in which speech occurs and the individual may experience impaired ability to discriminate words. Since a woman's speech is usually higher pitch than a man's, the individual may have more difficulty hearing a woman's voice. The individual may hold their hand up to their ear to amplify the sound, or remark, "*Say again.*" If the individual is self conscious, they may nod their head in agreement with the speaker, even when they did not fully hear what was said.
- The condition is permanent, and hearing aids are the only real treatment option. Severe cases that are not responsive to hearing aids have benefited from cochlear implants.

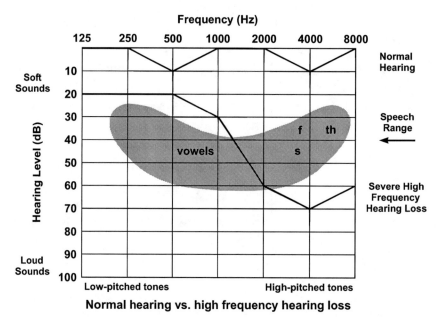

Normal hearing vs. high frequency hearing loss

Drug-Induced Ototoxicity (ICD: 389.9) (Merck Manual, p. 681)

- All drugs have side effects, and certain drugs are known to cause damage to the inner ear. Aminoglycoside antibiotic drugs, such as streptomycin, neomycin, and gentamycin are known to damage both the cochlea and vestibular apparatus. In countries where antibiotics are sold over the counter without prescription, two thirds of deaf mutism is caused by inappropriate use of antibiotics.
- Salicylates, quinine, and cancer medications are the other main categories of drugs that are ototoxic. However, any category of drug can be problematic under certain conditions, such as Heather Whitestone becoming deaf following a DPT shot. It is interesting to

note that the FDA does not require drug manufacturers to test how a new drug affects inner ear function prior to releasing the drug on the market.

- Once again, prevention is the key. Antibiotics can be life saving and should be taken when necessary. However, the patient should always to be told to be alert to ototoxic side effects. If the patient experiences ringing in the ears, hearing loss, or vertigo, they should stop taking the medication and call the prescribing physician immediately.

Tophi (Merck Manual, p. 460)

- Gout is a form of arthritis of that results in deposition of monosodium urate crystals, referred to as tophi. In addition to being deposited in and around the joints, these crystal aggregates may manifest on the external ear.
- Gouty tophi are small, white yellow, non-tender nodules located at the helix or antihelix. It is unlikely that you will discover an undiagnosed case of gout by observing a tophi nodule on the patient's ear. Gouty tophi may not manifest until ten years of chronic untreated gout.
- Treatment must be directed at the underlying systemic cause.

Darwin's Tubercle

- This painless nodule at the helix is sometimes mistaken for tophi. It is considered a normal variant.

Earlobe Crease

- A diagonal earlobe crease is a risk factor for coronary artery disease. These creases, also known as Frank's creases after their discoverer, are thought to be due to increased cholesterol (NEJM, 289:327-328, 1973).

External Ear Obstruction (ICD: 381.6) (Merck Manual, p. 669)

- The glands that line the external ear canal secrete a protective layer of wax. Normally this wax moves outward from the canal carrying dirt with it as skin cells slough off. When cerumen production is excessive, or if it is pushed inward in an attempt to remove the wax, cerumen impaction may result.
- Impacted ear wax is the most common cause of an air conduction deficit in adults. Wet and sticky cerumen is found in whites and blacks, and dry and flaky cerumen occurs in Orientals and Native Americans.
- Most people can successfully clean the cerumen with home measures. Over the counter products, such as Debrox, help to soften and remove impacted cerumen. However, some cases are very stubborn and you can perform a valuable service to your patient if you know the procedure for cleaning ears.

Perforated tympanic membrane (<u>Merck Manual</u>, p. 672)

- If the tympanic membrane is punctured from trauma, or ruptures as a consequence of untreated bacterial otitis media, it can heal with a persistent perforation. Surprisingly, your patient may not be aware of this, and small perforations may cause little hearing loss. They are however at increased risk for bacteria entering the middle ear.

Tympanostomy tubes (<u>Merck Manual</u>, p. 674)

- Children with recurrent acute otitis media may have tympanostomy tubes surgically implanted to relieve the pressure and facilitate drainage. This procedure is referred to as myringotomy.
- Tympanostomy tubes are usually recommended when otitis media does not respond to conservative treatment and persistent conductive hearing loss puts the child at risk for speech impediment. When possible, the child should be assessed via tympanometry and audiometry. Placement of tympanostomy tubes without proper cause does not meet medical 'standard of care' guidelines.
- The tubes normally fall out in 6-12 months and the tympanic membrane will heal with minimal scarring. Many of these children respond favorably with chiropractic adjusting and allergy management.

Tympanosclerosis

- When larger perforations of the tympanic membrane heal, they produce dense white patches. The injury may be the result of chronic inflammation or a consequence of tympanostomy tubes. Approximately one-half of children with tympanostomy tubes will develop tympanosclerosis.

Earache (ICD: 388.7) (<u>Merck Manual</u>, p. 667)

- Earache or otalgia can result from a number of different conditions, however it is most commonly the result of external ear (otitis externa) or middle ear (otitis media) infections. Other causes include dental pathology and TMJ dysfunction. Treatment must be directed to the cause.

External Otitis (ICD: 380.2)

Infection of the ear canal. (<u>Merck Manual</u>, p. 669)

- Otitis externa is an infection of the outer ear, usually caused by *Pseudomonas* or *Staphylococcus*. Because the condition is often associated with swimming, especially if the water is contaminated, it is frequently referred to as swimmer's ear.
- About 10% of external ear infections are fungal, usually caused by *Aspergillus* or *Candida* infection. Fungal infection in the ear canal and on the tympanic membrane presents with a white patch, similar to mold on bread.

- The individual will experience inflammation and pain of the outer ear. Upon inspection, the canal may appear swollen and red. A purulent foul smelling discharge may be present. Tugging on the pinna will be painful and there may be associated regional lymphadenopathy. If the canal becomes obstructed, conductive hearing loss will result.
- A preventive measure is to wash the ear canal with a 1:1 solution of alcohol and vinegar after swimming. The alcohol helps to dry the canal, and the vinegar lowers the pH which helps to prevent the growth of bacteria. Tea tree oil (melaleuca) is another self care remedy with potent antiviral, antibacterial, and antifungal properties.

Acute Mastoiditis (ICD: 383.0)

Bacterial infection in the mastoid process resulting in coalescence of the mastoid air cells. (Merck Manual, p. 675)

- The mastoid air cells are air filled sinuses within the mastoid process. With untreated acute otitis media, the bacterial infection can spread to the mastoid air cells.
- Clinically the condition presents with the same signs and symptoms of acute otitis media, with the addition of inflammation and palpatory tenderness over the mastoid processes. Hearing loss is common. Signs of a systemic infection, such as fever and an elevated white blood count, may also manifest.
- Initial medical treatment will likely be myringotomy and antibiotic treatment. If the condition is unresponsive, a mastoidectomy may be indicated. Untreated mastoiditis can progress to meningitis or intracranial abscess.

Keratinous Cyst (ICD: 706.2) (Wen; Sebaceous Cyst; Steatoma)

A slow-growing benign cyst containing follicular, keratinous, and sebaceous material and frequently found on the scalp, ears, face, back, or scrotum. (Merck Manual, p. 816)

- These benign tumors are the result of a blocked sebaceous gland. They are found most often on the scalp, ears, face, and back. They are often multiple, and painful if they become infected.
- Treatment is to lance the cyst and let it drain. If the dermatologist is unable to remove the cyst wall, it is likely that the cyst will recur.

Acute Otitis Media (ICD: 382.0)

A bacterial or viral infection in the middle ear, usually secondary to a URI. (Merck Manual, p. 673)

- Acute otitis media, also known as acute suppurative otitis media, is a bacterial infection of the middle ear. The condition is very common in infants and small children. It is estimated that by one year of age 50% of infants have experienced an episode of acute otitis media, and by three years of age 80% of children have had the condition. It is the most common reason for a visit to the pediatrician, and costs an estimated $3.5 billion in medical costs each year.

- Acute otitis media is usually preceded by an upper respiratory infection (URI). As we grow and the skull enlarges, the eustachian tube elongates and has a more downward slope. However in young children, this tube is much shorter and horizontal, which allows for easy migration of bacteria from the throat to the middle ear.
- Upon examination, the tympanic membrane is inflamed and presents with what is sometimes referred to as an 'angry red' appearance. The infection behind the eardrum will cause bulging and distort the cone of light reflex. The loss of tympanic membrane mobility produces an air conduction deficit. Tympanic membrane mobility can be measured via pneumatic otoscopy. The condition is painful, and if the tympanic membrane ruptures, there will be a foul smelling discharge, accompanied by a lessening of the pain. When a culture is obtained, the most common infective organism is *Streptococcus pneumoniae.*
- Medical treatment will be antibiotic medication initially. If the condition becomes recurrent, the MD will likely recommend tympanostomy tubes. Chronic infection will impair eardrum mobility and in turn compromise hearing. Because this is occuring while the child is learning language skills, speech may become affected, much as occurs with deaf children.
- Conservative management includes elimination of probable allergens, such as milk. If an infection is present, Tea Tree oil on a wisp of cotton in the ear has potent antibacterial, antiviral, and antifungal healing properties.

Secretory Otitis Media (Serous Otitis Media) (ICD: 381.4)

An effusion in the middle ear resulting from incomplete resolution of acute otitis media or obstruction of the eustachian tube. (Merck Manual, p. 674)

- When serous fluid accumulates behind the eardrum, this is referred to as secretory otitis media, or otitis media with effusion. The condition is usually chronic (greater than 3 months), and the fluid is not infectious. A child exposed to passive cigarette smoke from parents who smoke is at increased risk of otitis media with effusion.
- The symptoms of serous otitis media are less severe than with bacterial otitis media. The individual experiences a feeling of fullness and a popping or crackling sound with swallowing or yawning, which is why this condition is sometimes referred to as 'glue ear'.
- A conductive hearing loss is present, and an air fluid level may be visible behind the tympanic membrane.
- Diagnosis and treatment are similar to that for acute suppurative otitis media, except that antibiotics are only indicated when an infection is suspected. If the child has experienced bilateral effusion for three months and hearing is compromised (no better than 20 decibel hearing threshold level), the ENT specialist will likely recommend the placement of tympanostomy tubes.

Barotitis Media (Aerotitis Media) (ICD: 381.4)

Damage to the middle ear due to ambient pressure changes. (Merck Manual, p. 673)

- The eustachian tube allows for passage of air from the throat to the middle ear, thus equalizing the pressure on both sides of the eardrum. If the eustachian tube becomes swollen from either infection or allergies, this free passage of air is impaired.
- Most commonly the individual experiences difficulty with changes in air pressure experienced during air travel. When the airplane takes off and rises to altitude, the air within the middle ear will expand. Usually this air escapes easily down the eustachian tube. However, when the plane descends, the swollen eustachian tube does not allow the return of air to the middle ear. A similar phenomenon occurs while scuba diving referred to as ear squeeze.
- Self help measures include yawning, chewing gum, or expelling air while pinching the nose (Valsalva maneuver). If an individual knows that they are susceptible to this condition, it is often helpful to take Sudafed 30-60 minutes before the landing time.
- The blockage will cause the eardrum to bulge inward. If the air does not equalize, bleeding or even rupture of the tympanic membrane may result.

Cholesteatoma (Merck Manual, p. 677)

- Cholesteatoma is a malignant overgrowth of epidermal tissue through a perforation in the tympanic membrane. When an individual has recurrent eustachian tube blockage, the negative pressure in the middle ear may cause a retraction pocket of the eardrum, which can also develop into a cholesteatoma.
- Histologically, cholesteatoma is composed of dead skin cells. These necrotic cells exude enzymes which can damage surrounding tissue. This pocket of infection has a white or yellow-gray cheesy appearance and may produce a foul smelling discharge.
- Symptoms may include a feeling of fullness in the ear, hearing loss, and drainage from the ear. The condition may or may not be painful.
- The condition is typically unresponsive to antibiotic therapy alone. The individual needs surgical debridement of the infection, coupled with antibiotic therapy. Left untreated it can lead to bone erosion, brain abscess, and death.

Otosclerosis (ICD: 387)

A disease of the otic capsule and a common cause of progressive conductive hearing loss in an adult with a normal tympanic membrane. (Merck Manual, p. 677)

- Normal hearing occurs when vibrations are transmitted from the tympanic membrane via the malleus, incus, and stapes bones to the oval window of the inner ear. In about 10% of the population some degree of ankylosis of these three small bones occurs.

- Otosclerosis is hereditary and affects primarily Caucasians. It is much less common in Orientals and rare in Blacks. Fortunately only about 10% of affected individuals (1% of the general population) will develop symptoms. The condition is most prevalent in the 15-30 year old age group, and is the most common cause of hearing loss in young adults.
- Upon examination the individual will manifest signs of a conduction hearing loss: Weber lateralizes to the affected ear, and AC < BC on the Rinné test. As with most cases of hearing loss, some degree of tinnitus will probably manifest as the hearing worsens.
- If the hearing loss is mild, no treatment or hearing aids may be recommended. However, the condition is progressive, and surgery may become the only option to save the patient's hearing. Microsurgery techniques involve laser destruction of the stapes bone, followed by implantion of an artificial stapes prosthesis. This surgery has an approximately 80% success rate in restoration of hearing.

Vertigo (ICD: 386.2)

An abnormal sensation of rotary movement associated with difficulty in balance, gait, and navigation of the environment. (Merck Manual, p. 665)

- Vertigo is a symptom, not an anatomical diagnosis. Vertigo is experienced as a sensation of spinning, either the environment is spinning (objective vertigo) or the individual feels as if they are spinning (subjective vertigo).
- Patients with vertigo must be evaluated to determine the cause, such as benign positional vertigo, labyrinthitis and Meniere's disease.

Meniere's disease (ICD: 386.0)

A disorder characterized by recurrent prostrating vertigo, sensory hearing loss, tinnitus, and a feeling of fullness in the ear associated with generalized dilation of the membranous labyrinth (endolymphatic hydrops). (Merck Manual, p. 678)

- Meniere's disease was first described by French physician Prosper Ménière in 1861. The semicircular canals within the inner ear contain a fluid referred to as endolymph. With changes in head position, the motion of this endolymph fluid against hairlike nerve receptors is what supplies us with our sense of balance and equilibrium.
- For reasons that are not clear, some individuals produce too much endolymph fluid. This excess fluid creates a pressure that can cause a variety of symptoms such as vertigo, tinnitus, and hearing loss. When the vertigo is severe the individual may experience nausea and vomiting.
- While the condition is not common, it affects approximately 3 to 5 million Americans. There is a suggested inherited tendency toward

the condition, as about one half of individuals with Meniere's disease have a family history of the condition.

- The episodes may last from minutes to hours with three to ten attacks per month. There may be intervening periods where the vertigo abates, but the hearing loss and ringing in the ears persist. In about 75-85% of the cases, it occurs in only one ear.
- Medical treatment is primarily symptomatic, such as dramamine or transdermal scopolomine, to control the episodes of nausea.
- Natural alternative care should include adjusting, control of allergies, avoidance of caffeine and possibly restriction of salt in the diet. The herb ginger has documented effectiveness in the management of motion sickness.

Benign Paroxysmal Positional Vertigo (Benign Postural or Positional Vertigo) (ICD: 386.2)

Violent vertigo lasting < 30 sec and induced by certain head positions. (Merck Manual, p. 679)

- Benign Paroxysmal Positional Vertigo or BPPV is a very brief episode of vertigo brought on by a change of head position. Events such as laying down or rolling over in bed can trigger the vertigo.
- The condition affects women more than men in a 2:1 ratio. While it can appear at any age, the average age of onset is about 55. BPPV is the most common cause of vertigo, accounting for approximately 20% of all office visits related to vertigo.
- Otoconia are small calcium crystals attached to the nerve endings within the semicircular canals. If these crystals become dislodged, a change in head position can cause inappropriate stimulation of nerve endings within the canal.
- The condition is diagnosed by having the patient perform the Hallpike maneuver. A change of position from the seated to supine position with the head rotated to one side triggers vertigo, and the patient will manifest rotary nystagmus toward the affected ear.
- A variation of the Hallpike test, the Epley canalith repositioning procedure, creates a treatment. The following web site provides more information, including a demonstration of the Epley repositioning maneuver and home care:

  http://www.tchain.com/otoneurology/disorders/bppv/bppv.html

Herpes Zoster Oticus (Ramsay Hunt's Syndrome, Viral Neuronitis and Ganglionitis, Geniculate Herpes) (ICD: 0.53.1)

Invasion of the 8th nerve ganglia and the geniculate ganglion of the facial nerve by the herpes zoster virus, producing severe ear pain, hearing loss, vertigo, and paralysis of the facial nerve. (Merck Manual, p. 679)

- Shingles commonly presents as a band of vesicles between two ribs. While the varicella zoster virus typically remains dormant in the spinal dorsal nerve root ganglion, it also can remain dormant in cranial nerve ganglia. If the virus activates from CN VII or VIII, herpes zoster oticus can manifest.

- Herpes zoster oticus accounts for about 12% of all facial paralysis. While the symptoms are similar to Bell's Palsy, herpes zoster oticus is usually more severe and has a less favorable outcome than Bell's palsy. In addition to pain, the individual may experience vertigo and hearing loss. Most patients experience temporary paralysis, which they fully recover from within a few weeks. However, if the symptoms are severe, permanent paralysis is possible.
- As with shingles, it takes time for the body to recover from this viral infection. If administered early, antiviral drugs, such as acyclovir or famvir, can lessen the severity of the outbreak. These drugs are much less effective once the vesicles appear. The nutritional supplement Monolaurin is an effective and less costly alternative to these antiviral medications. Analgesics and antiinflammatory nutrients may provide symptomatic relief of the pain.

Acoustic Neuroma (ICD: 388.5) (Merck Manual, p. 683)

- Acoustic neuroma is a benign tumor of CN VIII. Because the tumor arises from an overgrowth of schwann cells, it is also referred to as a schwannoma. It is usually, but not always, slow growing. It affects about one in 100,000 persons and accounts for about 7% of all brain tumors. It is usually discovered in the 30-60 year age range.
- Because the tumor is slow growing, early symptoms may go unnoticed. The individual may experience tinnitus, a mild sensorineural hearing loss, or experience difficulty with balance. A CT or MRI will show the tumor.
- If the tumor is discovered early, and is not causing disabling symptoms, the initial management may be to adopt a wait and see attitude, putting surgery off until symptoms or a rapid growth of the tumor require intervention. When the tumor is small, stereotactic radiation therapy, or radiosurgery is used to halt tumor growth. Large tumors will require surgery. As with all brain surgery, the skill of the surgeon will affect how much damage occurs to structures adjacent to the tumor.

Nose

Septal Deviation and Perforation (ICD: 470) (Merck Manual, p. 684)

- A deviated septum can result from previous injury, such as a broken nose which healed in an abnormal position. Sometimes the nose will grow to an asymmetrical position not a result of trauma.
- Septoplasty is the term for surgical correction of a deviated septum. The main indications for surgical correction are nasal congestion and difficulty breathing, or correction of cosmetic deformity.
- Chronic cocaine use can lead to a perforated septum. Cocaine causes vasoconstriction and damages the vascular supply of the thin

epithelium of the septum. Small perforations may heal if the source of the irritation is removed.

Foreign body in nose (ICD: 932)

- On occasion, children push items such as peanuts or buttons up their nose. If the child is old enough to cooperate, block one of your nostrils and demonstrate a forceful exhalation with the mouth closed. When the child mimics your maneuver, they may be able to blow the item out.
- If the item is easily visible, it may be able to be retrieved with a pair of tweezers. All other cases should be referred to an ENT specialist.

Epistaxis (Nosebleed) (ICD: 784.7) (Merck Manual, p. 684)

- The nasal mucosa has a rich supply of blood via Kiesselbach's plexus. Trauma, inflammation, or congenital deformity such as an aneurysm may trigger the onset of bleeding. Spontaneous nosebleeds are known to occur upon ingestion of allergic foods.
- Most episodes of nosebleed can be controlled by holding the nose pinched for 5-10 minutes. If the bleeding persists in spite of conservative measures, medical care for administration of vasoconstricting medicine or cauterization may be necessary.

Fractures of the Nose (ICD: 802.0) (Merck Manual, p. 683)

- Trauma to the face can cause fracture of the nasal bones. Nasal fracture is the most common facial fracture, as well as one of the most frequently broken bones in the body. A nosebleed and periorbital ecchymosis (black eye) are common with this injury. There is disagreement among clinicians about whether an x-ray needs to be taken to assess the damage and position of the nasal bones. A CT scan may provide more useful information, especially regarding surrounding soft tissue injury.
- If the fracture is stable and not displaced, it will not need to be repositioned. The patient will only require supportive care during the healing process.
- When the fracture is displaced, cosmetic deformity and difficulty breathing can result, requiring manual reduction. If the swelling is not too great, it should be repositioned soon. When swelling is marked, the doctor may elect to wait 4-5 days for swelling to subside. If the doctor waits longer than 5-6 days it may become difficult to reposition the bones.
- A plastic splint is often used to protect the nose and maintain correct position during the healing process.

Rhinitis (ICD: 477.9)

Edema and vasodilation of the nasal mucous membrane, nasal discharge, and obstruction. (Merck Manual, p. 685)

- Rhinitis, or inflammation and drainage of the nasal mucosa can occur from a number of causes. Allergies are the most common cause. Approximately 20% of the population experience some degree of nasal symptoms due to allergy. The symptoms may be seasonal, due to cyclic variation of pollen, or perennial due to dust, molds, animal dander, and tobacco smoke. Non-allergic causes of rhinitis include the common cold and bacterial infections.
- Symptomatically, the individual experiences sneezing, congestion, and runny nose. Additionally, these same type of congestion symptoms may affect the eyes and throat. An individual with chronic allergies may manifest an 'allergic shiner' or a crease on the nose referred to as an 'allergic salute'.
- Upon examination, the nasal mucosa of an individual with allergic rhinitis may appear pale and boggy. When there is a nasal discharge that is yellow or green color, the individual probably has a secondary bacterial infection.
- A preventive treatment for rhinitis is to swab the nasal passages with a Q-tip soaked in 3% hydrogen peroxide. In addition to being an astringent which decreases congestion, hydrogen peroxide appears to inactivate pollen, mold, bacteria and viruses.

Polyps (ICD: 471)

Fleshy outgrowths of the mucous membrane of the nose. (Merck Manual, p. 686)

- Nasal polyps typically occur as a consequence of chronic inflammation of the nasal mucosa. Upon examination, they appear as smooth, fluid filled sacs hanging down from the nasal mucosa. If the polyps occur in a child with respiratory symptoms, a diagnosis of cystic fibrosis should be considered, as about 25% of CF children also experience nasal polyps.
- When the polyps are large the individual may experience anosmia and difficulty breathing, perhaps even marked enough to cause mouth breathing.
- Initial treatment will probably be corticosteroid nasal spray to shrink the inflammation. If this is ineffective, surgical removal of the polyps will probably be recommended. Unfortunately, this may be only palliative, as a large number of polyps grow back after surgery. Prevention of the cause of inflammation is the only true cure.

Anosmia (ICD: 352.0)

Loss of the sense of smell. (Merck Manual, p. 687)

- Rhinitis and nasal polyps are the most common cause of anosmia. Trauma which causes a tearing of the olfactory nerves at the cribriform plate can also cause permanent or temporary anosmia. It is estimated that 10% of major head injuries will result in anosmia. Viral and bacterial infections cause damage to nasal olfactory cells. One of the most common irritants to the sense of smell is tobacco smoke.

- Just as hearing and vision diminish as we age, olfaction also suffers, resulting in presbyosmia. Anosmia is a symptom, rather than an anatomical diagnosis. Treatment must be directed at the underlying cause.

Sinusitis (ICD: 461)

Inflammation of the paranasal sinuses due to viral, bacterial, or fungal infections or allergic reactions. (Merck Manual, p. 687)

- When an individual has allergies or an upper respiratory infection, the mucous membranes in the sinuses can swell and block the drainage of fluid. Usually the condition is self limiting, meaning it resolves in time with little or no treatment. If the condition persists longer than three months, the condition is referred to as chronic sinusitis.
- In addition to facial pain, the individual may experience nasal congestion and discharge, cough from post nasal drip, and perhaps even dental pain if the maxillary sinus is affected.
- Upon examination the sinuses will be tender to direct pressure and percussion. An absence of a red to orange glow upon sinus transillumination may suggest the sinus is filled with something other than air (or perhaps sinus agenesis when no pain is present).
- Initial medical management will involve nasal decongestant sprays and antibiotics if an infection is present. If these measures do not work, endoscopic sinus surgery can enlarge the sinus drainage openings.
- Many chronic sinusitis sufferers have found dramatic relief with nasal sprays containing colloidal silver.

Mouth & Throat

Angular Stomatitis (ICD: 266.0, 528.5) (Merck Manual, p. 46)

- Red sores at the corner of the mouth are referred to as angular cheilitis or stomatitis. This may be due to a nutritional deficiency of vitamin B2 (riboflavin), vitamin B3 (niacin), vitamin B6 (pyridoxine), or iron.
- Conditions that produce excess salivation, such as poorly fitting dentures, can create a warm moist environment at the corners of the mouth, which can also cause angular stomatitis.

Cleft Lip (ICD: 749.1)

- This is an obvious congenital defect that will almost certainly have been corrected prior to you seeing the patient. It occurs in about 1 in 1000 births, with slightly higher incidence in Asians, and slightly lower incidence in Blacks. The presence of a congenital defect should alert you to the possibility of other genetic abnormalities.

Lip Carcinoma (ICD: 140)

- Lip cancer is the most common site of cancer in the oral cavity. Approximately three quarters of individuals with lip cancer use tobacco (pipe, cigarettes, cigars, or chewing tobacco).
- Any lip sore that does not heal within a few weeks is suspect, and the patient should be referred to a dermatologist. Upon biopsy, most cases of lip cancer are identified as squamous cell carcinoma and usually occur on the lower lip.
- Surgical removal of the cancerous tumor is the most common treatment. If the tumor was large, cosmetic reconstructive surgery will be required. As with most forms of cancer, the earlier the condition is identified and appropriately treated, the more favorable the outcome. Early stage lip cancer has an 80-90% five year survival rate.

Herpesvirus Infections (ICD: 054.9) (Merck Manual, p. 756)

- A herpes simplex virus infection on the lips or mouth is referred to as a 'cold sore'. This is a very common condition affecting about 50% of adults. This highly contagious virus is often transmitted by kissing.
- Before the outbreak of sores, there is usually a prodromal period of several days, where the individual experiences a tingling, burning, or itching sensation. Once the clear vesicles appear, healing occurs within one to two weeks. When the individual first experiences the itching sensation, if they apply a drying agent such as a Q-tip soaked in 3% hydrogen peroxide, they may be able to abort the outbreak of vesicles.
- After the initial infection, the virus remains in your system, and may continue to manifest for the remainder of your life. However, the lesions are more likely to recur at times of stress. The amino acid lysine taken orally helps to prevent herpes outbreaks.
- In immunocompromised individuals with severe outbreaks, the MD will prescribe an antiviral drug, such as acyclovir (Zovirax).

Recurrent Apthous Stomatitis (Recurrent Apthous Ulcers; Canker Sores) (ICD: 528.2) (Merck Manual, p. 756)

- An apthous ulcer, or canker sore, typically appears as a small (< 1 cm), white circular lesion, with a red border. They may be located on the tongue, gum, cheek, or lip. A canker sore is a different lesion than the clear vesicles that occur with herpes simplex infection, or 'cold sores'. And unlike herpes cold sores, canker sores are not contagious.
- Canker sores occur in approximately 20% of the population. While the cause is unknown, they are thought to be a local reaction to irritation, such as eating acidic food, biting the tongue, etc.
- The lesions usually heal in 1-2 weeks with no treatment needed. The lesions can be quite painful, and topical anesthetic agents, such as anbesol or oragel, provide symptomatic relief.

- One study found that toothpaste containing sodium lauryl sulfate (SLS) was a contributory cause to recurrent apthous ulcers. The researchers speculated that SLS inhibits the normal mucin that protects oral mucosa from ulceration (Acta Odontol Scand. 1994;52:257-259).

Pharyngitis (ICD: 462)

Acute inflammation of the pharynx. (Merck Manual, p. 690)

- Inflammation of the posterior pharynx can result from a number of causes. Most commonly the condition is the consequence of a viral or bacterial upper respiratory infection, or allergies. Clinically, the condition is often associated with tonsillitis.
- Typically the sufferer is a child who presents with a sore throat, a feeling of a 'lump' or tickle in the throat, or difficulty swallowing. The child may also experience aching, malaise, or fever.
- About 15% of all pharyngitis cases are caused by Group A beta-hemolytic streptococci (GABHS) infection. Because strep throat can lead to rheumatic fever and acute glomerulonephritis, early diagnosis and treatment are essential. The following are the expected diagnostic criteria for strep throat:
    o tonsillar exudate
    o anterior cervical lymphadenopathy
    o temperature > 101°F
    o history of recent exposure to streptococcus
    o no cough
    o no rhinorhea
- The diagnostic protocol is to perform a rapid strep test. If the rapid strep test is positive, antibiotic treatment, usually penicillin, is begun immediately. If the rapid strep test is negative, a throat culture is performed, and antibiotic treatment is instituted if the throat culture is positive. Because the ASO (antistreptolysin O) titer does not rise for one to six months after an acute infection, the ASO test is not appropriate for evaluating an acute infection. Rather, it is used to identify previous infection, or individuals who may be a carrier.
- Echinacea and goldenseal, and gargling with warm salt water are effective self help preventive measures.

Tonsillitis (ICD: 463)

Acute inflammation of the palatine tonsils, usually due to streptococcal or, less commonly, to viral infection. (Merck Manual, p. 690)

- The tonsils are a collection of lymphatic tissue in the throat. While the exact function of the tonsils is not certain, they are known to contain white blood cells and immunoglobulins which help us to fight infection. Tonsillitis may develop following viral or bacterial infection in this tissue.

- While the condition can occur at any age, it is most common in children 5-15 years of age. Almost all children experience at least one episode of tonsillitis in their life.
- The most common presenting complaint is difficulty swallowing with a severe sore throat, lasting longer than 48 hours. Upon examination, the child will have a bright red sore throat. The tonsils will usually appear swollen with a white or yellow pustular exudate. Tonsillar enlargement is graded on how far toward the midline they protrude.
- Initial medical management is antibiotic therapy. Untreated tonsillitis can lead to a more serious condition, peritonsillar abscess. If a child experiences 6 or more episodes of streptococcal pharyngitis in a year, a tonsillectomy may be indicated. However, a recent study in the British Medical Journal found, "*Adenotonsillectomy has no major clinical benefits over watchful waiting in children with mild symptoms of throat infections or adnotonsillar hypertrophy.*" BMJ 2004;329:651.

Peritonsillar Cellulitis and Abscess (ICD: 465.9)

An acute infection located between the tonsil and the superior pharyngeal constrictor muscle. (Merck Manual, p. 691)

- If tonsillitis infection spreads to the adjacent peritonsillar tissue, an abscess or pocket of pus may result. The lay term for this condition is quinsy.
- Signs and symptoms are similar to streptococcal pharyngitis, however the soft tissue swelling of the soft palate may push the uvula to one side. Additionally the individual may experience trismus, or severe pain and muscle spasm with opening of the mouth.
- The abscess may rupture spontaneously. If it does not, incision and drainage of the abscess is indicated. Antibiotic therapy is required to avoid a systemic blood infection.

Oral Kaposi's Sarcoma (ICD: 176.2)

A multicentric vascular neoplasm caused by herpesvirus type 8 that has three forms: indolent, lymphadenopathic, and AIDS-related. (Merck Manual, p. 846)

- Oral lesions may be the first manifestation of AIDS. They often present as bruise like lesions on the hard palate.

Laryngitis (ICD: 464.0)

Inflammation of the larynx. (Merck Manual, p. 693)

- Laryngitis, or inflammation of the voice box, is usually the side effect of a viral upper respiratory infection. Chronic laryngitis may occur with overuse, such as with people who must speak or sing for long periods of time. Other possible diagnostic considerations are acid reflux, and throat cancer.

- The presenting symptom is hoarseness, or loss of voice. If the condition does not resolve with conservative care, laryngoscopic investigation of the vocal cords may be indicated.
- Treatment is primarily palliative. The individual must rest the voice to allow the inflamed vocal cords to heal. Warm fluids (chicken soup), and throat lozenges provide symptomatic relief. Obviously the individual should avoid irritants such as smoking or inhaling second hand smoke.

Croup (ICD: 464.0)

An acute viral inflammation of the upper and lower respiratory tracts, characterized by inspiratory stridor, subglottic swelling, and respiratory distress that is most pronounced on inspiration. (Merck Manual, p. 2333)

- The airways of a young child are very small and vulnerable to restriction. With the inflammation and mucous production that occurs with a viral upper respiratory infection, these airways may become partially blocked, resulting in croup. The condition typically occurs in an infant or young child (usually 6 months to 3 years of age).
- Symptomatically, the child may present with a cough which has a characteristic 'barking' sound. Respiration is labored and the child has more difficulty with inspiration, manifesting 'inspiratory stridor', more common at night. The child may have a low grade fever.
- Usually the child gets better in 5-7 days with supportive care, such as drinking warm fluids and breathing humidified air. Aspirin for pain relief should be avoided, because of the possibility of Reye's syndrome. Chiropractic treatment will aid with pain relief and mobilizing the body's innate healing response.
- If the child has a fever greater than 102°F, signs of dehydration, or the child is breathless with very labored breathing or faster than normal respiration, an immediate medical referral is indicated.

Teeth

Malocclusion (ICD: 524.4)

Deviation from the normal contact relationship of the maxillary and mandibular teeth. (Merck Manual, p. 764)

- Malocclusion literally means 'bad bite'. Normally, the upper and lower teeth meet with the biting surfaces touching each other. With deficient growth of the mandible an overbite develops, or with overgrowth of the mandible an underbite develops. Additionally, if bone growth around the tooth sockets is impaired, crowding of the teeth can develop, and the teeth may erupt at a twisted angle.
- An orthodontist will use braces, and in some cases surgery, to correct dental malocclusion. The braces gradually pull the teeth to a more correct location. The alveolar bone of the tooth socket will remodel to accomodate the new position. When dental crowding is present, the

dentist may need to extract teeth to make room for the remaining teeth. This process may take two years, although it is quicker in growing children.

- Dr. Weston Price is a dentist who for 35 years studied the effect of a 20th century diet on the physical health of native people on five continents. His work, *Nutrition and Physical Degeneration,* published in 1939 documents that native people on a traditional unrefined whole food diet suffered little of the chronic degenerative disease and dental abnormalities that occurs with a change to a 20th century refined food diet.

Caries (ICD: 521.0)

Tooth decay or cavities. (<u>Merck Manual</u>, p. 762)

- Infection or decay of a tooth is referred to as caries. It is considered the most common chronic disease, affecting most individuals at some time in their life.
- Dental caries is an entirely preventable condition. Plaque is the thin sticky film formed by saliva and food debris which covers the surface of the tooth. When the teeth are not cleaned regularly, *Streptococcus mutans* bacteria grow in this film and begin attacking the surface enamel of the teeth. In addition to poor dental hygiene, a diet high in sugar favors the growth of caries.
- Initially, dental decay appears as a white chalky spot on the tooth enamel. As the degeneration proceeds, the spot will turn brown or black, and lead to the formation of a 'cavity'.
- The dentist will drill and remove the decay, and apply a filling to the hole. More dentists are becoming aware of the danger of mercury amalgam fillings and will offer their patients composite restorations. In 2003 the Swedish government published a 33 page summary investigation into the hazards of mercury amalgam fillings. From this report:

"With reference to the fact that mercury is a multipotent toxin with effects on several levels of the biochemical dynamics of the cell, amalgam must be considered to be an unsuitable material for dental restoration."

"Every doctor and dentist should, where patients are suffering from unclear pathological states and autoimmune diseases, consider whether side-effects from mercury released from amalgam may be one contributory cause of the symptoms."

(http://www.dentalmaterial.gov.se/Mercury.pdf)

- Prevention is the key: regular dental hygiene, and avoidance of sugary foods in the diet. Application of topical fluoride to the tooth will harden the enamel, making it more resistant to decay. However, fluoridation of public water supplies is more controversial. If you have concerns in this area, drink distilled water, which does not contain fluoride. To educate yourself about the facts related to flouride visit:

http://www.fluoridealert.org
http://www.nofluoride.com

Gingivitis (ICD: 523)

Inflammation of the gingiva characterized by swelling, redness, change of normal contours, exudate, and bleeding. (Merck Manual, p. 766)

- When we are children, the most common dental problem is caries. As we age, gingivitis predominates. Approximately 75% of adults over 35 have gum disease.
- The predominant symptom will be bleeding gums. The individual will notice blood on their toothbrush when brushing their teeth. Additionally, halitosis or bad breath may be noticed, especially in the morning.
- The plaque that causes dental decay can become trapped in the gingival sulcus or 'pocket' between the tooth and gum. With poor oral hygiene, this plaque will harden and turn to tartar or calculus. This tartar buildup will serve as an ongoing source of infection and irritation to the surrounding gum.
- During examination, the dentist will measure the depth of the gingival pockets. If the depth of infection is not large, removal of the plaque and tartar is all that will be required. When the pockets are large, periodontal surgery to remove the diseased gum tissue may be required.
- Certain conditions, such as pregnancy and diabetes, place one at increased risk for periodontal disease. Untreated gingivitis can maintain a source of infection that places the individual at increased risk of heart disease. Various nutrients, such as Coenzyme Q10, are documented to improve periodontal health. Prevention is the key: daily brushing and flossing of the teeth.

Acute Nectrotizing Ulcerative Gingivitis (Trench Mouth; Vincent's Infection; Fusospirochetosis) (ICD: 523)

A noncontagious infection associated with a fusiform bacillus and spirochete, usually destroying the interdental papillae, and sometimes affecting the marginal and attached gingiva by direct extension. (Merck Manual, p. 767)

- Acute necrotizing ulcerative gingivitis (ANUG) is a much more serious form of periodontal disease than regular gingivitis. The term 'trench mouth' originated when soldiers living in poor hygienic conditions in trench warfare during World War I developed the condition.
- In addition to bleeding gums, the condition is very painful, and the characteristic foul breath is what gives rise to the term 'trench mouth'. Additionally, the individual may have a fever, malaise,

excessive salivation, painful swallowing, and there may be a gray white mucous film on the gums caused by decomposing gum tissue.

- The fusiform bacillus and spirochete infection seen with trench mouth is different than the *S. mutans* infection more typical of dental caries and uncomplicated gingivitis.
- Treatment is antibiotics and proper dental hygiene. Untreated trench mouth can become quite serious if the infection spreads to adjacent neck or jaw tissue.
- Rinsing the mouth with warm salt water water (about one teaspoon of salt to one cup of water) will help kill the bacteria and promote healing of normal tissue.

Periodontitis (ICD: 523.3)

Inflammation of the periodontium, which comprises the periodontal ligament, gingiva, cementum, and alveolar bone. (Merck Manual, p. 768)

- Periodontitis is similar to gingivitis except the condition is more severe, and the enlarged 'pockets' cause the gingiva to pull away from the tooth. Over time the gingival tissue degenerates and recedes, exposing the root of the tooth. This phenomenon is the origin of the phrase, *'long in the tooth'*.
- When the tissue that holds the tooth in place is severely compromised, the tooth becomes loose, and the individual is at risk of losing the tooth. Chronic dental infection may allow the spread of bacterial infection to other structures, such as the heart. In addition to good dental hygiene, a variety of nutrients, such as Vitamin C, CoQ10, and folic acid have documented benefit in improving dental health.

Gingival hyperplasia (ICD: 523.8)

- Gingival overgrowth can be seen as a side effect of long term use of anti-seizure medicine (Dilantin) and immunosuppression drugs (Cyclosporine). Other causes include puberty, pregnancy, and leukemia.

Lead line (ICD: 984.9)

- Lead poisoning is a systemic condition, which can demonstrate oral manifestations. During your examination of the oral cavity, be alert for a thin black line at the gum margin, which is a sign of lead poisoning.
- According to the CDC, approximately 80% of homes built prior to 1978 have lead based paint. If this paint peels and a child eats the paint chips, lead poisoning can result.
- Many of the symptoms are neurological, such as learning disabilities, hyperactivity, mental retardation, slowed growth, hearing loss, and headaches. The severity depends upon the magnitude of the poisoning.

- EDTA chelation therapy is the accepted medical treatment for lead poisoning.

Tongue

Candidiasis (ICD: 112.0) (<u>Merck Manual</u>, p. 755, <u>1037</u>)

- Oral candidiasis, also known as thrush, is usually a consequence of antibiotic therapy or immunosuppression. The thick white fungal patches are easily scraped off.

Leukoplakia (ICD: 702.8) (<u>Merck Manual</u>, p. 754)

- While similar in appearance to candidiasis, the white patches of leukoplakia are firmly adherent and do not easily scrape off. They may develop from chronic irritation such as with tobacco use, however the lesions are pre-cancerous and the patient should be referred for follow-up.

Hairy Tongue (ICD: 529.3) (<u>Merck Manual</u>, p. 754)

- While the cause of black hairy tongue is uncertain, it is thought to be related to poor oral hygiene. Upon examination, the filiform papillae are elongated and have a brown or black discoloration. The individual may be a smoker, or may have recently taken antibiotics. Unless a fungal infection is present, the lesions require no treatment other than good oral hygiene.

Atrophic Glossitis (ICD: 529.4) (<u>Merck Manual</u>, p. 754)

- A smooth glossy appearance to the tongue suggests a deficiency of certain B vitamins (riboflavin, niacin, folic acid, B6, and B12), or possibly iron. The tongue appears red and shiny due to the lack of the normal papillae. The patient may also experience dryness and burning of the tongue.

Fissured Tongue (ICD: 529.5) (<u>Merck Manual</u>, p. 754)

- Deep furrows on the tongue surface may present an appearance that is sometimes referred to as 'scrotal tongue'. Western medicine considers this condition a normal variant, or possibly due to dehydration. In Ayurvedic medicine, this condition is a sign of colon dysfunction. Since many colon problems can be prevented with more water and roughage in the diet, the Ayurvedic interpretation is reasonable.

Geographic Tongue (ICD: 529.1) (<u>Merck Manual</u>, p. 753)

- Geographic tongue presents with discrete areas of increased redness that are visible where the papillae are missing. Over time, these areas heal and new areas develop, presenting a changing map of reddened areas. The cause of this condition, also known as migratory glossitis, is unknown.

Ballon Assisted Craniofacial Adjusting (BACA) is a chiropractic technique that involves insertion of a small finger cot balloon attached to the squeeze bulb of a sphygmomanometer. It is carefully passed up the nasal meatus and the balloon is quickly inflated and then the pressure is immediately released. Because of the close proximity of this manipulation to the sphenoid bone, this technique is used as a method of cranial adjusting. This technique was first described by Dr. Joseph Janse in 1947. Children with recurrent middle ear infections which is beginning to impair normal hearing development may benefit from this or other methods of cranial adjusting. A summary of the technique can be found at: http://home.austin.rr.com/sberman/paper2.html.

Study Guide Objectives

o   Know the anatomical structures located in the external, middle, and internal compartments of the ear.
o   Know the anatomical landmarks of the external ear.
o   Know the anatomical landmarks of the typmpanic membrane.
o   What creates the 'cone of light'?
o   Know the functions of the middle ear.
o   What do tophi on the ear signify?
o   What does Darwin's tubercle signify?
o   A diagonal earlobe crease, also known as Frank's crease, is a risk factor for what health problem?
o   What ear conditions produce a foul smelling discharge?
o   What size speculum should you use when performing otoscopic examination of the ear?
o   What is the expected color of the tympanic membrane?
o   What does a bright red tympanic membrane signify?
o   What is tympanosclerosis?
o   What is otosclerosis?
o   A wen is another name for _____.
o   Know the differences between otitis externa, bacterial otitis media, and secretory otitis media.
o   What anatomical factors make children more at risk for middle ear infection?
o   What is the appearance of the tympanic membrane with serous otitis media?
o   What condition is sometimes referred to as 'glue ear'? Why?
o   Know how to perform and interpret the Weber and Rinné tests.
o   Know the expected results from the Weber and Rinné tests for conductive and sensorineural hearing loss.
o   Know the causes of sensorineural hearing loss.
o   Know the causes of conduction hearing loss.
o   When a person experiences hearing loss, which frequencies are most impaired?
o   What is the difference between objective and subjective vertigo?
o   Meniere's disease is a disorder characterized by recurrent episodes of what symptoms?

- What herb has documented effectiveness in the management of motion sickness?
- Ramsay Hunt syndrome is another name for what condition? Which cranial nerve is involved with this condition?
- When tinnitus is present, there is almost always some degree of _____.
- Know why children are at greater risk for middle ear infections.
- Know the purposes of the different tuning fork frequencies.
- Know the function of the structures in the nose, nasopharynx, and oral cavity.
- What is the most common cause of anosmia?
- What is coryza?
- What is epistaxis?
- What is angular cheilitis?
- Gingival hyperplasia is a side effect of what medical treatment?
- What does a thin black line at the gum margin signify?
- How can the doctor tell the difference between oral candidiasis and leukoplakia?
- What does a smooth glossy appearance of the tongue signify?
- What is the most commonly fractured facial bone?
- What do Koplik's spots signify?
- What are the diagnostic criteria for strep throat?
- What are the consequences of an untreated streptococcal throat infection?
- How many 'baby' teeth does a child have, and how many teeth does an adult have?
- Which cranial nerves provide sensory and motor function to the tongue?
- Know the locations of Stenson's and Wharton's ducts and which salivary glands they originate from.
- Know the changes that occur in the mouth with aging.
- What is trismus?
- Know the oral manifestations of HIV infection.

8 – Lungs & Respiratory

Anatomy & Physiology

The thoracic cage is a flexible structure that provides protection to the heart and lungs, while also allowing expansion and contraction of the lungs. The ribs are connected posteriorly at the costovertebral articulation. The upper seven ribs are attached directly to the sternum by costal cartilage. Ribs 8, 9, and 10 are attached only to costal cartilage, and the end of ribs 11 and 12 are 'floating', attached only to muscle.

It is important to know the names and location of external thoracic landmarks. The suprasternal notch is a shallow depression in the manubrium, or superior portion of the sternum. The union of the manubrium with the body of the sternum forms the manubriosternal angle, also known as the 'angle of Louis'. This helpful landmark, where the second rib attaches, and is a good place to start when counting rib interspaces. If we had Superman's x-ray vision, we would also see that the manubriosternal angle is where the trachea bifurcates into the two main bronchi. The inferior attachment of the costal cartilage forms the costal angle, with the xiphoid process at the apex of this angle. Usually the costal angle is less than 90 degrees. When the chest assumes a 'barrel' shape, as in emphysema, the costal angle increases.

When counting ribs posteriorly, we know that the medial spine of the scapula is usually over the 4th rib, and the tip or inferior angle of the scapula is near the 7th or 8th rib. The union of the 12th rib with the spine forms the costovertebral angle, which is helpful when assessing kidney pathology.

When describing areas on the chest wall, we often make reference to imaginary vertical lines:

- o midsternal line
- o midclavicular line
- o anterior axillary line
- o midaxillary line
- o posterior axillary line
- o scapular line
- o vertebral line

The base of the lungs rests upon the diaphragm at about the level of the T10 vertebra. With deep inhalation, the diaphragm drops down to about T12. The apex of the lungs extends a few centimeters above the medial edge of the clavicle. This is why palpation of the supraclavicular fossa during lymph node palpation is so important.

When performing lung auscultation, it is important to know and visualize the underlying lobes of the lung. The left lung has an upper and lower lobe separated by the left oblique fissure, which runs in an anterior and inferior direction from the T3 spinous process to the level of the 6th rib at the midclavicular line. Thus, most of the anterior chest is upper lobe, and most of the posterior chest is lower lobe. The right lung has three lobes. A right oblique fissure separates the upper and middle lobes from the lower lobe. The horizontal fissure runs from the right 5th rib at the midaxillary line to the 4th rib where it joins the sternum. The right middle lobe occupies a similar position in the right side of the chest as the heart does in the left side of the chest.

Adherent to the exterior surface of the lungs is the visceral pleura. Parietal pleura lines the inner surface of the thoracic cage, as well as the superior surface of the diaphragm. A small quantity of lubricating fluid separates these two layers, to allow for easy motion of the lungs with breathing.

After air enters the throat from either the nose or mouth, it passes to the trachea via the larynx. The epiglottis covers the larynx to prevent food or liquid from entering the windpipe. The trachea is anterior to the esophagus, and is palpable in the anterior neck. The trachea divides into the right and left main bronchi at about the level of the manubriosternal angle. Within the lung tissue the bronchi continue to branch into smaller airways until eventually the alveolar air sacs are formed. The ascinus is the functional respiratory unit where the exchange of carbon dioxide from the pulmonary arteries for oxygen to the pulmonary veins takes place.

The muscular diaphragm is the primary mechanism of respiration. When the diaphragm draws down, this creates decreased intrathoracic pressure, and the lungs expand to fill the void, which in turn draws air into the lungs. During inspiration, the ribs move in a 'bucket handle' motion, which results in increased transverse and anteroposterior diameter, as well as elevation of the sternum. The scalene and external intercostal muscles also assist with elevation of the ribs. Exhalation is primarily passive, and depends upon elastic recoil of flexible lung tissue to its' deflated shape. When this elasticity is lost with conditions such as emphysema, the internal intercostal and external oblique abdominal muscles may become the primary means of exhalation.

Respiration is under both voluntary and involuntary control. There is a respiratory control center in the brain stem that senses changes in blood carbon dioxide. When this level increases, the brain triggers an unconscious increase in the rate and depth of respiration.

Nature of the Patient

As with cardiac complaints, the age of the patient may make certain respiratory conditions more likely. An acute cough in a young person is most likely a viral upper respiratory infection. However, a chronic cough in an adult is usually a consequence of cigarette smoking.

Key History Questions

Do you have a cough?

- Is the cough acute or chronic?
    - o Acute onset suggests conditions such as upper respiratory infection or pneumonia.
    - o Chronic cough points to conditions such as bronchitis, emphysema, bronchiectasis, tuberculosis, or possibly cancer. A foreign body in the ear canal may stimulate a cough reflex and is a rare cause of chronic cough.
- Do you cough up any phlegm or sputum?
    - o Purulent sputum with the presence of fever suggests pneumonia or tuberculosis.
    - o Purulent sputum with no fever suggests chronic bronchitis or bronchiectasis.
    - o Bloody sputum suggests bronchogenic carcinoma. If there is chest pain with hemoptysis, think of pulmonary embolism. Foamy blood tinged sputum with difficulty breathing and an enlarged heart suggests congestive heart failure.

Do you experience shortness of breath?

- Is the shortness of breath episodic or most of the time?
    - o Episodic dyspnea accompanied with wheezing, but no fever or chest pain, points to asthma, possibly triggered by exposure to dust or pollen.
    - o If the condition is more or less constant with a gradual onset, suspect chronic diseases such as emphysema or congestive heart failure (CHF).

Do you experience chest pain with breathing?

- Chest pain that is increased with deep breathing points to conditions such as pleurisy, costochondritis, rib fracture or subluxation, and pneumothorax.
- All episodes of chest pain must rule out the possibility of serious, life threatening conditions such as myocardial infarction, pulmonary embolism or infarction, and dissecting aneurysm.

Do you have a history of lung problems?

- Previous episodes of asthma, bronchitis, pneumonia, or emphysema may have resulted in permanent damage to lung tissue.
- While most people experience some colds, unusually frequent or severe colds suggest immune deficiency.
- Family history of asthma, allergies, or tuberculosis may predispose your patient to weakness in this organ system.

Do you smoke?

- While we normally assess tobacco use during the personal/social history, for the purposes of a regional heart or lung examination, knowledge of your patient's smoking history constitutes a pertinent negative.
- As chiropractors, we are the leading <u>preventive</u> health care specialists. We should be interested in every factor where we can make a positive contribution toward our patient's health. Quitting tobacco is not easy. The Surgeon General has stated that nicotine is more addictive than crack cocaine. However, we must help our patients understand that quitting smoking is the single most important thing they can do to prevent life threatening illness.

Do you live or work around chemicals or dust that may affect your breathing?

- Many occupations carry increased risk of exposure to lung pollutants. Farmers may inhale pesticides or grain dust. Coal miners breath coal dust that causes pneumonoconiosis. Stone masons and potters breath dust that can cause silicosis. Some regions of the country are endemic for organisms that cause histoplasmosis and coccidioidomycosis.
- If you live or work around 'environmental tobacco smoke' (ETS), you are a 'second-hand' smoker, which carries increased risk for the same heart and lung disease that smokers suffer from.

Examination

Inspection

Most of the respiratory examination is performed standing behind the patient. First observe the shape of the chest wall. Normally the AP diameter is less than the lateral chest diameter in an approximate 1:2 ratio. With emphysema, the chest becomes barrel shaped, where AP = lateral chest diameter.

Observe the rate and depth of respiration. With some lung conditions, breathing is rapid (tachypnea) and labored. Normally the patient will be relaxed with their arms resting comfortably in their lap. With emphysema, the individual may assume a tripod position in an attempt to shift some of the weight of their chest to their arms. This individual may also manifest unconsciously perform 'purse lip' breathing to aid with exhalation. Severe COPD may manifest retraction of the rib interspaces on inhalation.

Observe the skin for any rashes or lesions. Herpes zoster manifests as painful vesicles in a line along the lateral chest wall between two ribs.

Palpation

Palpation of the chest wall should be performed to locate possible trigger points that may simulate lung pathology. When checking skin sensation we usually look for areas of decreased sensitivity. However, with herpes zoster, the patient will report <u>increased</u> skin sensation. They may even remark that it hurts where their shirt touches their chest.

If your patient is female, palpation of the anterior chest should be based upon clinical need. If she is complaining of pain in the pectoral area, by all means palpate for possible trigger points. However, if she has no complaints in this area, and you palpate near breast tissue, you may be opening yourself up to a perceived 'boundary violation'.

While standing behind the patient, place your thumbs at about the level of T10 with your fingers on the lateral chest wall. As you instruct the patient to take a deep breath, observe for symmetric chest expansion, also known as respiratory excursion. If one side fails to expand, it is probable that some pathology is present in the lung on that side.

Using either the metacarpalphalangeal ridge or the ulnar edge of your hand, place your hand on the chest wall and have the patient say "*ninety nine*". This test helps you to assess tactile fremitus. You may use either one hand or both hands simultaneously. Place your hand at sufficient locations to adequately assess all the lobes of the lungs. Very little is gained from assessing fremitus directly over the scapula, as this bone impedes sound transmission. Increased tactile fremitus occurs with conditions having increased fluid in the lung, such as pneumonia. Decreased tactile fremitus is felt with conditions such as emphysema or pneumothorax that cause increased air within the chest. Some conditions such as pleurisy or atelectasis create a barrier to sound transmission, and also result in decreased tactile fremitus.

During anterior palpation, we will also want to verify that the trachea is positioned midline. Place your thumbs or index fingers alongside trachea just above suprasternal notch to verify that the trachea is midline The trachea may be *pushed* toward the healthy side by tumor or pneumothorax. The trachea may be *pulled* toward the diseased side by pleural adhesions or a large atelectasis. Tracheal tugging, or a rhythmic downward pull in time with the heartbeat, suggests an aortic aneurysm.

Percussion

Percussion allows us to introduce a vibrating note to underlying tissue, as we feel and listen to the sound produced. Place your middle finger firmly on the skin, then strike your own finger with the middle finger of your dominant hand. Your striking finger is called the *plexor*, while the finger laid on the body surface is the *pleximeter*. Again, we must percuss sufficient locations to adequately assess all the lobes of the lungs. In practice, this amounts to every 4-5 centimeters, or every second or third rib interspace. Use a side to side comparison, rather than percussing down one side. If the patient rolls their arms forward, as if giving themselves a hug, this will rotate the scapula laterally to aid your percussion of the posterior lung fields. When percussing the anterior chest of a female, have her place her hands over her breasts and pull them to the side, and percuss just medial to her hands.

The expected percussion tone is resonant. Hyperresonance is found with conditions that manifest too much air in the chest, such as emphysema and pneumothorax. Conditions that cause increased density will result in a dull percussion note, such as with pneumonia, atelectasis, or lung tumor. During anterior percussion, we expect to hear tympany over the gastric air bubble in the left lower thorax, and a dull percussion note over the liver in the right lower thorax, and over the heart in the center of the chest.

A special percussion procedure is diaphragmatic excursion. Have the patient take a deep breath and hold it. On the posterior chest, percuss down from lung resonance to the dull percussion note once you are below the diaphragm and mark the spot. Then have the patient take a full breath out and hold it. Percuss from dullness up to resonance and mark the spot. Perform this on the opposite side of the chest. Diaphragmatic excursion should be 3-5 centimeters in an adult, although 7-8 centimeters would not be uncommon in a well conditioned athlete.

Note: Costovertebral percussion is a part of the abdominal examination, not the thoracic exam. However, in a routine examination of an asymptomatic patient, if you perform Murphy's kidney punch test here (or when the patient is in the prone position), it will save you time, and your patient having to change positions one extra time during the exam. When you ask your patient to change positions frequently during the examination, it becomes obvious to that you lack experience and have not thought of their comfort.

Auscultation

With the diaphragm of your stethoscope, listen to approximately the same locations you just percussed. Have the patient breath through their mouth, deeper than usual. You might say, "*Each time I place the stethoscope on your back take a deep breath in and out through your mouth. If you find yourself getting light headed, let me know and we can go more slowly.*"

Auscultation is performed last, because it is possible that percussion will loosen up lung secretions and make rales more easily heard. Three types of breath sounds are normally heard during auscultation:

Category	Location	Pitch	Amplitude	Duration
Bronchial	trachea	high	loud	I < E
Bronchovesicular	bronchi	moderate	moderate	I = E
Vesicular	periphery	low	soft	I > E

Abnormal breath sounds, such as crackles and wheezes, are referred to as adventitious breath sounds. When heard, proceed with voice sounds, also known as vocal resonance:

- Bronchophony - Listen with your stethoscope as the patient says "*ninety nine*". If the words are clear and distinct, consolidation of the lungs is present.
- Egophony - Listen with your stethoscope as the patient says "*eeee*". If you hear "*aaaa*", like the sound made by a bleating goat, the lungs have consolidation.
- Whispered pectoriloquy - Listen as the patient whispers "*one, two, three*". Again if you hear the words clearly and distinctly through your stethoscope, lung consolidation is present.

Voice sounds are a confirmatory test, usually performed only when adventitious lung sounds are heard. In most cases, the usual cause for abnormal voice sounds is lung consolidation.

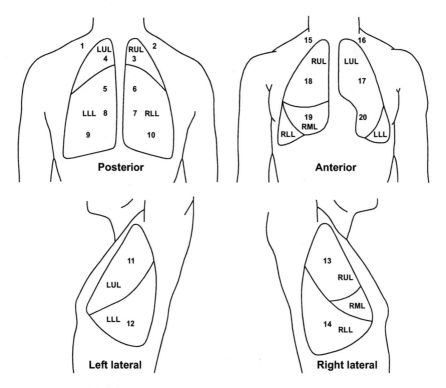

The numbered areas above are examples of appropriate locations for performing tactile fremitus, percussion, and auscultation. Have male patients remove their shirt. Female patients will be in a gown. Tactile fremitus and percussion can be performed over the gown. Auscultation should be directly on the skin. For female patients, when the examination is adjacent to breast tissue, have the patient place her hand as a boundary between her breast and the area being examined, to avoid what might be misperceived as a 'boundary violation'.

An excellent online article on lung auscultation is:
http://omj.med.jhu.edu/bedside/vol3/nov97.shtml

Summary of Physical Examination

- Assessment of respiratory conditions includes:
    o Observation of general appearance for pallor, cyanosis, dyspnea, and use of accessory muscles of respiration.
    o Measure vital signs: temperature, pulse, respiration, blood pressure.
    o Inspect the shape and symmetry of the chest.
    o Palpate for chest wall tenderness, symmetry of respiratory excursion, tracheal shift.
    o Percuss lung fields.
    o Auscultate for normal breath sounds and the presence of adventitious lung sounds.
    o Auscultate heart sounds.
    o Auscultate for bowel sounds and bruits. Examine the abdomen for masses and tenderness.
    o Examine the extremities for edema, cyanosis, diminished pulses, and digital clubbing of fingernails.
    o EENT examination (if URI suspected).

Diagnostic Studies

- AP & lateral chest x-ray
- Spirometric pulmonary function testing (PFT)
    o All smokers > 45 years old should be tested with spirometry (CHEST 2000; 117:1146-1161)
- Lab
    o CBC, sed rate, chemistry panel
    o Cardiac enzymes (if cardiac dysfunction is suspected)
    o Thyroid panel (if hyperthyroidism is suspected)
    o Microscopic sputum examination
- ECG (if cardiac dysfunction is suspected)

Sample Documentation

The thorax was oval with AP < lateral diameter. Respirations were 16 per minute, relaxed and even. No rashes or lesions were noted on the chest wall. Upon palpation, no areas of tenderness or hypersensitivity were elicited. Chest expansion was full and symmetric. Tactile fremitus was equal bilaterally. The trachea was midline. The lungs were resonant to percussion in all areas. Diaphragmatic excursion was 5 cm bilaterally. Upon auscultation, the lungs were clear, and breath sounds were vesicular over the lung fields. No adventitious lung sounds were heard. Spoken voice sounds were not performed.

Abnormal Findings

Deformities of the Thorax

- Barrel chest: When charting a normal thoracic examination, we record: AP < lateral diameter (1:2 is the approximate normal ratio). When a patient is barrel chested, we record AP = lateral diameter. This condition is caused by chronic over-inflation of the lungs, usually the result of chronic obstructive pulmonary disease (COPD).
- Pectus excavatum: This condition, also called funnel chest, is characterized by a marked depression of the sternum. It is usually congenital, and is not thought to be clinically significant.
- Pectus carinatum: Pectus carinatum, or 'pigeon chest', is characterized by a forward protrusion of the sternum. It also is usually congenital, and is not thought to be clinically significant.
- Scoliosis: While a mild degree of scoliosis may be 'normal', when viewed from behind the thoracic spine should be straight up and down. A lateral curvature, more common in teenage girls, may result in vertebral body rotation, and unequal hip and shoulder levels. Severe scoliosis (> 45 degrees) may interfere with lung function. Adams test is the screening test for functional scoliosis.
- Kyphosis: When viewed from the side, the thoracic spine presents a convex curvature posteriorly. An pronounced posterior curvature, or kyphosis, may be the result of osteoporosis and compression fracture of the anterior vertebral bodies. When seen in post-menopausal women, it results in the 'dowager's hump'. Severe kyphosis may restrict lung function.

Adventitious Lung Sounds

- Crackles: By underlining a few letters, we can see the alternative term for crackles - rales. If you want to simulate the sound of rales, moisten your thumb and index finger and pull them apart in front of your ear. If we visualize the pathology, this is exactly what we are hearing under our stethoscope in a patient with rales - the sound of mucous pulling apart. As such, rales occur during the inspiration phase of respiration. Early rales, that begin with the start of inspiration and do not last into late inspiration, are from chronic bronchitis and asthma. Late rales are more indicative of pneumonia, early congestive heart failure, or interstitial fibrosis. Fine, high pitched sounding rales are described as sibilant, whereas coarse, low pitched rales are sonorous. Coarse rales indicate copious mucous in the lungs from pneumonia or pulmonary edema.
- Wheeze: Wheezes are high pitched squeaking sounds that occur when air is forced past narrowed passageways. As such, it tends to occur more with exhalation, although it can occur on inhalation. Wheezes indicate airway obstruction such as with asthma or emphysema. Low pitched sonorous wheezes are called rhonchi, which suggest obstruction of larger airway passages, such as with

tracheobronchitis. A high pitched wheeze that occurs with inspiration is called stridor, and suggests trachea or larynx airway obstruction, such as with croup.

- Pleural friction rub: Pleuritis, or inflammation and loss of the normal fluid lubricating the lung membranes can cause a coarse low pitched sound, similar to the sound of two pieces of leather being rubbed together. The sound is on both inspiration and expiration, and is loudest on the anterolateral chest wall where the lung tissue is most mobile.

Common Respiratory Conditions

The Common Cold (ICD: 460)

*An acute, usually afebrile, viral infection of the respiratory tract, with inflammation in any or all airways, including the nose, paranasal sinuses, throat, larynx, and sometimes the trachea and bronchi. (*Merck Manual*, p. 1277)*

- The common cold is an upper respiratory infection (URI) usually caused by either rhinovirus or coronavirus. About 10-15% of colds are caused by influenza viruses, which result in longer lasting and more severe colds.
- While colds affect all age groups, young children average twice as many colds per year as adults, probably due to their close proximity to other children. Hand washing is especially important, as the virus can survive on the hands for several hours.
- Predominant common cold symptoms are sneezing, watery eyes, sore throat and a general malaise. Flu symptoms are similar but more severe. The entire body aches, and the individual usually has a headache. Nausea and vomiting may occur. The cough is usually non-productive, unless a secondary bacterial infection has developed. In the elderly and individuals with compromised immune function, influenza may prove life threatening.
- Uncomplicated common cold will have a normal heart and lung examination. Cervical lymph nodes may be enlarged. The primary findings will be inflammation of the nasal and pharyngeal mucous membranes. If a fever is present, it is low grade. However, with flu, a fever usually is present.
- Common cold is a self limiting condition, requiring only supportive care. Drink plenty of fluids (chicken soup), and rest in bed. Over the counter remedies for relief of malaise and nasal congestion may prove helpful.
- If given early enough in adequate doses, Vitamin C may abort an impending cold, or lessen the severity of symptoms. Zinc throat lozenges also have documented effectiveness with the common cold. For severe viral infections, the supplement Monolaurin may prove helpful.

Acute Bronchitis (ICD: 466.0)

Acute inflammation of the tracheobronchial tree, generally self-limited and with eventual complete healing and return of function. (Merck Manual, p. 582)

- The inflammation of acute bronchitis is usually a complication of a prior upper respiratory infection. Exudates from the nasal and pharyngeal infection travel down the respiratory tract to produce further irritation. Other causes include irritation from dust or fumes, such as cigarette smoke.
- Upper respiratory infection symptoms usually precede the bronchitis symptoms. The patient may feel a burning pain in the upper chest. The hacking cough is usually dry and nonproductive. When the condition is marked, the cough may become productive, and there may be a fever. Upon auscultation the lungs are clear, or there may be wheezing, especially after a cough.
- The treatment is symptomatic, i.e. bedrest and fluids. The patient may wish to use OTC remedies for fever and malaise. If the sputum is purulent, a secondary bacterial infection may require antibiotics.

Pneumonia (ICD: 486)

An acute infection of lung parenchyma including alveolar spaces and interstitial tissue. (Merck Manual, p. 601)

- Pneumonia is an inflammation, and usually an infection, of the lung parenchyma. This 'lower respiratory infection' frequently follows a cold or the flu. Decreased body resistance may allow the 'normal flora' bacteria of the throat to enter the lungs and become infective. Fungi, viruses, or even inhalation of chemical irritants are other possible causes.
- The alveoli air sacs fill with bacteria, blood cells, fluid, and cellular debris, causing 'consolidation'. The infection may be limited to a single lobe, resulting in 'lobar pneumonia'. When the involved area is large, hypoxia and cyanosis may result. If both lungs are affected, this is called 'double pneumonia'. When body resistance is low, pneumonia can be quite lethal. It is the most frequent complication of hospitalization, and is the sixth leading cause of death.
- The patient will appear ill, and may manifest fever and chills. The respiratory rate will be increased, and breathing is labored. Palpation reveals increased tactile fremitus. The lungs will be dull to percussion over the fluid filled lung parenchyma. Upon auscultation there will be inspiratory rales, with bronchophony over areas having consolidation. The chest x-ray will show increased density from consolidation and an 'air bronchogram' sign.
- Many of these patients require hospitalization. Antibiotics and respiratory therapy to bring up the phlegm may be needed. Less severe cases may be able to be managed with herbal expectorants and postural drainage (Encyclopedia of Natural Medicine, p. 299).

Tuberculosis (ICD: 011)

A chronic, recurrent infection, most commonly in the lungs. (<u>Merck Manual</u>, p. 1193)

- Tuberculosis, or TB, is caused by *Mycobacterium tuberculosis*. The condition is usually confined to the lungs. When it is found at other sites, such as the meninges, lymph nodes, or genitourinary tract, this is considered a metastasis of the primary lung site. Without treatment tuberculosis is often fatal. Worldwide, it is the leading cause of death from infectious disease.

- The organism is spread via microscopic airborne droplets. While the organism is highly infective, the host resistance of individuals who inhale the TB organism plays a critical role. Even individuals living in close quarters with someone having the disease display a surprising amount of resistance. Once infected, the body's immune response is usually able to wall off the bacteria. Only about 10% of individuals with a positive tuberculin skin test will manifest symptoms of the active disease, 90% will be asymptomatic.

- Individuals with a mild case of TB may remark that they are "*not feeling well.*" As the condition progresses, a cough that "*does not go away*" may develop. If the individual is a smoker or has had a recent cold, they may discount their symptoms. Eventually, the cough becomes productive of yellow or green phlegm. They may develop a fever and night sweats. Upon examination, rales in the upper posterior chest may be heard. A chest x-ray is usually diagnostic.

- While it was once thought this condition might be eradicated, it has rebounded significantly in the last twenty years. Many factors are thought to contribute to this resurgence. Individuals with AIDS have lowered resistance to the TB organism. The poor and homeless often live in close contact with other infected individuals. This, coupled with their poor nutritional status, increases their susceptibility to the TB organism. Many of these same individuals are unable to comply with the six to twelve months of antibiotic treatment needed to control the infection.

Pleurisy (ICD: 511)

Inflammation of the pleura, usually producing an exudative pleural effusion and stabbing chest pain worsened by respiration and cough. (<u>Merck Manual</u>, p. 642)

- Pleural effusion is a sign rather than a condition. Excess fluid collects in the intrapleural space for a variety of reasons, such as infection, lung cancer, congestive heart failure, etc. Gravity shifts the fluid to the lowest portions of the lung, where the fluid accumulation compresses the adjacent lung tissue.

- While the pleural membranes adherent to the viscera are insensitive, the parietal pleura adherent to the chest wall are very pain sensitive. Pleuritic chest pain, usually severe, is described as a 'stabbing' sensation, that is worse with a deep breath. In order to minimize motion, the individual's breathing may be rapid and shallow. They may have a dry nonproductive cough. Other symptoms, such as lower extremity edema or fever, may be present as a consequence of the underlying cause of the pleural effusion.

- Upon examination, there will be decreased respiratory excursion on the side of effusion, and tactile fremitus will be decreased. The area of effusion will percuss dull to flat. While fluid within the lungs results in increased breath sounds, pleural effusion serves as a barrier to sound, thus breath sounds are decreased to absent over the fluid accumulation. A pleural friction rub while not frequent, is characteristic when heard.

- A chest x-ray is the primary method of confirming the diagnosis. Blunting of the costophrenic angles will be observed. With massive pleural effusion (> 1000 ml), the mediastinum will shift away from the side of effusion.

- Treatment is geared toward the underlying cause. However, emergency measures to drain the excess fluid may be required.

Pneumothorax (ICD: 512)

Free air between the visceral and parietal pleura. (Merck Manual, p. 649)

- Normally, only a small amount of lubricating fluid is found in the pleural spaces. When air enters this space from a rupture of lung tissue (spontaneous pneumothorax), or when air enters the chest wall following injury (traumatic pneumothorax), air expansion can cause partial or complete lung collapse. Pneumothorax may occur in a young, previously healthy individual.

- If the pneumothorax is developing slowly, initially the chest pain may be minimal. As the condition progresses, the chest pain becomes sharp, and is made worse with movement or a deep breath. The pain may be severe enough that it radiates to the shoulder. In order to minimize chest movement, breathing may be rapid and shallow.

- Upon examination, chest expansion is decreased on the affected side. Tactile fremitus is decreased or absent, and when the air expansion is large the trachea will deviate away from involved side. Over the areas of air expansion, the chest is hyperresonant to percussion. Breath sounds are decreased or absent over the intrapleural air expansion. A chest x-ray is diagnostic, especially on a view taken with full expiration. There will be obvious signs of radiolucency adjacent to areas of increased lung density, and there may be a mediastinal shift away from a large pneumothorax.

- Pneumothorax is a medical emergency, requiring immediate referral. Untreated pneumothorax can lead to cardiac arrest.

Chronic Obstructive Airway Disorders

Asthma (ICD: 493)

A pulmonary disease characterized by reversible airway obstruction, airway inflammation, and increased airway responsiveness to a variety of stimuli. (Merck Manual, p. 556)

- Asthma is a hypersensitivity reaction usually triggered by airborne allergens such as dust, animal dander, or pollen. It affects 5% of the population and is most common in children under ten. The initial onset of an asthma attack is characterized by a narrowing of the bronchial airways as a result of bronchospasm and tissue inflammation. A study in the British Medical Journal (2000;55:266-270), found that heavy use of the OTC painkiller Tylenol is associated with increased incidence and severity of asthma attacks.
- During an attack the individual appears anxious and experiences wheezing, labored breathing, and 'air hunger' as a result of difficulty with exhalation. The chest will feel 'tight' and the individual may cough. They will usually sit, often in the tripod position, and the use of accessory muscles of respiration may be visible.
- Upon examination, tachypnea and tachycardia are likely. Tactile fremitus is decreased. Percussion of the lungs may disclose hyperresonance. Upon auscultation, breath sounds are decreased, and a high pitched wheeze is heard on expiration. Impairment of peak expiratory flow rate with pulmonary function testing is diagnostic. The CBC will typically show eosinophilia.
- When severe, the condition can be life threatening. Medical management involves bronchodilator medicine (Ventolin inhaler) during an attack, and identification of possible allergens.
- Chiropractic thoracic adjusting is very effective in curtailing an acute episode. After the initial phase subsides, secretion of excess mucous into the air passages is a consequence of histamine release from mast cells. This inflammation and edema increases airway resistance, resulting in prolonged expiration. Cayenne pepper (tabasco sauce) has fibrinolytic activity that helps thin the mucous and promote expectoration.
- An excellent two part summary of asthma was published in July and August 2003 by the American Chiropractic Association. At the time this book was printed these articles were available online at: http://www.acatoday.com/media/releases/asthma.shtml

Chronic Obstructive Pulmonary Disease (COPD) (ICD: 496)

A disease characterized by chronic bronchitis or emphysema and airflow obstruction that is generally progressive, may be accompanied by airway hyperreactivity, and may be partially reversible. (Merck Manual, p. 568)

- COPD is a category of obstructive pulmonary conditions that are chronic and typically irreversible (see fig 68-1 in Merck Manual p. 569). As such, it includes individuals with irreversible asthma as well as emphysema (COPD type A) and chronic bronchitis (COPD type B).
- COPD is very common, the fourth leading cause of death in the US. Approximately two-thirds of adult males and one-fourth of females will have emphysema at death.
- Most cases of emphysema are the result of a lifetime of cigarette smoking. Destruction of elastic pulmonary connective tissue results in

permanent enlargement of the alveoli air sacs. While muscular contraction of the diaphragm produces lung expansion, lung contraction is passive, requiring elastic recoil of lung tissue. The lack of normal lung resiliency accounts for many of the signs seen with emphysema.

- The patient with emphysema is sometimes characterized as a 'pink puffer'. Chronic lung hyperinflation greatly increases the work of breathing. The individual has dyspnea and uses the accessory muscles of respiration to aid with expiration. They may assume the tripod position and unconsciously perform 'purse lip' breathing. Upon observation, the chest may have a barrel shape, due to chronic over inflation of the lungs. In contrast to the patient with chronic bronchitis, the individual may be thin, without cyanosis or edema. Radiographic examination will show increased radiolucency of the lung parenchyma, a narrow heart shadow, and a flat diaphragm.

- When chronic bronchitis is the more prominent condition, the patient may present as a cyanotic 'blue bloater'. This individual shows signs hypoxia typical of pulmonary hypertension and right ventricular hypertrophy (cor pulmonale). This individual may appear similar to the congestive heart failure patient, manifesting dyspnea on exertion, pitting edema of the legs, and may be overweight, in contrast to the thin emphysema patient. When sputum production and diminished expiratory flow rate are present, the condition is more likely COPD, rather than CHF.

- Upon examination, chest expansion will be decreased. Measurement of chest circumference is a surprisingly good predictor of forced vital capacity readings on pulmonary function testing. Lung examination signs are as expected with hyperinflated lung parenchyma: decreased tactile fremitus, hyperresonant percussion, and decreased breath sounds on auscultation. Prolonged expiration, possibly as long as six seconds, with an expiratory wheeze is likely.

- The first intervention for both medical and natural therapeutics is the same: <u>Stop Smoking!</u> A bronchodilator inhaler (Ventolin) may help with the dyspnea. Supplemental oxygen may be required when hypoxia is marked. When the condition is severe, the individual will probably be given steroid anti-inflammatory medicine. Lung transplantation is now a medical management option. In fact, COPD is now the most common diagnosis for which lung transplantation is carried out.

- Many times there are natural therapeutics agents that serve similar functions to the drugs, at less cost, and with few if any side effects. Quercetin and other flavonoids help moderate excessive histamine release which is a part of the inflammatory response. L-cysteine and cayenne help thin respiratory mucous. Bromelain is a potent herbal anti-inflammatory. Magnesium is a smooth muscle relaxant and will help promote bronchodilation.

- An online review article on COPD:
    http://www.nejm.org/content/2000/0343/0004/0269.asp

Bronchiectasis (ICD: 494)

Irreversible focal bronchial dilation, usually accompanied by chronic infection and associated with diverse conditions, some congenital or hereditary. (Merck Manual, p. 584)

- The bronchial airways contain small hair like cilia that sweep particles toward the larger airways where they can be expelled. When this process is interfered with, mucous may build up, which in turn may damage the airways, causing them to enlarge. The initial cause of the damage may be allergies or recurrent respiratory infections.
- Most cases are acquired, however a specific underlying cause is identified in less than half of the cases. While bronchiectasis may occur congenitally, this is rare. Cystic fibrosis is an inherited condition where mucous which is normally slippery, becomes thick and sticky. Because they have difficulty coughing up mucous, bronchiectasis is common in children with cystic fibrosis.
- The predominate symptom is a chronic cough with sputum, which is often purulent and foul smelling. Hypoxia may result in clubbing of the fingernails.
- Upon examination, lung auscultation usually reveals crackles, usually in the lower portion of the lungs. The chest film may show increased bronchovascular markings. A CT will confirm dilated airways.
- Medical treatment includes bronchodilator medicine, antibiotics for infection, and respiratory therapy. Postural drainage will facilitate elimination of bronchial secretions.

Atelectasis (ICD: 518)

A shrunken, airless state affecting all or part of a lung. (Merck Manual, p. 590)

- Atelectasis or a collapsed lung is usually the result of bronchial obstruction by a mucous plug. Lack of air in and out of the alveoli causes shrinkage of lung tissue supplied by that bronchus. The uninvolved tissue expands and shifts toward the collapsed area. With a large collapse, the heart and trachea will shift toward the lesion.
- A small atelectasis may be asymptomatic. When the collapse is larger, symptoms of tachypnea, dyspnea, and chest pain manifest. Cyanosis and a fever may be present.
- Upon palpation there is decreased tactile fremitus over the affected area, and diminished chest expansion on that side. Percussion is dull over the airless area. Auscultation discloses decreased or absent breath sounds over the collapsed lung.
- A chest x-ray confirms the diagnosis. The collapsed lung will display increased density. The mediastinum will shift toward the collapse, and the diaphragm will be elevated on the affected side.
- Medical treatment may involve bronchoscopy to remove the bronchial obstruction. Deep breathing is encouraged to reinflate collapsed lung tissue. 'Middle lobe syndrome' is a form of chronic recurrent atelectasis due to bronchial compression by the

surrounding lymph nodes. Chronic atelectasis usually leads to chronic pneumonia. Antibiotics are usually required to treat an infection. If the collapsed lung does not reinflate, it may have to be removed surgically.

Pulmonary Embolism (ICD: 415.1)

Sudden lodgment of a blood clot in a pulmonary artery with subsequent obstruction of blood supply to the lung parenchyma. (Merck Manual, p. 593)

- Just as a blood clot to the brain may cause a stroke, if a blood clot becomes lodged in a lung blood vessel, pulmonary embolism will result. Most blood clots originate from the legs. Recent surgery, fracture, trauma, or other conditions that lead to immobilization are considered to be a pre-embolic condition. Heart disease, hypertension, and cigarette smoking all favor the formation of blood clots.
- When the blockage is small, symptoms may be mild, such as dyspnea. With a large lung embolism, the pain may be severe and 'knife-like', with hemoptysis. Pulmonary embolism causes hypoxia, and hypoxemia can in turn cause tachycardia. When a patient has unexplained tachycardia, pulmonary embolism should be considered a possibility.
- Pulmonary embolism can be missed by good diagnosticians. It is now even called the 'great masquerader' because it can cause symptoms that mimic other conditions. Pulmonary embolism can cause: shock, chest pain, stroke, asthma, atrial flutter, pleural effusion, anasarca (leg edema), antibiotic resistant pneumonia, hyponatremia, and liver congestion.
- Auscultation may disclose decreased breath sounds, crackles, wheezes and a possible friction rub. If there is no lung infarction, the x-ray may be normal. The ECG will show evidence that the right side of the heart is working harder.
- Medical treatment involves blood thinners (Coumadin) and thrombolytic drugs to facilitate breakdown of the clot. While lung tissue does not 'die' as quickly as brain and heart tissue when deprived of circulation, early intervention is still key.

Bronchogenic Carcinoma (ICD: 162.9)

A highly malignant primary lung tumor that accounts for most cases of lung cancer and has a very poor prognosis. (Merck Manual, p. 651)

- Lung cancer is the leading cause of cancer death in the US for both men and women. Worldwide it claims about one million lives each year. Since 90% of lung cancer is the direct result of cigarette smoking, most of these deaths are entirely preventable.
- Symptoms include a hacking 'smoker's cough', chest pain, dyspnea, hemoptysis, and weight loss. With severe hypoxia, clubbing of the fingernails may be seen. If the cancer is a superior sulcus (Pancoast)

tumor, it may affect sympathetic nerves and manifest symptoms of Horner's syndrome.

- Upon examination, the supraclavicular lymph nodes may be enlarged. Chest percussion over the tumor may be dull. Breath sounds may be normal to diminished. The chest x-ray will show a mass and possibly a wide mediastinum.

- Unfortunately, at the time of initial diagnosis three quarters of lung cancers have already metastasized. This accounts for their poor prognosis. Treatment for cancer may consist of: surgery, radiation, and chemotherapy.

Chest Wall Pain

Costochondritis (ICD: 733.6)

- Costochondritis is an inflammation of the cartilage connection between the ribs and sternum. It may be considered an atypical form of arthritis. The pain is commonly felt at the 2nd to 5th costosternal articulations, and usually involves more than one joint.

- Typically it develops as a consequence of physical activity, such as moving furniture. Individuals with a chronic cough, such as a smokers cough, are at risk for developing this condition. Women who carry a heavy bag on one shoulder may also experience costochondritis.

- The pain may be intense, and may occasionally radiate to the shoulder and arm. Because it is aggravated by exercise, it may be confused with cardiac pain. The pain is increased with taking a deep breath. This is an important differential, because unless there is also lung pathology, cardiac pain is <u>not</u> made worse with deep breathing.

- Upon examination, there will be palpable tenderness at the costosternal articulation. When there is localized swelling in addition to the tenderness, the condition is referred to as Tietze's syndrome.

- The condition responds well to conservative chiropractic care, but keep in mind, your patient may have more than one condition. It would not be unusual for this individual to have a concurrent subclinical heart condition. An ECG and lab testing of cardiac enzymes would be a prudent step to safeguard your patient's health, as well as your peace of mind.

Herpes Zoster (ICD: 053)

An infection with varicella-zoster virus primarily involving the dorsal root ganglia and characterized by vesicular eruption and neuralgic pain in the dermatome of the affected root ganglia. (Merck Manual, p. 1294)

- Herpes zoster, more commonly known as shingles, manifests as a painful rash. The vesicles follow the course of a single nerve, usually located in the dermatomal band between two ribs (zoster is latin for 'belt').

- The infection is caused by the same virus that causes chickenpox, usually in childhood. After the infection resolves, the virus remains

152

dormant in the dorsal root ganglia. When immune function is compromised, the virus may again become active. While cancer or HIV infection may be the cause for this reappearance, in most cases it manifests as a consequence of the normal decline in immunity that occurs with aging.

- About 10-20% of adults will experience at least one episode during their life, usually after age 50. Prior to an outbreak, the individual experiences pain at the site where the vesicles will erupt. While the vesicles usually heal within a few weeks, many people experience burning skin hypersensitivity referred to as 'postherpetic neuralgia'.
- The diagnosis is established primarily by the characteristic appearance of the vesicles. However, during the two to three days prior to the eruption of the blisters, the condition is easily misdiagnosed. The description of the pain may provide the needed clue, "It hurts to have my shirt rub against the skin." When a patient experiences pain from an ordinarily nonpainful stimulus this is referred to as allodynia.
- Antiviral drugs, such as Zovirax (acyclovir) or Famvir, if started early in the outbreak, may lessen the severity of symptoms. These drugs are however quite expensive, and the antiviral nutritional supplement Monolaurin is also quite effective, at substantially less cost. Supplemental intake of the amino acid lysine, and avoiding foods high in arginine (nuts, seeds, chocolate) is also recommended.

Study Guide Objectives

- Know the normal anatomy of the respiratory tract.
- Know the mechanics of respiration.
- Know the common thoracic deformities.
- The trachea bifurcates into the right and left main bronchi at the level of what structure on the anterior chest?
- What is the significance of the costal angle?
- What is another name for the manubriosternal angle?
- Where are the apices of the lung assessed during your examination of the anterior and posterior chest?
- Know the locations of the fissures and lobes of the lungs.
- Which phase of respiration is active vs. passive? What implication does this have for conditions such as emphysema?
- Know the appropriate history questions for examination of the thorax and lungs.
- What is the significance of pink foamy sputum?
- Why do we perform auscultation last when examining the lungs?
- What is the significance of increased skin sensation during palpation of the posterior chest?
- What lung conditions manifest increased tactile fremitus?
- What lung conditions manifest decreased tactile fremitus?
- Know which lung conditions cause tracheal deviation and which direction the trachea is pushed or pulled.
- What is the normal expected tone during lung percussion?

- Which lung conditions cause hyperresonance during lung percussion?
- What is the significance of a dull sound elicited with lung percussion?
- Know how to perform diaphragmatic excursion.
- Know the types and characteristics of the three normal breath sounds.
- What examination finding would cause you to perform bronchophony, egophony, and whispered pectoriloquy?
- Know the types and characteristics of adventitious breath sounds.
- Know the significance of an altered AP to lateral chest diameter ratio.
- Know the pathologic changes that occur with the various lung and thoracic conditions discussed.
- What is the medical term for 'funnel chest'?
- What is the medical term for 'pigeon chest'?
- What is the screening test for functional scoliosis?
- What is another name for rales?
- The common cold is an upper respiratory infection caused by which organism?
- What are the differences between the common cold and influenza?
- What is lung consolidation?
- What are the expected examination findings with pneumonia, specifically tactile fremitus, percussion, breath sounds, etc?
- Upon lung auscultation of a TB patient, where might rales (crackles) be heard?
- Why is TB so difficult to treat?
- What are the causes of pleural effusion?
- Which is more pain sensitive: parietal or visceral pleura?
- How is pleuritic chest pain typically described?
- What causes blunting of the costophrenic angle on a chest x-ray?
- What are the mechanisms that cause lung collapse in pneumothorax?
- When an individual experiences an asthma attack, which phase of respiration do they have difficulty with?
- What is the most likely cause of emphysema?
- What are the expected examination findings with emphysema, specifically tactile fremitus, percussion, breath sounds, etc?
- Which type of COPD is referred to as a 'pink puffer'?
- Which type of COPD is referred to as a 'blue bloater'?
- An individual with COPD has difficulty with which phase of respiration?
- Which nutrient is a smooth muscle relaxant helpful in promoting bronchodilation?
- Which lung condition causes a chronic cough with purulent 'foul smelling' sputum?
- What does clubbing of the fingernails indicate?
- What lung condition is common in children with cystic fibrosis?
- What is the mechanism that causes lung collapse in atelectasis?
- What are the tracheal shift differences between atelectasis and pneumothorax?

- o What are the predisposing factors toward pulmonary embolism?
- o X-ray is diagnostic for most lung conditions. Which lung conditions manifest a normal chest x-ray?
- o What is the most likely cause of lung cancer?
- o What is a Pancoast tumor and why does it manifest Horner's syndrome?
- o What is an important differential to distinguish cardiac pain from costochondritis?
- o What is Tietze's syndrome?
- o What childhood infection predisposes an individual to shingles?
- o What is allodynia?

9 – Heart & Cardiovascular

Anatomy & Physiology

The heart is located slightly left of midline within the chest, in the mediastinum between the two lungs. It is positioned roughly from the second intercostal space and the right sternal border (the 'base' of the heart), to the fifth intercostal space at the left midclavicular line (the 'apex' of the heart). The apex is where the apical impulse is usually palpable on the chest wall during systole. The heart is rotated within the chest, positioning the right side of the heart more anteriorly, and the left side of the heart more posteriorly. This rotation accounts for the apparent reversal of the aortic and pulmonic valve sites on the chest wall during heart auscultation.

The 'great vessels' are found superior to the base of the heart. The superior and inferior vena cava carry unoxygenated venous blood to the right atrium. Blood leaving the right ventricle (still unoxygenated) exits the pulmonary artery for the lungs. Once oxygenated, this blood travels to the left atrium via the pulmonary veins. Finally, blood exits the left ventricle via the aorta to supply oxygen rich blood to the body.

The heart has three layers. The tough fibrous pericardium is composed of two layers separated by pericardial fluid that facilitates easy motion of the heart. The myocardium is the thick muscular wall of the heart that contracts during systole to pump the blood. The endocardium is a thin layer that lines the valves and chambers to provide for smooth laminar flow of blood.

The valves of the heart are located at the entrance and exit points of the ventricles. Blood enters the ventricles from the atria via the atrioventricular or AV valves. The right AV valve is the tricuspid valve, and the left AV valve is the mitral valve. Blood exits the ventricles via the semilunar valves. On the right is the pulmonic valve preventing back flow of blood from the pulmonary artery to the right ventricle. On the left is the aortic valve preventing backflow of blood from the aorta to the left ventricle. While the AV valves mark the exit point of the atria, there are no valves at the entrance to the atria. As such, restriction of blood flow within the heart may cause blood to back up from the right side of the heart to the peripheral circulation and from the left side of the heart to the lungs.

The cardiac cycle is a sequence of events marked by electrical and mechanical changes that result in pressure changes that cause opening and closing of the valves. Systole and diastole are the two phases of the cardiac cycle. During diastole, the ventricles are relaxed and slowly fill with blood. The AV valves are open and the semilunar valves are closed. Toward the end of diastole, just before systole, the atria contract. This presystolic atrial contraction, referred to as the 'atrial kick', increases by about 25% the blood entering the ventricles.

Systole begins with contraction of the ventricles. Increased intraventricular pressure causes the AV valves to close and the semilunar valves to open. The S1 heart sound is heard when the AV valves close, and marks the beginning of systole. At the end of ventricular contraction, the pressure within the ventricles falls sufficiently that the pressure below the semilunar valves is now less than above the valves. This closes the semilunar valves, preventing retrograde flow of blood from the aorta and pulmonary artery back into the ventricles. The S2 heart sound is heard when the semilunar valves close, and marks the end of systole and beginning of diastole. The atrial blood pressure is now greater than ventricular pressure, so the AV valves open once again to begin the next cycle of ventricular filling.

While the right side of the heart pumps blood only to the lungs, the left side of the heart must pump blood to the entire body. As such the left side of the heart is larger and the heart sounds produced when the mitral and aortic valves close are louder than the tricuspid and pulmonic valve closure sounds. The aortic and pulmonic valves normally close simultaneously. However, during inspiration decreased intrathoracic pressure causes the pulmonic valve (P2) to close slightly later than the aortic valve (A2), which creates the phenomenon known as physiological splitting of S2.

S1 and S2 are 'normal' heart sounds produced when the heart valves close. Extra heart sounds may be heard during auscultation which usually signifies pathology of some kind. S3 is an extra sound that is produced by ventricular filling in early diastole. If the normal heart creates a *LUB-dup, LUB-dup* sound, a heart with an S3 sound might be heard as *LUB-duppa, LUB-duppa*. It is a soft, low pitched sound. Since it is low pitched, it is best heard with the bell of the stethoscope. Later in diastole, just before the next S1, a presystolic S4 sound may be heard.

Heart murmurs are the sound created by turbulence within the normally smooth flow of blood through the heart. When heart murmurs occur in young healthy people, they are probably 'innocent'. However, in older adults this turbulence is usually caused by valvular heart disease.

When electrodes are placed on the chest, an electrocardiogram or ECG, can trace the flow of electrical current through the heart. The sinoatrial or SA node is the 'pacemaker' of the heart which sends an electrical current to both atria. The AV node is located low in the septum between the two atria. It picks up the electrical impulse and transmits it to the bundle of His and to both ventricles via the right and left bundle branches. The waveform produced on the ECG has specific peaks that correspond to specific cardiac events:

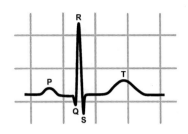

P wave	atrial depolarization
PR interval	the delay that occurs as the electrical impulse travels from the SA node to the AV node and then to the ventricles
QRS complex	depolarization of the ventricles
T wave	ventricular repolarization

As a part of the cardiac examination, we assess the carotid artery and jugular venous pulses in the neck. The carotid artery is located just lateral to the trachea, in the groove between the trachea and the SCM muscle. The external jugular vein is located superficial and lateral to the SCM muscle.

Nature of the Patient

While heart disease is now occurring at an earlier age, it is still a condition that takes time to develop, and is unlikely in a patient under 30. When a young person experiences pain similar to angina, a chest wall syndrome or esophagitis is the more likely cause.

Key History Questions

Your first task with a patient who presents with chest pain is to determine: Is this a medical emergency, i.e. a heart attack? When in doubt, send your patient for a second opinion. It is unwise to adopt a 'wait and see' attitude with potential heart problems. Clot busting drugs (streptokinase and t-PA) are available, and if administered within the first few hours of a heart attack, substantially reduce myocardial injury.

Do you experience chest pain or tightness?

- When did this pain begin and how long did it last?
  - o A single episode of acute chest pain suggests an acute MI, pulmonary embolism or pneumothorax.
  - o Chronic chest pain points to chronic coronary insufficiency, esophagitis, hiatal hernia, or possibly a chest wall syndrome, such as a rib subluxation.
- What is the character and location of the pain?
  - o The pain of an acute myocardial infarction is frequently described as crushing substernal chest pain, as if an elephant was stepping on the chest. The patient is unable to localize their pain with a single finger. Rather, they may hold a clenched fist over their chest when describing the pain (Levine's clenched fist sign). The chest pain may radiate to the jaw or left shoulder and arm.

- A patient with pulmonary embolism may experience a gripping or stabbing pain, more common on the right than the left, and they may be able to localize their pain with a single finger.
- Pneumothorax pain occurs at the lateral thorax and is described as sharp or tearing.
- Pneumonia pain may have a more burning quality, located over a larger area of lung involvement, and with associated cough, fever, and sputum production.
- While chest pain of gastrointestinal origin may also be substernal, it tends to have more of a burning quality, occurring after ingestion of food.

- Is the pain precipitated by certain activities?
  - Angina chest pain may be brought on by physical activity or emotionally stressful situations.
  - Chest pain of gastrointestinal origin usually occurs in relation to meals.
- Are there any other associated symptoms of cardiac dysfunction?
  - Sweating (diaphoresis); cold, clammy skin; ashen gray or pale skin
  - Rapid heart beat (tachycardia), or heart skips beats (palpitations)
  - Swelling of lower legs
  - Dizziness, nausea, vomiting
- What makes the pain better?
  - Angina pain usually lasts a only few minutes, and is relieved by rest or with sublingual nitroglycerin.
  - If the pain is relieved with antacids, you should consider gastrointestinal conditions, such as esophagitis or hiatal hernia.
  - Chest pain that is relieved by lying down may suggest mitral valve prolapse.
- What makes your pain worse?
  - Chest pain made worse with deep breathing suggests a chest wall problem, such as rib subluxation or fracture, or costochondritis (Tietze's syndrome). Deep breathing also aggravates pneumothorax or pleurisy pain.
  - Deep chest pain that is made worse with movement may point to pericarditis.
  - Chest pain that occurs after eating and is made worse with laying down points to reflux esophagitis.

Do you have any shortness of breath?

- Decreased cardiac output of heart disease can cause a pooling of blood in the lungs, which in turn impairs lung function.
  - The individual may experience shortness of breath (SOB), or shortness of breath on exertion (SOBOE), also referred to as

160

dyspnea on exertion (DOE). When there is exercise intolerance, try to quantify the impairment in terms of time or distance walked.

- o Paroxysmal nocturnal dyspnea (PND) is typical of congestive heart failure. The recumbent position increases the pooling of intrathoracic blood, and the weakened heart has difficulty with the work load. Respiratory distress may awaken the person after a few hours of sleep, where they have to stand and get some fresh air. To compensate, the individual may need to sleep with their torso propped up with pillows. If so, we document the number of pillows they must use, e.g. two pillow orthopnea.

Do you have a cough?

- The presence of an associated cough with cardiac disorders points to lung involvement. Frothy, blood tinged sputum suggests congestive heart failure. A pulmonary embolism may also manifest with hemoptysis. If the sputum is purulent and there is a fever, pneumonia is the likely cause.

Do you tire easily?

- Fatigue that worsens with activity or at the end of the day suggests decreased cardiac output. When the fatigue is worse with <u>inactivity</u>, and improves with exercise, anxiety or depression is the likely cause.

Have you noticed any swelling of your legs or feet?

- Dependent edema is a sign of congestive heart failure. The swelling is typically worse after a day of activity, and is better after a night's rest with legs elevated.

Do you have to get up at night to urinate?

- Tissue edema is a feature of congestive heart failure. The horizontal position while sleeping facilitates resorption of this excess fluid, which must then be excreted by the kidneys.

Do you have a personal or family history of heart trouble?

- Chronic hypertension increases the workload on the heart, as it pumps against this peripheral resistance, which in turn can lead to the cardiac enlargement typical of congestive heart failure.
- Previous strep throat infections may predispose to rheumatic heart valve defects.
- You must document all previous heart related treatment, e.g. current and previous blood pressure and heart medications, electrocardiograms (ECG), cholesterol checks, angioplasty or other heart surgery.
- *With your blood relatives (parents, grandparents, brothers and sisters), do any of them have, or have they ever had?*

- o high blood pressure
- o stroke
- o heart attack
- o diabetes
- o obesity

Cardiac Risk Factors

- Many of the questions we ask during the personal/social history relate to risk factors for coronary heart disease:
  - o Diet: A diet high in fat and low in fruit and vegetables contributes toward atherosclerosis.
  - o Alcohol: In addition to causing liver problems, chronic alcohol abuse can also hasten the development of atherosclerosis.
  - o Smoking: While we typically consider tar and nicotine to be the culprits with tobacco, cigarette smoke also contains carbon monoxide. Carbon monoxide ties up the oxygen sites on red blood cells and reduces the ability of your blood to carry oxygen. A lack of oxygen to cardiac muscle is what precipitates myocardial infarction (MI).
  - o Exercise: The heart is a muscle, and the aphorism 'use it or lose it' applies here. Studies show a 30% reduction in coronary artery disease in those who exercise regularly, in comparison to people with a sedentary lifestyle.
  - o Stress: Type A behavior refers to individuals who are tense, compulsive about time, and place unrealistic expectations on themselves or others. Research has shown that Type A personalities have a greater risk of heart attack and stroke.

Examination

Inspection

With the patient in the supine position, observe for the presence of jugular venous pulsations. Because there is no valve to prevent backflow of blood from the right atrium, the jugular venous pulse represents an indirect measurement of the central venous pressure (CVP) of the right side of the heart. Central venous pressure is important enough in some patients hospitalized for congestive heart failure that the patient may have a central venous line placed in the subclavian vein in order to provide ongoing assessment of the CVP.

To assess jugular venous pressure, position your patient supine with the head and chest elevated. Jugular venous pulsations are normally visible with approximately 30-40 degrees elevation of the head of the table. Tangential lighting is helpful when trying to see the pulsations. When the CVP is high, the torso may need to be elevated to 60 degrees. Place one edge of a straight edge object at the site of visible jugular pulsations. Place the other end over the sternal angle of the breast bone. Keeping this straight edge perfectly horizontal, measure with a ruler how far above the sternal angle the free edge of the straight edge is positioned above the sternal angle.

Jugular venous pressure is not routinely measured. However, when congestive heart failure is suspected, the jugular venous pressure should be assessed. If the measured distance is greater than 3 cm, congestive heart failure of the right side of the heart is probable. When congestive heart failure is present, jugular venous distention can be made more pronounced by applying firm pressure under the right costal margin. This maneuver, referred to as the hepatojugular reflex, causes emptying of the liver sinusoids and will cause the jugular venous pulse to become more prominent.

Inspect the precordium of the chest. With thin individuals you may be able to see the apical impulse of cardiac contraction. When visible, the apical impulse is usually seen at the 4th or 5th rib interspace at the mid clavicular line. Patients with cardiomegaly may have a very pronounced apical impulse that is referred to as a lift or heave.

Palpation

One at a time, palpate each carotid pulse. Assess the contour and amplitude of each pulse. Diminished pulse strength occurs with vascular occlusion and decreased cardiac output. Increased carotid pulse amplitude is felt with hyperkinetic states.

Palpation of the precordium is to feel for cardiac thrills, the vibration produced by heart murmurs, and to identify the PMI, or point of maximal impulse. With the pads of your fingers palpate the same locations you will be listening to with your stethoscope:

Locations for Cardiac Auscultation

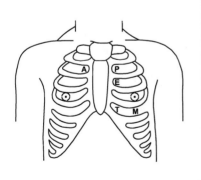

Aortic valve	right 2nd intercostal space at sternal border
Pulmonic valve	left 2nd intercostal space at sternal border
Erb's point	left 3rd intercostal space at sternal border
Tricuspid valve	lower left sternal border (4th or 5th intercostal space)
Mitral valve	left 5th intercostal space at the midclavicular line

When present, a thrill might produce a vibration similar to a cat purring. It is the vibration produced by turbulent blood flow within the heart.

While you are palpating the mitral valve area, attempt to locate the PMI. With one finger, try to localize the point where the apical impulse is felt most strongly. This point is usually small and located near the mitral valve area. If the PMI is large, spanning more than one rib interspace, cardiac enlargement is probable. When the PMI is displaced laterally, toward the anterior axillary line, this also suggests cardiac enlargement, most likely left ventricular hypertrophy.

Percussion

Percussion of the heart is not routinely performed. Cardiac enlargement is more accurately predicted with a chest x-ray. In the absence of an x-ray, percussion may be performed to assess hypertrophy of the heart. The left border of the heart is normally percussed at the midclavicular line. The right border of the heart should not extend beyond the right border of the sternum.

Auscultation

With the diaphragm of your stethoscope, listen to the five traditional valve areas listed above. Use a Z pattern, starting at either the mitral area and progressing toward the aortic area, or vice versa. Do not 'jump' the stethoscope from area to area, rather 'inch' your stethoscope to the next point, listening to more than just the five points along the Z. It takes practice to hear heart sounds. A quite room is essential. As you are listening try to assess:

- Rate and rhythm
- S1 and S2 (relative intensity varies with location of stethoscope)
- Splitting of S1 or S2
- Extra heart sounds in systole (ejection click or midsystolic click)
- Extra heart sounds in diastole (opening snap, S3, or S4)
- Systolic or diastolic murmurs

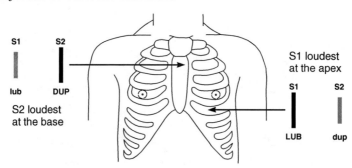

The diaphragm of the stethoscope is for listening to high pitched sounds, such as S1, S2, aortic and mitral regurgitation murmurs, and pericardial friction rubs. In order to hear low pitched sounds, such as S3, S4, and mitral stenosis murmurs, switch the stethoscope to the bell and briefly listen to the heart sounds a second time. On a routine physical examination, with no signs or symptoms of cardiac dysfunction, many doctors listen with only the diaphragm of the stethoscope.

Most of the cardiac exam can be conducted with the patient in the supine position. If the patient has cardiac complaints, or when you hear murmurs, listen to the heart with the patient in two additional positions.

- Left lateral decubitus - this position uses gravity to shift the heart closer to the mitral valve site and may enhance the sound of S3, S4, and mitral stenosis murmurs.
- Seated, lean forward, and exhale - this position raises the base of the heart and may enhance the sound of aortic and pulmonic valve murmurs.

With the bell of the stethoscope, auscultate for carotid artery bruits at the same location you palpated the carotid pulse. A bruit is a soft whooshing sound created by blood moving through a narrowed artery. This low pitched pulsatile sound is relatively difficult to hear. Have the patient take a breath and hold it while you listen, otherwise tracheal breath sounds make it impossible to hear the bruit. Be careful to press only hard enough to seal the stethoscope to the skin. If you press too hard, this can create an artificial bruit. If this is a screening examination, one site on each side is probably sufficient. However, if you suspect the presence of atherosclerotic plaque in the arteries, listen to three locations on each side:

- At the base of the neck in the supraclavicular area
- Midcervical lateral to the thyroid cartilage
- High in the neck, inferior to the angle of the jaw

Be aware that if the patient has a heart murmur, this can transmit sound into the left lower neck that might be confused for a bruit.

Summary of Heart Auscultation

Heart auscultation requires practice and a quite room. In time, your ears will become more attuned to hearing the subtleties of heart sounds. The key is to listen to many normals, so that when you hear abnormal, it sticks out like a sore thumb. While you may be uncertain about what you hearing, you know 'something' is not right, and needs to be referred for more definitive diagnosis. In this area, you may be more similar to your medical colleagues than you suspect. A study of family practice and internal medicine residents (not medical students), found that physicians could correctly identify twelve commonly encountered cardiac events only 20% of the time (JAMA 1997;278:717-722). As medical science becomes increasingly reliant on sophisticated technology such as echocardiography, the mastery of general physical examination skills suffers.

Summary of Physical Examination

Assessment of cardiovascular conditions includes:

- Observation of general appearance for sweating, pallor, cyanosis, and increased respiratory effort.
- Measure vital signs: temperature, pulse, respiration, blood pressure.
- Palpate for chest wall tenderness, symmetry of respiratory excursion, tracheal shift.
- Percuss lung fields.
- Auscultate for normal breath sounds and the presence of adventitious lung sounds.
- Auscultate heart sounds.
- Auscultate for bowel sounds and bruits. Examine the abdomen for masses and tenderness.
- Examine the extremities for edema, cyanosis, and diminished pulses.

Note: By convention, when the patient is in the supine position, the doctor stands on the right side of the patient. This probably developed because most doctors are right handed. It is uncertain whether your Part IV National Board exams use this as a grading criterion. In your own practice, find a routine that works for you and does not involve frequent changes from one side of the table to the other.

Diagnostic Studies

- ECG
- Treadmill stress ECG
- 24 hour Holter monitoring with heart rate variability (HRV) analysis
- Lab
    - CBC, sed rate, chemistry panel (a routine chemistry panel usually includes HDL and LDL cholesterol).
    - A recent study in the New England Journal of Medicine (http://content.nejm.org/cgi/content/short/347/20/1557) found: "*These data suggest that the C-reactive protein level is a stronger predictor of cardiovascular events than the LDL cholesterol level.*"
    - Cardiac enzymes: CK-MB, AST, LDH, Troponin I
    - Amylase and Lipase, if pancreatic disease is suspected
- Echocardiography
- Plain chest film
- Endoscopy, if esophagitis is suspected

Sample Documentation

Carotid artery pulses were strong and symmetrical. No carotid artery bruits were auscultated. Jugular venous pressure was not measured. No abnormal pulsations or lifts were observed upon inspection of the precordium. The point of maximal impulse (PMI) was palpated at the left

5th intercostal space at the midclavicular line. No thrills were palpable. Upon auscultation, the apical heartbeat was regular and rhythmic. S1 was heard loudest at the apex, and S2 was loudest at the base of the heart. Physiological splitting of S2 was noted at the pulmonic point during inhalation. No clicks, murmurs, or extra heart sounds were heard.

Abnormal Findings

Rate and Rhythm Abnormalities

- Tachycardia: Heart rate > 100. This rate is usually exceeded with exercise and is not pathological under those circumstances. However, a resting heart rate of 100 may be cause for concern. Sudden onset gives rise to the adjective paroxysmal, e.g. paroxysmal atrial tachycardia (PAT). Heart rate greater than 150-200 is referred to as fibrillation, an irregular spasmodic contraction of the myocardium.
- Bradycardia: Heart rate < 60. In well conditioned athletes, bradycardia is a consequence of superior cardiac function. In individuals with poor cardiac function, bradycardia may indicate a 'heart block' of the electrical impulse to the ventricles.
- Sinus Arrhythmia: Sinus arrhythmia refers to the normal speeding up of the heart rate with inspiration, and slowing down with expiration. A new technique in cardiology, heart rate variability (HRV) is an objective measure of this function, and may turn out to be the earliest predictor of heart disease, even better than a stress ECG. An intact nerve supply to the heart is the essential requirement for normal heart rate variability. Can chiropractic adjustments have a positive effect on heart disease? Of course they can!

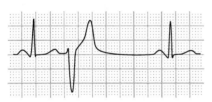

- Premature Contractions: Premature contractions may arise from the atria or ventricles and requires an ECG to determine the site of the conduction defect. In general, atrial rhythm defects are less serious than ventricular defects. While premature ventricular contractions (PVC's) in young healthy individuals may be a 'normal variant', PVC's in older patients are clinically significant and may be a sign of impending myocardial infarction (MI).

Split and Extra Cardiac Sounds

- Splitting of S2 is a normal event referred to as physiological splitting. Normally the aortic and pulmonic heart valves close synchronously. During inspiration, decreased intrathoracic pressure causes a slight delay in the closure of the pulmonic valve. It is only heard at the pulmonic valve area at the end of inspiration. It is not heard during exhalation, and disappears if you ask the patient to hold their breath.

If the normal heart sound at the pulmonic area is *lub-DUP, lub-DUP,* physiological splitting of S2 might sound like *lub-DRUP, lub-DRUP.*

Physiological Splitting of S2

Exhalation		Inhalation				Exhalation	
S1	S2	S1	S2	S1	S2	S1	S2
			A₂ P₂		A₂ P₂		
lub	DUP	lub	DRUP	lub	DRUP	lub	DUP

- Fixed splitting (inspiration and expiration), or paradoxical splitting (expiration) of S2 are abnormal.
- Ejection click: A short high pitched click immediately after S1 suggests stenotic valves, either aortic or pulmonic depending on where the click is heard loudest.
- Mid-systolic click: A short high pitched click heard in mid to late systole is indicative of mitral valve prolapse. If the chordae tendinea are too long, the valve leaflets balloon up or prolapse into the left atrium. Heard best at the heart apex, this condition is also known as a click-murmur syndrome and floppy valve syndrome, and may be accompanied by a mitral regurgitation murmur.
- Opening snap: We normally hear the valves when they close, and they are silent when they open. The S2 sound is produced by closing of the aortic and pulmonic valves, marking the end of systole. Almost immediately, the mitral and tricuspid valves open, to allow rapid filling of the ventricles. In the presence of stenotic AV valves, usually the mitral valve, a sharp, high pitched snap is sometimes heard at the lower left sternal border, followed by the low pitched diastolic rumble of mitral stenosis.
- S3: S3 is the sound of ventricular filling. It may be physiologic in children. However when the patient is over 40, it is probably pathologic. An abnormal S3 is referred to as a ventricular gallop, and represents decreased compliance of the ventricles, and may be the earliest sign of heart failure. It is best heard at the heart apex using the bell, with the patient in the left lateral position.
- S4: S4 is similar to S3, except it is heard later in diastole, just before the next S1. It also is heard best with the bell at the heart apex, and the patient in the left lateral position. While it can be physiologic or normal in an athletic heart, a pathologic S4 is referred to as an atrial gallop, and is related to stiffness of the ventricular myocardium to rapid filling. When both S3 and S4 are present, a quadruple rhythm or summation sound gallop may be heard.
- The combination of S3 and S4 extra heart sounds produces a 'gallop rhythm':
- Pericardial friction rub: Inflammation of the membranes surrounding the heart may give rise to a high pitched scratchy sandpaper like

sound, best heard with the diaphragm. The sound is present during both systole and diastole. If the sound disappears when the patient holds their breath, the sound is from a pleural, rather than pericardial friction rub.

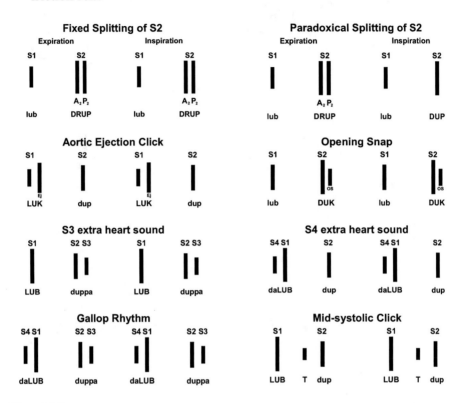

Heart Murmurs

Normally, the flow of blood through the chambers of the heart is silent. When the flow is turbulent, a soft, blowing sound may be heard on the chest wall. In children or well conditioned athletes, a forceful heart contraction can produce this turbulent sound. The increased blood volume associated with pregnancy can also cause a 'normal' murmur. However, when heart murmurs are not physiologic or 'innocent', valvular defects are the usual cause. Knowing the phase of the cardiac cycle (systolic vs. diastolic), sound pattern (regurgitant murmurs tend to fill the entire phase, while stenotic murmurs usually have start and end points within a phase), and where on the chest they are heard best, help you to diagnose which valves are producing the murmur:

- Aortic Stenosis: Mid-systolic, crescendo-decrescendo murmur heard loudest at the second right intercostal space (ICS).
- Pulmonic Stenosis: Systolic, crescendo-decrescendo murmur heard loudest at the second left ICS.

- Mitral Regurgitation: Pansystolic murmur heard loudest at the heart apex.
- Tricuspid Regurgitation: Pansystolic murmur heard loudest at the lower left sternal border.
- Mitral Stenosis: A low pitched diastolic rumble heard best at the heart apex with the patient in the left lateral position. It is almost holodiastolic, and is usually accentuated at the beginning by an opening snap after S2. Mitral stenosis affects females more than males (2:1), and almost all cases are rheumatic in origin.
- Tricuspid Stenosis: A diastolic rumble heard best at the lower left sternal border, louder with inspiration.
- Aortic Regurgitation: A high pitched decrescendo diastolic blowing sound heard best with the diaphragm at Erb's point. If you have the patient sitting, leaning forward, and breath held in exhalation, this will bring the valve closer to your stethoscope. About 2/3 of aortic regurgitation murmurs are a consequence of rheumatic heart disease, and affects males more than females (3:1).
- Pulmonic Regurgitation: The pulmonic valve is located very close to the aortic valve and will have the same timing and characteristics of the aortic regurgitation murmur.

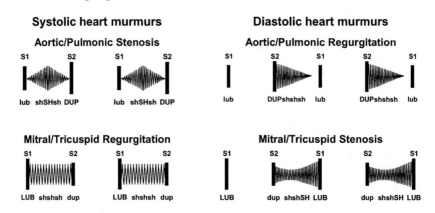

Congenital Heart Defects

Some heart defects are present at birth, and may require surgical correction:

- Patent Ductus Arteriosus (PDA): In fetal circulation there is a connection between the aorta and the left pulmonary artery. When this shunt fails to close, a continuous 'machinery' like murmur may be heard in both systole and diastole.
- Atrial Septal Defect (ASD): If the foramen ovale fails to close, a persistent connection between the atria may cause a systolic ejection murmur.

- Ventricular Septal Defect (VSD): An abnormal opening between the ventricles causes a loud holosystolic murmur.
- Tetralogy of Fallot: Ventricular septal defect combined with pulmonic stenosis, right ventricular hypertrophy and an over-riding aorta comprise the Tetralogy of Fallot. The shunting of blood away from the lungs results in a loud systolic ejection murmur and severe cyanosis.
- Coarctation of the Aorta: Constriction of the descending aorta, usually just distal to the ductus arteriosus, results in decreased circulation to the lower extremities. In a high percentage of cases, VSD (33%), PDA (66%), and aortic valve defects (75%) are also present with coarctation of the aorta. Upper extremity blood pressure readings 20 mm higher than lower extremity readings are diagnostic.

Common Cardiovascular Conditions

Arterial Hypertension (ICD: 401.9)

Elevation of systolic and/or diastolic BP, either primary or secondary. (Merck Manual, p. 1629)

- Hypertension, or increased blood pressure is very common, affecting an estimated 50 million Americans. When high blood pressure persists for an extended period of time, it in turn produces 'target organ' damage. In the United States, heart disease is the leading cause of death, and stroke the third leading cause of death.
- The clinical definition is systolic blood pressure of 140 or greater, or diastolic pressure of 90 or greater. In a small percentage of cases, hypertension has an identifiable cause, such as kidney disease. However, in 85-90% of the cases, no cause is found, and the condition is considered 'essential' hypertension.
- While the cause of hypertension is unknown, the condition is more common in individuals over age 60 and among African Americans. Other risk factors include smoking, dyslipidemia, and diabetes mellitus.
- Elevated blood pressure produces damage in multiple systems of the body, and is a direct contributing factor to conditions such as retinopathy, stroke, myocardial infarction, kidney disease, and peripheral artery disease. Therefore, physical examination should include assessment of 'target organ' structures that may suffer the effects of hypertension:
  - Fundoscopic examination for papilledema, AV nicking, hemorrhages and exudates
  - Auscultation of possible carotid artery bruits
  - Auscultation of the heart for tachycardia, murmurs, clicks, or extra heart sounds
  - Abdominal examination for renal or aortic bruits, and palpation for enlarged kidneys or a pulsatile abdominal aorta

- o Peripheral extremity examination for edema or diminished pulses
- Laboratory examination should include routine urinalysis, a CBC, and a chem profile to include electrolytes, C reactive protein, BUN, creatinine, uric acid, glucose, and lipids. An ECG to assess ventricular hypertrophy should also be performed.
- Because hypertension may be symptom free, many of these individuals are unaware that they have high blood pressure. This is why periodic monitoring of blood pressure is critical for early detection.
- Nearly 75% of individuals with hypertension are not controlling the condition. However, almost all authorities agree that unless the condition is severe, conservative non-drug measures should be the initial treatment intervention. Lifestyle and dietary measures might include:
  - o Quitting cigarette smoking is important for all forms of cardiovascular disease, including hypertension. Nicotine is a stimulant and each cigarette smoked causes a transient rise in blood pressure.
  - o Weight loss of as little as 10 pounds reduces blood pressure in overweight individuals.
  - o Excessive alcohol intake is a risk factor for hypertension, and can negate the effectiveness of antihypertensive therapy.
  - o Regular aerobic exercise is a must. Sedentary individuals have a 20-50% increased risk of hypertension.
  - o General dietary advice for management of hypertension should include a diet high in fruit and vegetables, and low in saturated animal fat.
  - o While sodium restriction is good advice for most people, it is especially important in individuals with hypertension. African Americans and diabetic patients appear to be more sensitive to salt than others. It is important to remember that three quarters of most salt intake comes from processed food, not from salt added at the table.
  - o In addition to restricting sodium, most people do better with increased potassium in the diet. Potassium is a diuretic and many studies have documented the relationship of increased blood pressure with inadequate potassium intake.
  - o Calcium and magnesium are two additional minerals with documented benefit in the management of hypertension.
  - o Relaxation therapy and biofeedback have a powerful effect on reducing the stress that can spike blood pressure. Have your patient purchase an at home blood pressure device. In addition to controlling for the 'white coat' error of hypertension measurement, the biofeedback of self monitoring actually serves to lower blood pressure.
  - o Therpeutic fasting has proven to exert a powerful effect on blood pressure reduction, often more effective than weight

loss, sodium restriction, etc. For more information read *"Medically Supervised Water-only Fasting in the Treatment of Hypertension"* (JMPT June 2001) by Alan Goldhamer, DC.

- When blood pressure is not adequately controlled by conservative measures, pharmaceutical intervention may be required to prevent the potentially life threatening complications of sustained hypertension. These drugs may include:
  - o Diuretics
  - o Beta adrenergic blockers
  - o Alpha adrenergic blockers
  - o Calcium channel blockers
  - o Angiotensin converting enzyme (ACE) inhibitors
  - o Angiotensin II receptor blockers

Coronary Artery Disease

Angina Pectoris (ICD: 413)

A clinical syndrome due to myocardial ischemia characterized by precordial discomfort or pressure, typically precipitated by exertion and relieved by rest or sublingual nitroglycerin. (Merck Manual, p. 1662)

- Angina, a brief episode of substernal chest pressure or discomfort, usually brought on by exercise, is an early sign of myocardial ischemia. It affects 5 million Americans, men more than women. Once the physical activity is stopped, angina pain usually lasts less than ten minutes. If the pain persists for more than 15-20 minutes, call 911, the individual may have had a heart attack.
- Exertional, also called stable angina, is consistently triggered by physical activity, and rapidly recedes with rest. If an atherosclerotic plaque shifts, the attacks may become more frequent, severe, and longer lasting, or occur while at rest. The condition is now referred to as 'unstable' angina.
- Physical examination is usually normal. If an ECG is run during an angina episode, ST depression and possibly T wave inversion may be seen. The individual may appear apprehensive, and display increased blood pressure and heart rate.
- Natural therapy for angina should be targeted at diminishing the atherosclerotic plaque:
  - o Diet and exercise regimens such as the Pritikin program have documented effectiveness with coronary artery disease.
  - o Carnitine enhances the ability of heart muscle to utilize oxygen.
  - o Pantethene helps to reduce triglycerides and increase HDL cholesterol levels.
  - o Coenzyme Q10 is present in every cell of your body and is especially important for cells that are oxygen deficient.
  - o Vitamin E is an antioxidant that prevents free radical damage, thought to initiate atherosclerosis.

- o Magnesium is a smooth muscle relaxant. It works much like nitroglycerin to promote vasodilation, especially important with Prinzmetal angina, that is characterized by vasospasm.
- o The herb Hawthorn (Crataegus) helps to lower blood pressure and cholesterol, and improve oxygenation of heart muscle.

Myocardial Infarction (ICD: 410)

Ischemic necrosis usually resulting from abrupt reduction in coronary blood flow to a segment of myocardium. (Merck Manual, p. 1668)

- In the progression of coronary artery disease from stable angina, to unstable angina, the next step is myocardial infarction. A larger atherosclerotic plaque has become lodged in a coronary artery and is blocking circulation to a region of myocardium. Platelet aggregation contributes to this process, which is the logic behind taking an aspirin tablet at the onset of acute chest pain.
- While most heart attack victims experience episodes of angina in the days and weeks prior to their attack, about 20% of heart attacks are 'silent', which means that their first perceived symptom is an MI. Heart disease is the leading cause of death in America. Each year almost 1 million people will experience a heart attack. Of these, about one quarter will die, many before receiving any medical help.
- The sudden onset of MI pain may occur when the patient is at rest. The pain is described as crushing substernal chest pain. The individual may hold a clenched fist against their chest when describing their pain (Levin's sign). As with angina, the pain may radiate to the neck and either shoulder. Many of these patients have previously taken nitroglycerin for angina, but with this episode, it does not relieve their pain.
- Upon examination, the individual may be pale or sweating, and experiencing nausea and shortness of breath. They may be apprehensive with an impending sense of doom. The pulse may be weak and thready. Blood pressure is variable, it may be high if there is concomitant hypertension, or it may be low if they are approaching heart failure.
- Cardiac monitoring is essential for individuals suspected of having a heart attack. An inverted T wave, ST elevation, and a deep Q wave are commonly seen with MI. Rhythm abnormalities are very common. If PVC's are seen, heart failure may be imminent. Cardiac enzymes are elevated. (What is the sequence that these enzymes peak?)
- Prevention is the key! Your guidance should be the same as for angina, but more aggressive. Intravenous EDTA chelation therapy is a safe and effective alternative to coronary bypass surgery. The American College for Advancement in Medicine (ACAM) is the organization that trains and certifies doctors to perform chelation. To find a doctor in your area who performs chelation therapy visit the website: http://www.acam.org.

Heart Failure

Congestive Heart Failure (ICD: 428.9)

Symptomatic myocardial dysfunction resulting in a characteristic pattern of hemodynamic, renal, and neurohormonal responses. (<u>Merck Manual</u>, p. 1682)

- Congestive heart failure (CHF) is a chronic condition that develops as a consequence of some underlying pathology, such as sustained hypertension, coronary artery disease, or myocardial death of heart attack. While the heart has not yet 'failed', it is a much less efficient pump. As such, blood flowing to the heart may back up, or become 'congested'.
- Either or both sides of the heart may be affected. When the left side is functioning poorly, fluid will accumulate in the lungs, causing wheezing and shortness of breath. Hypofunction of the right side of the heart leads to edema and fluid accumulation in the extremities. When fluid accumulation is marked, ascites will manifest. Right ventricular hypertrophy caused by lung disease is referred to as cor pulmonale.
- The patient may appear pale, with gray or cyanotic skin. The individual may be weak and fatigued due to decreased cardiac output, and appear anxious due to their 'air hunger'. They are usually uncomfortable laying flat, which worsens the fluid accumulation in their lungs, and need to be propped up in bed in order to sleep (orthopnea). Lung congestion may awaken them at night with paroxysmal nocturnal dyspnea (PND). The cough is productive, usually frothy pink.
- Physical examination may disclose a swollen abdomen due to ascitic fluid accumulation. Jugular venous distention (JVD) may be visible. The ankles usually show dependent, pitting edema. Upon auscultation, heart rate will be increased and an S3 gallop may be heard. Crackles and wheezing will be heard on lung auscultation. The liver and spleen may be palpably enlarged from venous congestion.
- With venous pooling and decreased cardiac output, blood pressure decreases. As the kidneys attempt to compensate for this decreased cardiac output, sodium and water are conserved, which in turn worsens the tissue edema. In addition to assessing cardiac enzymes, kidney function must be assessed (BUN, creatinine).
- On the ECG, axis deviation may be present if the CHF is caused by previous myocardial infarction. A chest x-ray will show cardiac enlargement, sometimes twice normal size. Echocardiography will document the decreased cardiac output.
- Medical treatment is symptomatic: diuretics for the fluid retention, and heart medicine to strengthen cardiac contraction.
- Natural alternative treatment should be tailored toward resolving the underlying conditions of hypertension and coronary atherosclerosis.

Hypertrophic Cardiomyopathy (ICD: 425.1)

Congenital or acquired disorders characterized by marked ventricular hypertrophy with diastolic dysfunction in the absence of an afterload demand (eg, valvular aortic stenosis, coarctation of the aorta, systemic hypertension). (Merck Manual, p. 1697)

- Hypertrophic cardiomyopathy (HCM) is an abnormal thickening of the heart myocardium. About one-half of the cases are genetically inherited. With acquired forms of HCM, the cause of left ventricular hypertrophy (LVH) is undetermined.
- You have probably seen stories in the news where a seemingly healthy young person dies suddenly during strenuous exercise, such as when 23 year old basketball star Hank Gathers died suddenly in 1990. Many of these individuals probably suffer from the congenital form of HCM. When warning symptoms are experienced, the most common symptom is shortness of breath, followed by angina type chest pain. The individual may experience associated symptoms of dizziness, 'graying out', or fainting. Whereas nitroglycerin usually relieves angina, it may actually aggravate hypertrophic cardiomyopathy.
- Upon examination, the ECG will show a left axis deviation typical of left ventricular hypertrophy. Because the cardiac muscle hypertrophies inward, a chest x-ray is unlikely to disclose cardiac enlargement. Echocardiography will show the characteristic encroachment of the left ventricular chamber. (Merck Manual, p. 1695)
- The condition appears to worsen during puberty. HCM is a chronic condition that has no cure. Symptomatically, heart medications are used to slow the heart rate, which prolongs the period of diastolic filling. Of primary importance is to counsel the individual to avoid strenuous or competitive sports. About 4% of individuals with the condition die each year. The poorest prognosis is with individuals that manifest symptoms at a young age.

Heart Palpitations (ICD: 785.1)

Palpitations are the perception of heart action by the patient. (Merck Manual, p. 1603)

- We are usually not aware of our heart beating. During strenuous exercise or times of stress our heartbeat becomes more noticeable. If there is increased awareness of an irregular, skipped, or rapid heartbeat, while at rest, this is referred to as palpitations.
- Most palpitations are harmless, the consequence of anxiety, too much alcohol or coffee, or a lack of sleep. If anxiety and nervousness are the predominant complaints, thyroid function should be checked.
- When palpitations are accompanied by chest pain, light-headedness, fainting or shortness of breath, there may be more serious underlying pathology. Cardiac rhythm defects will usually <u>not</u> appear on a

standard ECG, which runs for just two minutes. Twenty four hour Holter monitoring is required to locate the source of the defect.

- Arrhythmias may be atrial or ventricular in origin. In general, atrial rhythm defects are not life threatening. However, while usually life threatening, atrial rhythm defects can predispose to clot formation. It is estimated that 15% of strokes are caused by atrial fibrillation. Ventricular rhythm defects, such as premature ventricular contractions (PVC's) often are life threatening.

Valvular Heart Disease (Merck Manual, p. 1753-1763) (ICD: 396)

- The heart ventricles have valves that allow blood to enter from the atria, and valves where blood exits to the aorta and pulmonary artery. Congenital defects, aging, or infections may cause valvular defects. When the valves do not open fully, they are stenotic, and may cause a back up of blood typical of congestive heart failure. If the valves do not close fully, the valves are incompetent, which causes regurgitation of blood in a direction opposite the normal flow, also known as insufficiency.
- Normally, the flow of blood through the chambers of the heart is silent. Valvular defects cause a turbulence in this laminar flow, causing murmurs. Knowing the phase of the cardiac cycle (systolic vs. diastolic), sound pattern (regurgitant murmurs tend to fill the entire phase, while stenotic murmurs usually have start and end points within a phase), and where on the chest they are heard best, help you to diagnose which valves are producing the murmur.
- Some heart murmurs are 'innocent' or functional. These murmurs are generally mid systolic and barely audible. If the patient is experiencing symptoms, such as fatigue, palpitations, dyspnea on exertion (DOE), dizziness, or fainting, the murmur is most likely pathologic.
- Damaged heart valves are at risk for infection, and may require antibiotics after dental care in order to prevent endocarditis. Most valvular heart defects do not require treatment. However, when the impairment of blood flow becomes severe, surgery to repair or replace the damaged valve may be necessary.
- Valvular heart defects, especially mitral valve prolapse, have been shown to improve with magnesium and CoQ10 supplementation.

Mitral Valve Prolapse (ICD: 424.0)

A bulging of one or both mitral valve leaflets into the left atrium during systole, commonly producing a crisp systolic sound or click and a delayed or late systolic mitral regurgitation murmur. (Merck Manual, p. 1753)

- Mitral valve prolapse (MVP) is one of the most common cardiac problems, affecting approximately 5-25% of the general population. The condition affects females more than males. Quite often the condition is initially discovered in young thin individuals. It is also associated with pectus excavatum and kyphoscoliosis.

- Quite often the condition is asymptomatic, and is only discovered on a routine physical examination. When the condition becomes symptomatic, the patient may experience chest pain, palpitations, fatigue, and shortness of breath. If the condition is pronounced, and the heart has to work harder to compensate for retrograde flow of blood, cardiac enlargement may eventually result.
- When the chordae tendinea are too long, the valve leaflets balloon up or prolapse into the left atrium. This produces a short high pitched mid-systolic click that is heard best at the apex of the heart. If there is also backflow or regurgitation past the mitral valve, a murmur will result. As such, this condition is also referred to as a click-murmur syndrome and floppy valve syndrome.
- Definitive diagnosis requires echocardiography, which allows visualization of the protruding mitral valve leaflets. While chest x-rays are not specifically indicated, a routine film may disclose an elongated heart silhouette with a narrow AP diameter.
- When mitral regurgitation becomes severe, surgical repair may be needed. Because bacterial endocarditis is 4-5 times more common in patients with MVP, prophylactic antibiotics may be recommended prior to dental surgery.
- The condition is made worse when blood volume is low. As such, both caffeine and alcohol, which are diuretics, should be avoided. Magnesium and CoQ10 have documented symptomatic benefit with MVP patients.
- Dysautonomia refers to an imbalance between the sympathetic and parasympathetic nervous system. Mitral valve prolapse has a known association with dysautonomia. Do you think chiropractic adjustments might benefit MVP?

Pericarditis (ICD: 420)

Inflammation of the pericardium, which may be acute or chronic and may result in pericardial effusion. (Merck Manual, p. 1768)

- An acute inflammation of the pericardial sac may occur from a variety of infective organisms, such as streptococcus or coxsackievirus. However, autoimmune inflammatory disorders, such as RA and lupus may also cause pericarditis. Pericarditis also occurs in 10-15% of individuals who have had a heart attack (Dressler's syndrome).
- If the fluid accumulates more quickly than can be absorbed by the body, a life threatening condition known as cardiac tamponade may develop. Cardiac tamponade interferes with the filling of the heart during diastole, and will probably result in diminished blood pressure and pulse during inspiration, known as pulsus paradoxus.
- When the individual has epigastric prominence due to marked pericardial effusion, this is referred to as Auenbrugger's sign.
- Upon examination, the individual will likely appear anxious and their breath will be shallow as a consequence of the pain. Their substernal

chest pain varies from dull to sharp, and from mild to severe. It is worse with motion and laying down, and better with sitting up and leaning forward. By contrast, the pain from an MI is <u>not</u> aggravated by thoracic motion.

- Fever and tachycardia will likely be present. A pericardial friction rub is heard about 60-70% of the time. The CBC and sed rate will show signs of inflammation. A chest x-ray may show effusion with an increased size of the heart shadow. The ECG shows ST elevation, as an MI does, but with no pathologic Q waves.
- Medical treatment will include supportive care, and antibiotics if there is a bacterial infection. When fluid accumulation is marked, emergency pericardiocentesis will be required.

Aortic Dissection (ICD: 441)

A tear in the aortic intima through which blood surges into the aortic wall, stripping the media from the adventitia. (Merck Manual, p. 1779)

- <u>A dissecting aortic aneurysm is an acute surgical emergency.</u> The condition may occur in individuals with Marfan's syndrome, an inherited disorder characterized by loss of normal connective tissue elasticity. A tear within the wall of the aorta may allow the formation of a false channel. Under pressure the aorta may rupture.
- The predominant symptom is immediate excruciating pain at the anterior chest or between the shoulder blades. According to William Osler, *"spontaneous tear of the arterial coats is associated with atrocious pain."* The patient may describe their pain as *"being torn in half"*. The intensity of the pain is maximal at the onset, whereas conditions such as MI, pulmonary embolism, and pneumothorax will have increasing pain as the condition worsens. Upon examination, hypertension is probable, and about two thirds of patients will have peripheral pulse deficits. If blood is leaking from the aorta, left pleural effusion may occur. If this fluid leaks into the pericardial space, cardiac tamponade may result.
- The ECG will be normal, unless the dissection has also caused a heart attack. Cardiac enzymes will also be normal, with the possible exception of LDH, which is liberated with tissue damage anywhere in the body. A plain chest film may demonstrate a wide mediastinum, however a CT or MRI will probably be ordered.
- It is important that this condition is not misdiagnosed as an MI, because thrombolytic therapy is contraindicated. The mortality rate for surgical repair of aortic dissection is about 15%.

Study Guide Objectives

o Know the normal anatomy of the heart.
o Know the position of the heart valves during each phase of the cardiac cycle.
o Know the characteristics and factors that affect the intensity of the S1 heart sound.

- Know the characteristics and factors that affect the intensity of the S2 heart sound.
- Know the locations where individual heart valves are heard most loudly.
- What causes the apparent reversal of where the aortic and pulmonic sounds are heart?
- Know which heart valve defects cause systolic murmurs.
- Know which heart valve defects cause diastolic murmurs.
- Know what causes physiological splitting of S2.
- Know the basics of what creates the various components on the ECG tracing.
- How do streptococcal infections relate to cardiac function?
- Know the appropriate history questions for a cardiovascular exam.
- What is Levine's sign?
- What are the associated symptoms of cardiac dysfunction?
- Chest pain that is relieved by laying down suggests what condition?
- What causes paroxysmal nocturnal dyspnea?
- Why does congestive heart failure cause nocturia?
- Know the risk factors associated with coronary heart disease.
- What is the significance of jugular venous distention?
- What is the cause of a cardiac thrill?
- What is the significance of a laterally displaced PMI?
- Why is percussion not part of the routine cardiac examination?
- Why do we 'inch' the stethoscope during cardiac auscultation?
- Which part of the stethoscope is most useful during routine cardiac auscultation: the bell or the diaphragm?
- Why would you listen to the heart with the patient in the left lateral decubitus position?
- How would you accentuate the sound of an aortic or pulmonic valve murmur?
- Why should the patient hold their breath during auscultation of the carotid arteries?
- What is the threshold for tachycardia and bradycardia?
- What is sinus arrythmia?
- Which is more serious: atrial or ventricular rhythm defects?
- What is the significance of premature ventricular contractions?
- What does a mid-systolic click signify during cardiac auscultation?
- How do you distinguish a pericardial from a pleural friction rub?
- What are the components of Tetralogy of Fallot?
- What is 'essential' hypertension?
- What are the 'target organs' that are damaged by sustained hypertension?
- What are the dietary and lifestyle measures recommended in the management of hypertension?
- What are the clinical differences between angina and myocardial infarction?
- What are some of the main ECG findings seen with myocardial infarction?

- What are the clinical differences between left sided vs. right sided heart failure?
- Right ventricular hypertrophy caused by lung disease is referred to as _____.
- What are the early warning symptoms of hypertrophic cardiomyopathy?
- What is the age range typical of hypertrophic cardiomyopathy?
- Which diagnostic test is used to assess the severity of cardiac rhythm defects?
- In which phase of the cardiac cycle are 'innocent' heart murmurs most likely: systolic or diastolic?
- Definitive diagnosis of mitral valve prolapse requires _____.
- Which nutrients have documented benefit for mitral valve prolapse?
- What is dysautonomia?
- Which body position worsens the pain of pericarditis?
- What inherited condition is associated with aortic dissection?
- Which cardiac condition is associated with immediate excruciating pain that is at maximum intensity at the onset?
- Why is it important that aortic dissection not be misdiagnosed as myocardial infarction?

10 – Breast & Axilla

Anatomy & Physiology

The female breast is an accessory reproductive organ, comprised of glandular tissue that produces milk for newborn babies. While breast tissue in males is rudimentary, about 1% of all breast cancer is found in males.

The breasts lie over the anterior chest wall musculature, extending from about the 2nd rib superiorly to the 6th rib inferiorly, and from the lateral edge of the sternum medially to the mid axillary line laterally. We often describe breast anatomy in terms of quadrants. The upper outer quadrant contains the tail of Spence which extends into the axilla. The glandular tissue of the breast converges at the nipple. Surrounding the nipple is the areola which contains small raised sebaceous glands, also called Montgomery's tubercles.

The internal glandular tissue of the breast is comprised of 15 to 20 lobes, which drain into lactiferous ducts. The milk is stored in the lactiferous sinus, until it exits the nipple during nursing. The weight of the breast is supported by Cooper's suspensory ligaments that attach to the chest wall. When cancer is present, contraction of these ligaments may produce dimpling. Surrounding and overlying the glandular tissue, adipose tissue comprises most of the bulk of the breast.

An extensive network of lymphatic ducts drains the breast. About three quarters of the drainage is to the axillary lymph nodes near the tail of Spence. The axillary lymph region can be visualized as a pyramid with four sides meeting at the apex: lateral brachial nodes, posterior subscapular nodes, midaxillary central nodes, and anterior pectoral nodes. A lesser amount of drainage occurs via the supraclavicular, infraclavicular, and internal mammary lymph nodes.

During adolescence, hormonal changes stimulate breast maturation. Breast development typically begins around age ten, but it may begin as early as eight, or as late as thirteen years of age. Tanner described five stages of sexual maturation. When these stages occur earlier or later than expected, it _may_ suggest hormonal hypo or hyperfunction.

During pregnancy, hormonal changes initiate growth of breast tissue during the second month after conception. As the breasts enlarge, they may become more nodular. The nipples enlarge and become more erectile. As breast tissue expands, the areola also enlarges and becomes darker in color. Mongomery's tubercles hypertrophy and become more prominent. As vascular circulation increases, a blue network of mammary veins may become visible underneath the skin. Later in the pregnancy, the breast may begin secreting colostrum, a precursor to breast milk that contains protein and lactose, but not the fat found in breast milk.

With menopause, the glandular and adipose tissue atrophies, resulting in decreased size and elasticity of breast tissue.

Nature of the Patient

Fibroadenoma is a condition primarily of young women in their late teens or twenties. The incidence of benign fibrocystic breast disease increases with age and is most common between age 30-50, and is rare after menopause. Breast cancer is rare under age 30. Two thirds of all breast cancer occurs after age 50.

Key History Questions

Do you have any pain or tenderness in your breasts or underarm area?

- Is there a known cause? Trauma or a poorly fitting bra can cause breast pain.
- Is the pain localized to a single spot or does it cover the entire breast? Most benign breast lesions are painless. Some degree of premenstrual breast tenderness is common and may be more pronounced in women taking birth control pills (BCP). Unilateral breast pain may be caused by inflammation or infection. Bilateral pain and tenderness suggests benign breast disease, also known as fibrocystic breast disease.

Have you noticed a lump or thickening in your breasts or underarm area?

- How long have you had this lump? Glandular breast tissue has a certain degree of nodularity or lumpiness. If this has been present for years, it may represent what is 'normal' for her. However, this highlights the importance of breast self examination (BSE). A new change in the pattern of nodularity or lumpiness is cause for concern.
- Swollen axillary lymph nodes may indicate infection (mastitis) or carcinoma in breast tissue, both of which require prompt referral. While most chiropractors do not perform breast examinations on their patients, the addition of axillary lymph node palpation to your routine physical examination is recommended.

Have you had any discharge from the nipple?

- Bloody discharge is unlikely to be benign. Unilateral bloody discharge suggests carcinoma or Paget's disease of the breast (carcinoma of the mammary ducts).
- Unilateral non-bloody discharge with a palpable breast mass suggests an abscess or early carcinoma.
- If the discharge is milky and bilateral, order a serum prolactin. If prolactin is high, a pituitary tumor is possible.

Do you have any rash on the breast or underarm area?

- Paget's intraductal carcinoma starts with a rash at the nipple and areola. Eczema or contact dermatitis are benign causes of a breast rash, but rarely start at the nipple.
- A rash in the underarm area may be a contact dermatitis reaction to underarm deodorant.

Do you experience swelling of your breasts?

- Unilateral breast swelling with associated tenderness is most likely due to infection, such as an abscess, or mastitis. The presence of an associated fever increases the likelihood of an infection.
- Bilateral breast swelling prior to menses is most likely benign, due to fibrocystic changes.
- Non-tender breast swelling may be cystic or carcinoma. Transillumination may help to differentiate these conditions.

What is your menstrual history?

- The following factors often supply valuable clues to hormonal imbalance:
    o Age at menarche
    o Age at menopause
    o Length of menstrual cycle
    o Duration and amount of menstrual flow
    o Premenstrual breast symptoms
- When was your last menstrual period? Bilateral breast pain with a missed period points to pregnancy.

Do you have a personal or family history of breast cancer?

- A mother or sister with breast cancer constitutes a high risk factor.

Have you had previous breast surgery or biopsies?

- You need to be aware of previous needle biopsies, mastectomy, or breast augmentation surgery.

Do you perform monthly breast self-examination (BSE)?

- Early detection of breast tumors while the tumor is still small, via BSE and mammography, reduces cancer mortality. While mammography can detect tumors too small to be palpated, it does not detect all palpable lumps, or lumps that develop since the last mammogram. This is why we must stress the importance of monthly BSE to our female patients. Instructions you can give your patient on how to perform breast self examination can be found in many places, such as the American Cancer Society website: http://www.cancer.org.

Examination

Always respect your patient's modesty, and expose the breasts only as needed during the examination. As you perform the exam, explain what you are checking for. This will help teach what she should be checking during breast self examination, and help dissipate some of her nervousness during this sensitive exam.

Breast examination begins with inspection. This is performed with the arms in several positions. With the patient seated and the arms resting comfortably in the lap, observe the overall symmetry of breast contour. It is not uncommon for one breast to be larger than the other, more typically the left breast. Observe the skin for evidence of dimpling or retraction. Note any areas of swelling or discoloration. The skin should be smooth and free of peau d'orange texture. The nipples should be symmetrically positioned and not deviated or pointing in different directions. Note any bleeding, ulceration, or discharge at the nipple. Nipple inversion may be a normal variant. It is important to determine if this has been present for many years or is a recent change. Occasionally you will observe supernumerary nipples visible along the track of the 'milk line'.

We next have the patient perform three maneuvers to provide further visualization of breast retraction:

- Arms raised overhead
- Arms pressed downward on hips, or hands pressed together. Both of these maneuvers help to contract the pectoralis muscles.
- Leaning forward with hands on knees, or arms supported by the doctor. This position is primarily for women with larger, more pendulous breasts.

During each of these three positions observe for any dimpling, skin retraction, or fixation of breast tissue to the chest wall. After breast inspection, have the woman replace her gown. Next, perform axillary lymph node palpation. When examining the left axilla, use the fingers of your right hand to palpate. To relax the muscles, lift the elbow with your opposite hand. Using a light circular motion, press the lymph nodes against the underlying tissue to assess that the nodes are: small, movable, soft, and nontender. Abnormal lymph nodes may be: enlarged, fixed, hard, or painful. Assess all four quadrants of the axillary 'pyramid', and repeat the procedure for the other axilla.

Breast palpation is best performed with the patient in the supine position. Have the patient remove one arm from the gown, leaving the opposite breast covered. Place a small pillow or rolled up towel under the shoulder blade, and have the patient position her arm resting above her head. Both of these maneuvers help to flatten the breast tissue against the chest wall. You may choose either of three methods: circular (spiral), wedge, or vertical strip method. The important thing is to be consistent and thorough, and not miss any tissue.

With the spiral method, you may begin at the nipple and work in increasingly larger circles to the tail of Spence, or you may begin at the tail of Spence and palpate in a spiral pattern toward the nipple. Approximately one half of all breast cancer is found in the upper outer quadrant. For this reason, your palpation of this quadrant and the tail of Spence must be thorough. If a woman has large, pendulous breasts, you may find it helpful to use a bimanual technique, using one hand to support the breast and your dominant hand to palpate. Finally, using your thumb and forefinger, gently compress the areola toward the nipple, checking for discharge.

If any breast lesions are palpated, the breast mass must be described in terms of:

- Location: Using a clock position, describe how many centimeters from the nipple.
- Size: Height, width, and thickness in centimeters.
- Shape: Round, oval, regular or irregular.
- Consistency: Soft, firm, hard.
- Movable: Movable or fixed to chest wall.
- Borders: Well circumscribed?
- Tenderness: Tender upon palpation?

Sample Documentation

The left breast was slightly larger than the right breast, otherwise they were symmetrical at rest and with motion. No rashes or lesions were visualized. The contour was smooth, without dimpling or retraction. The nipples were everted and without discharge. Upon palpation, the breast tissue was firm and homogenous. No masses or palpable tenderness was elicited. No palpable lymph nodes were found in the supraclavicular, infraclavicular, or axillary regions.

Diagnostic Studies

- Breast ultrasound is a less invasive way to distinguish cystic from solid breast lumps.
- Breast mammography should be performed on all palpable breast lumps, as well as an annual screening procedure for women at high risk for breast cancer.
- Fine needle biopsy should be performed on all suspicious breast lumps.
- Serum chemistry examination may include:
  o Beta hCG pregnancy test
- Tumor markers
  o CA 15-3, CA 27.29, & CEA (breast carcinoma)
- When carcinoma is found, a CT, MRI, or bone scan may be performed to investigate possible metastasis.
- CT or MRI of the head, if a prolactin secreting pituitary adenoma is suspected.

Abnormal Findings

- Dimpling of breast tissue: Fibrosis, probably caused by cancer, pulls on the suspensory ligaments of the breast. This may cause tissue retraction and a shallow dimple. Skin dimpling may be more noticeable on palpation of breast tissue, which highlights the importance of observation, in addition to what you feel, during palpation.

- Nipple retraction and deviation: Nipple 'inversion', if it has been present for years and is not fibrotic, may be normal for her. However, a recent retraction or deviation of the nipple may represent fibrotic pulling from an underlying tumor.

- Fixation of breast to chest wall: This is observed when your patient leans forward. If one breast fails to move with this maneuver, there may be an underlying fibrosis that is fixing the breast tissue to the chest wall.

- 'Orange Peel' skin texture: Carcinoma can block the lymphatic drainage of the breast and cause edema. This edema results in a characteristic 'peau d'orange' texture, where the hair follicles are more prominent. It tends to occur more at the lower portion of the breast.

- Paget's Intraductal Carcinoma: This condition appears as a dry, red, scaling of the tissue surrounding the nipple, which may appear similar to eczema. However, unlike eczema, intraductal carcinoma is usually unilateral. Unless there is a known cause, such as with breast feeding, any dermatitis of the nipple is cause for concern.

- Plugged milk duct: When a woman is breast feeding her baby, it is not uncommon for a milk duct to become clogged. The condition usually resolves spontaneously, although manually expressing any remaining milk to fully empty the breast may help.

- Mastitis and abscess: Nursing mothers can develop an infection within the breast. Other signs such as fever, flu like symptoms, and an increased WBC count may be present. Medical treatment with an antibiotic is indicated. Untreated mastitis can lead to the formation of a pus pocket within the breast, or breast abscess. At this point, surgical incision and drainage may be necessary.

- Galactorrhea: A milky discharge not associated with pregnancy is cause for concern, and may be from a prolactin secreting pituitary tumor.

- Gynecomastia: Transient mild gynecomastia can occur in boys due to the hormonal changes at puberty. In the elderly, decreased testosterone levels may also produce breast enlargement.

- Breast carcinoma in males: Approximately 1-2% of breast cancer occurs in males. Because of the lack of breast tissue to obscure the mass, these tumors are usually detected early. Most of these tumors are directly under the nipple. As such, a routine male physical examination should check for nipple retraction and mobility. The examination takes only a few seconds and is a valuable preventive health screening measure. You might say to your patient, "*While breast cancer in males is not common, about 1-2% of all breast cancers occur in men, so it is important make sure there is no tissue hardening in this part of your chest.*"

Common Breast Conditions

Fibroadenoma (Merck Manual, p. 1974)

- Fibroadenoma is the most common benign tumor of the breast. It usually occurs during the early years of menstruation and becomes much less common after age 30. While the cause of these breast lumps is not known, a high fat diet is thought to play a role.
- These lumps are not tender and may not be noticed until discovered with breast self examination or during an annual checkup.
- Upon examination, fibroadenoma palpates as a single firm well defined mass that is freely mobile. It may feel like a "small slippery marble". The lump does not produce dimpling or breast retraction signs. In contrast to fibrocystic breast disease, the lump does not vary with the menstrual cycle. The lump is usually single and unilateral, however about 25% of the time the condition is bilateral.
- While a trained physician can usually feel that this lump is non-cancerous, a breast biopsy will still be performed. While a fibroadenoma is not thought to be precancerous, surgical removal of the lump may be advised.

Fibrocystic Breast Disease (Merck Manual, p. 1973)

- Fibrocystic breast disease is also known as benign breast disease. The condition is very common, affecting an estimated 60% of women during their lifetime.
- While the exact cause is not known, the symptoms are worse premenstrually, therefore hormonal fluctuations are thought to play a part in this condition. An alteration of the estrogen to progesterone ratio during the luteal phase of the menstrual cycle causes hyperplasia of the epithelial lining of the mammary ducts and cyst formation.
- While the condition may be asymptomatic, it usually causes bilateral breast tenderness one to two days prior to the onset of menses. The breasts may be engorged and swollen with cystic fluid accumulation.
- Upon examination, multiple soft round fluctuant masses are palpated which are freely movable. Occasionally a breast discharge will manifest, which should be sent for cytology.
- Medical management may involve needle aspiration to verify that the palpated mass is cystic, with laboratory evaluation of the aspirated fluid. A similar low tech method is transillumination of the cystic mass.
- While fibrocystic breast disease is not thought to increase the risk of breast cancer, the lumpiness that is present may complicate the early detection of breast cancer.

- Benign breast disease is best managed with conservative measures. Fibrocystic breasts are thought to be more sensitive to adrenergic hormones. As such stress reduction and restriction of methylxanthines (caffeine and chocolate) may help with reduction of symptoms. Vitamins E and B6 seem to help normalize hormonal fluctuations. Thyroid function should be investigated.

Breast Cancer (Merck Manual, p. 1974)

- Breast cancer is the second most common cause of cancer death in women (lung cancer is #1 in both sexes). About one in eight women will develop breast cancer during their life, and one half of these women will die from the disease. The risk for breast cancer continues to increase after age 30, with 60 being the average age at diagnosis.
- Several factors are considered to be 'high risk' factors for breast cancer: a personal history of previous breast cancer, atypical hyperplasia noted on previous breast biopsies, and a first degree relative (mother or sister) with breast cancer. Other factors such as early menarche, late menopause, nulliparity, obesity, or a second degree relative (aunt or grandmother) with breast cancer are considered to be 'moderate' risk factors. However, these guidelines should not be given undue importance. About 70% of breast cancer occurs in women with no risk factors other than being over age 50.
- About 9 out of 10 breast lumps are noticed first by the woman herself, which stresses the importance of breast self examination (BSE). The majority of these lumps turn out to be benign, however certain signs are cause for concern:
  - o Recent onset of breast pain
  - o An unusual increase in the size of one breast
  - o Dimpling of breast tissue
  - o Nipple retraction
  - o Nipple discharge, rash, or ulceration
  - o An 'orange peel' texture to an area of the breast
  - o A lump or swelling in the underarm area
- Upon examination, the physician should inspect for asymmetry of contour, and dimpling, puckering, or other signs of retraction. Have the patient perform several maneuvers which will provide further visualization of possible breast retraction:
  - o Arms raised overhead
  - o Arms pressed downward on hips, or hands pressed together, which help to contract the pectoralis muscles
  - o Leaning forward with hands on knees, or arms supported by the doctor (this position is primarily for women with larger, more pendulous breasts)
- With the patient in the seated position, palpate the axillary, supraclavicular, and infraclavicular lymph node areas.
- With the patient in the supine position, palpate the entire breast, with special attention to the upper, outer quadrant.

- Any questionable lump should be investigated with a mammogram, and possibly a fine needle biopsy. The American Cancer Society recommends a baseline mammogram at age 40, every one to two years between age 40-49, and annual mammography after age 50.
- Prevention is the key with cancer:
  o Don't smoke and limit your use of alcohol
  o Exercise regularly and maintain a healthy body weight. A recent study in the <u>Archives of Internal Medicine</u> (Oct 25, 1999;159:19:2290-6) showed that exercising 7 hours or more per week may decrease a woman's risk of developing breast cancer by nearly 20%.
  o Eat a healthy diet which is low in fat and high in phytoestrogens
  o Perform monthly breast self examination (BSE)
  o While all x-rays cause some genetic damage, mammography is a relatively low dose of radiation, and can detect tumors that are much smaller than can be felt by palpation
- CA 15-3, CA 27.29, and CEA are tumor markers that many preventive minded physicians perform as a screen for women wishing an early warning of breast cancer tendency. This however is controversial, as orthodox medicine does not consider tumor markers suitable for detection of cancer. Rather they are intended to monitor the status of previously diagnosed cancer.

It is important to be aware of the differences between the three types of breast masses. Some of the highlights are:

- Benign fibrocystic breast disease is very common, affecting 50% of all women to some degree. It presents as bilateral breast tenderness, usually with increased tenderness prior to the menstrual period. Fibroadenoma is usually not tender. While the conventional wisdom is that breast cancer is a painless condition, the presence of tenderness does not rule out malignancy. Newer research suggests that about one-quarter of palpable breast cancer is associated with pain or tenderness.
- The palpable mass of carcinoma is usually irregular, hard, and fixed, with poorly defined margins. Fibroadenoma and benign breast disease palpate as round, rubbery, and mobile, with well defined margins. The nodularity of fibrocystic breast disease may make it more difficult to palpate carcinoma changes.
- Carcinoma causes retraction signs, dimpling, and nipple retraction or deviation. Fibroadenoma and benign breast disease do not.

Study Guide Objectives

o Know normal breast anatomy.
o What are Montgomery's tubercles?
o What are the breast changes that are normal with pregnancy?

- What is colostrum?
- Know the age ranges typical for fibroadenoma, fibrocystic breast disease, and breast cancer.
- Know the appropriate history questions for a breast exam.
- Know which breast conditions manifest bilaterally vs. unilaterally.
- What is the significance of a bloody discharge from the breast nipple?
- When should you order a serum prolactin test?
- What is the significance of a rash at the nipple and areola?
- Why is it important for a woman to perform monthly breast self examination even if she is receiving periodic mammograms?
- Know the components of the breast exam.
- What are the three maneuvers a woman should perform during the inspection phase of the breast examination?
- What is the purpose of these three maneuvers?
- What is the optimum patient position for breast palpation?
- What are the three methods of breast palpation?
- Know the items to document when describing a breast mass.
- What causes retraction signs in breast contour?
- What is the difference between nipple inversion and nipple retraction?
- What causes 'peau d'orange' skin texture?
- What is the significance of a milky breast discharge not associated with pregnancy?
- What causes gynecomastia?
- Approximately what percentage of breast cancer occurs in males?
- Know the pathologic changes that occur the various breast conditions discussed.
- Know the palpation findings present with fibroadenoma, fibrocystic breast disease, and breast cancer.
- During which phase of the menstrual cycle is fibrocystic breast disease most likely to be symptomatic?
- Know the risk factors for breast disease.
- What is the most significant risk factor present in women who develop breast cancer?
- Approximately what percentage of breast lumps are discovered by the woman herself (rather than by the physician)?
- Know the signs of concern that a woman may notice during her monthly breast self examination.
- Which breast quadrant is most at risk for breast cancer?

11 – Abdomen & GI disorders

Anatomy & Physiology

The abdominal cavity is bounded superiorly by the muscular diaphragm and inferiorly by the pelvis. The spinal column and paravertebral musculature form the posterior margin and the external abdominal musculature form the lateral and anterior margins of the abdomen. The visceral organs within the abdominal cavity are 'hollow' organs (stomach, gallbladder, small intestine, large intestine, and bladder) or 'solid' organs (liver, spleen, pancreas, kidneys, adrenal glands, uterus, and ovaries). As an interesting aside, Chinese acupuncture considers the hollow organs to have *Yang* characteristics and solid organs to have *Yin* characteristics.

For ease of description, imaginary vertical and horizontal lines are drawn through the umbilicus to divide the abdomen into four quadrants. A less intuitive mapping method divides the abdomen into nine regions. However, when describing pathology that is found on the midline, it is helpful to use three of these regional descriptors: epigastric, periumbilical, and suprapubic.

Visceral pain is often poorly localized. The patient may only be able to specify a regional quadrant for their pain. Your knowledge of anatomy helps you to visualize the structures contained in that quadrant that might be the source of their pain:

Right Upper Quadrant (RUQ)
Liver
Gallbladder
Duodenum
Head of the pancreas
Right kidney and adrenal gland
Hepatic flexure of the colon
Ascending and transverse colon

Left Upper Quadrant (LUQ)
Stomach
Spleen
Left lobe of liver
Body of pancreas
Left kidney and adrenal gland
Splenic flexure of the colon
Transverse and descending colon

Right Lower Quadrant (RLQ)
Appendix
Cecum
Right ovary and fallopian tube
Right ureter
Right spermatic cord

Left Lower Quadrant (LLQ)
Part of descending colon
Sigmoid colon
Left ovary and fallopian tube
Left ureter
Left spermatic cord

Midline
Aorta
Uterus
Bladder

Nature of the Patient

As with heart and lung complaints, many gastrointestinal conditions are the consequence of chronic degenerative changes. As such, diverticulitis, acute abdominal aneurysm, and carcinoma are much less likely in a young person. Appendicitis, while it can occur at any age, is most likely in teenage males. Cholecystitis is most likely in middle aged females. Peptic ulcer affects both sexes and all ages, but is most common in middle aged males. While gallstones can lead to pancreas dysfunction, most patients with pancreatitis have a history of chronic alcohol ingestion.

Key History Questions

Do you have a loss of appetite?

- Some gastrointestinal conditions, such as pancreatic and liver cancer manifest first as anorexia. Unexplained weight loss is a 'red flag' danger signal. Appetite is often lost with acute febrile conditions such as flu. Chronic alcohol ingestion also suppresses appetite and results in poor dietary choices.

Do you have difficulty swallowing?

- Dysphagia points to esophageal disorders such as reflux esophagitis, esophageal stricture or spasm, and possibly carcinoma.

Do you have difficulty with certain foods? What symptoms do you experience when you eat them?

- Heartburn after meals suggests peptic ulcer or gastroesophageal reflux disease (GERD).
- Lactose intolerance is common, affecting 30-50 million Americans. Approximately 75% of Blacks and 90% of Asians lack the lactase enzyme needed to digest milk sugar. Symptoms may include gas, bloating and diarrhea within a few hours of eating foods containing lactose. As we age, digestive efficiency decreases, and many people benefit from switching to lactose reduced milk or cultured milk products and cheese, which are naturally low in lactose.
- Food intolerance is far more common than suspected, and can result in a wide range of symptoms. Many clinical ecologists maintain that the majority of undiagnosed disease is due to food intolerance.

Do you have any abdominal pain?

- Literally dozens of conditions cause abdominal pain. Many of them are serious, requiring immediate referral. The answers from your chief complaint history help narrow the possibilities:
  - *Where is your pain?* While visceral abdominal pain may be hard to localize, your patient can usually point to a specific quadrant. Visualize the anatomy and structures contained in that region.

o *Does your pain radiate from that point?* Referral patterns may be helpful, for example the pain of a kidney stone typically radiates to the flank, groin, and in the case of males, the testicles. However, don't be fooled into expecting every case to be typical. For example, gallstone pain may or may not radiate to the right scapula.

o *When did you first notice this pain?* Acute onset points to acute inflammation, such as from appendicitis or gastroenteritis (food poisoning). However, acute pain may also be the result of exacerbation of a chronic subclinical condition, such as diverticulitis or gall bladder dysfunction. Chronic recurrent abdominal pain indicates pathogenesis that develops over time, such as peptic ulcer, renal calculus, or inflammatory bowel disease.

o *Is your pain getting better or worse?* Acute abdominal pain that is worsening warrants a surgical consult, unless a benign cause, such as food poisoning, is easily discernible.

o *Does your pain have any relationship to meals?* Chronology and timing of pain provides valuable clues about where along the gastrointestinal tract the pain originates. Pain that begins soon after eating, or possibly just before meals, suggests gastric ulcer. When pain develops two to three hours after eating, allowing time for the food to pass from the stomach to the small intestine, duodenal ulcer may be the cause. Cholecystitis pain typically awakens the individual at night with a gnawing RUQ pain, after eating a high fat meal three to five hours earlier.

o *What is the quality of your pain?* Intermittent, crampy pain suggests obstruction of a viscus, such as with intestinal blockage or a kidney stone. Viscus pain is related to peristalsis, and the individual may be writhing from the pain. Peritoneal irritation, such as with appendicitis, pancreatitis, diverticulitis, or a ruptured ectopic pregnancy causes diffuse constant pain. This individual avoids any motion, which worsens their pain. Peptic ulcer pain is frequently described as burning or gnawing.

o *How severe is your pain?* A rigid, 'board like' abdomen with severe pain may indicate an 'acute abdomen', a general term for acute surgical emergencies.

o *What makes your pain better and worse?* Duodenal ulcers may manifest as pain that is relieved by meals, whereas eating may provoke rather than relieve gastric ulcer pain. The individual may experience temporary relief from antacids with both conditions. Gallbladder pain usually manifests after eating high fat foods. Abdominal pain that decreases following a bowel movement suggests disease of the large intestine, however if the pain remains, the small intestine may be the source of pain.

  o *Are there any other symptoms you feel might be associated with your abdominal pain?* Nausea and vomiting are common to gallbladder, pancreatic, and intestinal complaints. Menstrual irregularities must be investigated in all females with abdominal pain. Frequent painful urination points to bladder, kidney, or prostate dysfunction. Discolored stool warrants investigation for occult gastrointestinal bleeding.

Have you experienced nausea or vomiting?

- The most likely cause of nausea and vomiting is food poisoning. For this reason, you should always ask, "*What have you eaten in the last 24 hours, and did anyone else you ate with experience similar symptoms?*"
- When a significant amount of pain is experienced, we begin to consider appendicitis, pancreatitis, cholecystitis, or kidney stones. If there is also a fever, an infectious organism may be involved. When the individual is young we suspect appendicitis, whereas the other conditions are unlikely in a young person.
- When a surgeon is trying to differentiate food poisoning from appendicitis they may ask, "*Which came first, the vomiting or your pain?*" Typically with appendicitis the pain develops first, and when the pain becomes severe, the vomiting begins. If the vomiting came first, appendicitis is unlikely.
- Remember to ask, "*Is there any blood in what you bring up?*" Hematemesis suggests peptic ulcer (gastric or duodenal), or possibly esophageal varices.

How are your bowel movements?

- Constipation may indicate a complete or partial intestinal obstruction. If the constipation alternates with diarrhea, irritable bowel syndrome (IBS) is the most likely cause.
- If there is blood mixed with the stool, ulcerative colitis or colorectal carcinoma may be present. If a rectal mass is also palpable, the patient must be referred for investigation of colorectal carcinoma.
- Diarrhea is frequent, watery bowel movements, probably in excess of three per day. Acute episodes are probably caused by viral or bacterial infection. Nausea, vomiting or fever may be associated. You should inquire if they have been traveling or camping where they might have drunk contaminated water. When the diarrhea is chronic, consider conditions such as irritable bowel syndrome, ulcerative colitis, or Crohn's disease.
- *What is the color of your stool?*
  - o Black, tarry stool suggests upper GI bleeding, most likely from an ulcer. Iron supplementation also causes black stool, but without the tarry consistency.
  - o Red blood in the stool is from lower GI bleeding, most likely hemorrhoids.

- o Pale, foul smelling stool that floats, suggests gallbladder dysfunction.

Have you had any abdominal problems prior to this current episode?

- The past health history must document all previous episodes of appendicitis, ulcer, hepatitis, gallbladder attacks, colitis, etc. You must also be aware of previous surgeries or diagnostic studies such as upper or lower GI imaging. Abdominal surgery often leaves scar tissue adhesions, which predisposes toward bowel obstruction in later years.

What prescription (Rx) and over the counter (OTC) medicines are you taking?

- Just about every drug in the PDR lists gastrointestinal side effects. Diarrhea is common when taking antibiotics. Many of your patients will be taking nonsteroidal anti-inflammatory (NSAID) medicine, such as aspirin or ibuprofen. While NSAID's are very effective at relieving inflammation, they also cause ulcers. Every day thousands of people arrive at the emergency room with GI bleeding caused from these drugs.

Do you drink? Do you smoke?

- Alcohol is a known risk factor for many conditions, especially liver and pancreatic disease. Alcohol in combination with certain drugs, such as Tylenol, is toxic to the liver. (<u>Postgraduate Medicine</u>, April 1999)
- In addition to causing lung cancer, smoking is a risk factor for peptic ulcer. Getting your patients to quit smoking is one of the best preventive health measures they can take. <u>In the US, the combined total of deaths from AIDS, alcohol, car accidents, murder, suicide, illegal drugs, and fire is less than the number of deaths caused by cigarette smoking.</u>

What is your diet like?

- Quite obviously, dietary factors have a profound influence on abdominal complaints. Management of your patients' food allergies may be the key element in their recovery. Helping your patient to make more sensible dietary choices has an enormous impact on lessening their risk for future disease.
- Computer analysis of a seven day diet diary, while time consuming, reveals a surprising amount of information. The 'hard copy' documentation of how many teaspoons of sugar their food contains, and graphs of their nutrient deficiencies helps you 'sell' the dietary changes they must make.

Examination

All of the abdominal examination, with the exception of costovertebral percussion (Murphy's test), is performed with the patient in the supine position. Several maneuvers help to relax the abdominal musculature:

- Pillow under the patient's head
- Patient's knees bent or a large pillow under the knees
- Patient's arms relaxed at the side of the abdomen
- Warm hands and stethoscope

Prior to beginning your abdominal examination, it would be wise for your patient to empty their bladder. Abdominal palpation can be painful when the bladder is full.

Proper draping requires a second gown, in addition to the gown the patient is wearing. Place the drape gown over the patient's legs and pelvic region. Have the patient slide the upper gown to just below the breast area. Then ask them to slide the lower gown down until it is just below the level of the ASIS's. With both of these gown repositioning maneuvers, it is best to let the patient move the gowns. If the doctor repositions the gown, this might be misconstrued as a 'boundary violation'.

Inspection

While observing from the side, note the contour of the abdomen. The terms used to describe abdomen contour are: scaphoid, flat, rounded, and protuberant. Lack of abdomen symmetry may manifest with ventral abdominal hernias. If you suspect a hernia, have the patient perform a partial sit-up to see if this accentuates the bulging. Conditions causing hemoperitoneum, such as pancreatitis, may manifest a bluish discoloration around the umbilicus, referred to as Cullen's sign.

As you observe, note the presence of any scars, rashes, lesions, or striae. Striae are 'stretch marks' that occur with minute tears in the elastic connective tissue of the skin. Usually this is from pregnancy or obesity. Recent striae are pink to purple blue. As the tissue heals, it turns a silvery white. Cushing's syndrome causes skin fragility and is a less common cause of striae. The striae produced from Cushing's syndrome remain a darker purple color.

It is important to note surgical scars, as most abdominal surgeries produce varying degrees of intraabdominal adhesions, which may predispose toward intestinal blockage later in life. The abdominal veins are normally only slightly visible. When they become prominent and dilated suspect portal hypertension and cirrhosis.

With thin individuals, the pulsatile abdominal aorta may be visible. Very prominent pulsation of the aorta may manifest with hypertension or abdominal aortic aneurysm. Normally peristalsis is not visible. When peristalsis is pronounced, suspect gastroenteritis or intestinal blockage.

While performing abdominal inspection, note the general demeanor of your patient. A patient with obstruction of a viscus is unable to find a position of comfort and may be moving from side to side. When peritonitis is present, the patient will lie very still, as any motion makes their pain worse.

Auscultation

Abdominal auscultation is to evaluate the presence of bowel sounds and vascular bruits. In the abdominal region we perform auscultation prior to percussion or palpation because these more vigorous maneuvers might possibly alter the bowel sounds you will hear. Additionally, if a bruit is heard over the abdominal aorta this should alert you to the possibility of an aneurysm and the need to exercise caution during abdominal palpation. Vascular bruits are a low pitched sound that requires you to listen with the bell of your stethoscope. High pitched bowel sounds are heard best with the diaphragm.

When assessing bowel sounds, we must listen at least once in each quadrant. Hyperactive bowel sounds, or 'stomach growling', are called borborygmi and occur with conditions that cause increased peristalsis, such as food poisoning. If you do not hear bowel sounds, you must listen for five minutes before you determine that bowel sounds are absent. It is unlikely that this individual will be in your office, as they will probably be in a great deal of pain and will have enough sense to go to the emergency room.

Bruits are not normally heard. Their presence suggests the possibility of atherosclerotic plaque in the arteries, especially when hypertension is also present. We listen for bruits in seven locations:

- Abdominal aorta - approximately midway between the umbilicus and xiphoid process.
- Renal arteries - lateral and inferior to where you listened to the aorta, essentially in the middle of each upper abdominal quadrant.
- Iliac arteries - inferior to the umbilicus at approximately the midclavicular line, essentially in the middle of each lower abdominal quadrant.
- Femoral arteries - over the palpable femoral pulse in the inguinal region.

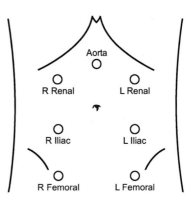

While rare, it is possible you might hear 'friction rubs' over the liver or spleen. Friction rubs are produced by conditions that cause inflammation of the peritoneal membranes, such as cancer or infection. A venous hum may be heard over periumbilical region with cirrhosis and portal hypertension.

Percussion

Gently percuss the abdomen to assess general tympany in all four quadrants. Increased abdominal gas will manifest as hyperresonance. If dullness is percussed, attempt to determine the borders of the area of dullness. We also perform additional percussion techniques to assess the size of the liver and spleen.

The liver is thinner at the medial edge gets progressively thicker toward the lateral margin. By convention, we assess the liver span at the midclavicular line. When percussing inferior to the liver, you will hear tympany. Percuss up until the tone becomes dull. Percuss down from the resonance of the lung until you reach the dull liver tone. When percussing the chest of a female, have her cup her breast laterally and percuss inferior to her hand. The normal span of the liver for an adult is 6-12 cm at the midclavicular line.

The normal spleen is too small to localize with either percussion or palpation. To assess splenic enlargement, percuss the left anterior axillary line at the lowest rib interspace. This will normally elicit a tympanic percussion note. Then have the patient take and hold a deep breath, and percuss this same location again. The percussion note should remain tympanic. If the percussion tone changes to a dull percussion note, the spleen may be enlarged and you may be able to percuss the borders of splenic enlargement. An enlarged spleen may be detected by percussion prior to being large enough to be palpable. If splenic enlargement is suspected, deep palpation should be performed with care, as an enlarged spleen is friable and easily damaged.

Costovertebral percussion is also part of the abdominal examination, although you must wait until completion of the supine portion of the exam, when the patient sits up. Place one hand over the costovertebral angle, then with your closed fist strike your own hand. Perform three separate blows starting lightly, with progressively more force with the second and third blow. Pause briefly with each blow to give the patient time to say "ouch" before you deliver a more forceful blow. This test, called Murphy's kidney punch, introduces a jarring vibration to the kidneys. If inflammation is present, pain will result.

Palpation

Abdominal palpation should be performed in two stages, light and deep. Some texts describe three passes of palpation, although two is usually adequate. Superficial or light palpation is performed to assess muscular guarding and involuntary rigidity. It also gets the patient used to your touch and helps to relax the abdominal muscles for deep palpation. Most doctors sit or stand at the right side of the patient, and begin their palpation in the right lower quadrant and continue in a clockwise pattern. However, if the patient presents with abdominal pain, always begin your palpation at the quadrant most distant from the area of complaint.

A second pass of deeper palpation is used to assess organomegaly and tenderness. You may be surprised at which structures are normally palpable in the abdomen. The free edge of the liver may be palpable in some individuals. If the liver is felt more than 2 cm below the costal margin, the liver may be enlarged and you should order a chem screen to assess liver enzymes. The pulsatile abdominal aorta is usually palpable, unless obesity is marked. The bladder is not usually palpable unless urinary retention is present. A non-gravid uterus is not normally palpable with routine abdominal palpation. Portions of the large intestine may be palpable, especially if fecal stasis is present. The stomach, spleen, pancreas, gallbladder, small intestine, and kidneys are not normally palpable.

When palpating if you place all of your fingers flat on the abdomen and distally depress the fingertips, this is usually more comfortable to your patient, than if your hand is at an angle with only the fingertips pressing on the skin. If obesity is marked, you may need to use both hands, one on top of the other in order to press deeply enough. Note any areas of tenderness and organomegaly. If a mass is palpated, record the size, location, consistency, and mobility. If an abdominal mass is palpated have the patient perform a partial sit-up to determine if the mass is intraabdominal or within the body wall. If the mass is still palpable it is in the body wall. If you no longer feel the mass during the partial sit-up the mass is intraabdominal. This test is referred to as Carnett's maneuver.

Once general abdominal palpation is complete, we attempt specific bimanual palpation of certain structures:

- Liver - Using either your fingertips or the radial edge of your index finger, attempt to palpate the free edge of the liver. An alternative method is the 'hooking technique' where the doctor stands at the shoulder of the patient and places the palms of the hands on the lower rib margin and hooks the fingers over and under the costal margin. The free edge of the liver may or may not be felt. If it is felt, it should not extend beyond 2 cm below the rib margin, and the consistency should be soft to firm and nontender.
- Spleen - Attempt to palpate the spleen by placing one hand underneath the ribcage and your palpating hand just inferior to the left costal margin. It may take several cycles of the patient breathing to relax the abdominal muscles. When the patient inhales, hold your palpating hand steady. When the patient exhales, attempt to increase the depth of your palpation.
- Kidneys - The method of kidney palpation is similar to that used for spleen palpation. The kidneys are retroperitoneal, so the palpation

must be quite deep. The right kidney is displaced lower than the left by the liver. The kidneys are not normally palpable unless they are enlarged. Normal size kidneys <u>may</u> be palpable in a child or very thin adult.

- Abdominal aorta - Place the radial edge of each hand alongside the expected location of the abdominal aorta, slightly left of midline just superior to the umbilicus. Gently increase the palpating pressure until you feel the aortic pulsations. In an adult the palpated width should be between 2.5 and 4 cm and should pulsate in an anterior direction. If the aortic pulse is wide or pulsates in a lateral direction, your patient should be referred for investigation of a possible abdominal aortic aneurysm. The key is that an aortic aneurysm is expansile, pushing the two hands apart.
- The following is a summary article on abdominal aortic aneurysm: http://www.medscape.com/CPG/ClinReviews/2001/v11.n09/c1109.01. kett/mig-pnt-c1109.01.kett.html

While not strictly a part of the abdominal examination, inguinal lymph node and femoral pulse palpation are most easily performed as a part of the abdominal examination. When examining male patients, ask the patient to take their hand and *"push your privates to one side"*, to ensure your palpating hand will not inadvertently create a 'boundary violation'. Start at the ASIS and palpate down the inguinal ligament toward the symphysis pubis. About two thirds the distance toward the symphysis, you should palpate a strong femoral pulse. Almost always you will palpate lymph nodes in the inguinal region. If you are not palpating any, try again, they are probably there. This is normal and expected, provided the palpated lymph nodes are small, movable, soft, and nontender. Abnormal lymph nodes may be enlarged, fixed, hard, and painful.

If you suspect appendicitis, there are several additional procedures you may perform:

- Rebound tenderness - At a site away from the most tender quadrant, with your fingers perpendicular to the abdominal wall, very slowly press your fingers about two inches in, or until the patient voices their discomfort. At this point <u>quickly</u> pull your hand away from the body. This maneuver will create a rebound vibration in the abdomen. Rebound tenderness, also called Blumberg's sign, suggests peritoneal inflammation, such as with appendicitis. If rebound palpation of the LLQ creates RLQ pain, this is called Rovsing's sign, typical of appendicitis.
- Iliopsoas muscle test - Position the patient's straight leg elevated approximately 30 degrees and slightly abducted. While stabilizing the left ASIS, place a downward pressure over the patient's right knee. The patient must contract the psoas muscle to resist this motion. If an inflamed appendix is positioned near this muscle, this motion will increase their pain.

- Obturator test - With the patient's right leg flexed at the hip and knee, internally rotate the femur. If this motion, which stretches the obturator muscle increases the right lower quadrant pain, we suspect appendicitis.

If gallbladder dysfunction is suspected, perform the inspiratory arrest test. With the pads of your fingertips, slowly press into the right upper abdominal quadrant. Slowly increase your depth until the patient voices mild discomfort. Then while holding your fingers immobile, have the patient take a deep breath. If they abruptly stop their inspiration, this is considered Murphy's inspiratory arrest sign for gallbladder dysfunction. As originally described by Dr. Charles Murphy in 1903, "*The diaphragm forces the liver down until the sensitive gallbladder reaches the examining fingers, when inspiration suddenly ceases as though it had been shut off.*" If the gallbladder is palpable, this is referred to as Courvoisier's sign, and may be associated with obstructive jaundice.

If ascites is suspected, perform the 'fluid wave' test. Have the patient place the ulnar edge of their hand on the midline of the abdomen. Place your palpating hand on one side of the flank. With your opposite hand tap the opposite flank firmly. If you feel the tap with your palpating hand, a large amount of abdominal ascites is likely present. If the abdominal distention is due to air or excess body fat, you should not feel the tap.

Shifting dullness is another test for ascites. With the patient in the supine position, attempt to percuss the air fluid level on the flank of the abdomen. Then have the patient roll on their side, and percuss again. If ascites is present, the fluid level and the region where you percuss dullness will shift toward the umbilicus. The shifting dullness test is not sensitive for small amounts of ascites fluid accumulation. Abdominal ultrasound is more reliable than either of these two methods for assessing ascites.

Summary of Physical Examination

- Observation of general appearance: Is the patient lying very still not wanting to move? This suggests conditions such as appendicitis or peritonitis. If they are restless, frequently shifting position in an attempt to find a position of comfort, this suggests obstruction of a viscus, such as with gallstones, kidney stones, or intestinal obstruction.
- Measure vital signs: temperature, pulse, respiration, blood pressure. If the temperature is elevated, you must investigate the source of possible infection. If an individual with abdominal pain has hypotension, blood loss must be investigated.
- Abdominal inspection: A rigid 'board like' abdomen has a high likelihood of being an 'acute abdomen' requiring a surgical consultation. Ecchymosis of either the umbilicus or flank points to hemoperitoneum, possibly caused by pancreatitis. Board question:

What are the names for umbilical ecchymosis and flank ecchymosis? Abdominal distention may simply reflect obesity, but you should always be mindful of the other 'F' causes of distention: fluid, feces, fetus, flatus, fibroid, full bladder, false pregnancy, and fatal tumor. If the umbilical veins are prominent and dilated, this is referred to as 'caput medusa', a sign of portal hypertension. Lastly, are there surgical scars? Previous abdominal surgery often causes adhesions that later predispose toward intestinal blockage.

- Auscultation: Absent bowel sounds point toward peritonitis or adynamic ileus. Hyperactive bowel sounds suggest gastroenteritis or early intestinal obstruction. Obviously, the presence of an abdominal bruit requires further investigation.
- Percussion: Percuss a few times in each abdominal quadrant to assess general tympany of bowel sounds. Specific percussion is helpful to assess organomegaly of the liver and spleen. Costovertebral percussion (Murphy's test) indicates kidney pathology, such as infection or inflammation from a kidney stone.
- Palpation: If the abdomen is tender, begin palpation at a quadrant away from the location of pain. Then work toward the painful area. Always begin with light palpation to assess muscular rigidity. Involuntary guarding is a sign of peritoneal irritation. Deep palpation will allow you to feel the size, shape, consistency, and mobility of suspected organomegaly. Rebound tenderness is a confirmatory test for peritonitis. If deep palpation over the gall bladder causes abrupt cessation of breathing (inspiratory arrest) this is referred to as Murphy's sign. Abdominal palpation is not complete without palpation of the borders of the pulsatile abdominal aorta, and palpation of the inguinal lymph nodes.
- If appendicitis is suspected, the following confirmatory tests may be performed: Obturator test, Iliopsoas muscle test, Markle's heel jar test, and Rovsing's sign.
- Any woman who presents to her MD with abdominal pain will probably receive a pelvic examination, especially if the pain is in the lower abdomen.
- When an older male presents with urinary symptoms, in addition to abdominal or back pain, a prostate exam is indicated.
- Another confirmatory test for appendicitis is a digital rectal examination (DRE). There may be right sided rectal tenderness when an inflamed appendix is positioned low in the pelvic bowl.
- Palpate lower extremity pulses. Decreased leg pulses and blood pressure should alert you to the possibility of a leaking abdominal aneurysm.

Diagnostic Studies

- Lab
  - o CBC, sed rate, chemistry panel, UA
  - o Amylase and lipase, if pancreatitis is suspected

- o   Beta hCG, if pregnancy is suspected
- X-ray
  - o   Plain abdominal film (KUB)
  - o   Upper GI series
  - o   Lower GI series
- Abdominal ultrasound
- MRI & CT
- Flexible sigmoidoscopy

Sample Documentation

Upon inspection the abdomen was rounded and symmetric. No striae, lesions, or abdominal pulsations were visible. A well healed 3 cm appendectomy scar was noted in the right lower quadrant. Upon auscultation, bowel sounds were present in all quadrants. No vascular bruits were heard. Upon percussion, tympany was the predominant tone in all quadrants. The liver span was 10 cm at the right midclavicular line. Splenic dullness was not audible at the anterior axillary line at the lowest rib interspace with either phase of respiration. Tests for ascites were not performed. Upon palpation, the abdominal wall was supple without involuntary rigidity. No masses or organomegaly were noted. The patient experienced mild discomfort upon deep palpation of the left lower abdominal quadrant. Femoral pulses were 2+ bilaterally. Small, moveable, nontender lymph nodes were palpable in the inguinal region bilaterally. No tenderness was elicited upon percussion of the right or left costovertebral angles.

Common Gastrointestinal Conditions

Gastroesophageal Reflux Disease (GERD) (ICD: 530.81)

Reflux of gastric contents into the esophagus. (Merck Manual, p. 232)

- Upward reflux of acid stomach contents into the esophagus causes heartburn typical of GERD. It is estimated that one third of Americans experience heartburn at least once a month, and 7% experience heartburn daily. While GERD may be associated with hiatal hernia, not all cases of hiatal hernia experience esophageal reflux.
- GERD usually produces heartburn, a bitter or sour taste in the mouth from reflux of stomach contents. If the acid reflux is more than minimal, the individual will probably experience dysphagia and laryngitis.
- The burning sensation in the lower chest may alarm the individual that they are having a heart attack. Or the opposite may occur, an individual with a history of dyspepsia, may dismiss cardiac pain as being heartburn.

- Many individuals with GERD have concurrent peptic ulcer disease that should be investigated. If the condition is not responsive to conservative symptomatic treatment, endoscopy may be indicated.
- Eating too large a meal, or laying down after meals may trigger esophageal reflux. As such, conservative treatment begins with having the patient eat smaller, more frequent meals, and not laying down for several hours after a meal. Antacids, or H2 acid blockers (Zantac) are used to decrease stomach acidity.
- While many people experience relief with antacids or drinking milk, in the long run this may be counterproductive. Sipping a cup of warm water mixed with a tablespoon of vinegar can neutralize the excess acid, without triggering the production of more stomach acid.

Hiatus Hernia (ICD: 553.3)

Protrusion of the stomach above the diaphragm. (Merck Manual, p. 233)

- Hiatal hernia is a protrusion of the upper part of the stomach into the chest cavity. Approximately one in four older adults have this condition. Small hiatal hernias do not usually cause symptoms. Large herniations are likely symptomatic, due to associated esophageal reflux.
- Predominant symptoms are belching, heartburn (especially when bending over or lying down), difficulty swallowing, and chest pain. Pregnancy and obesity may contribute to a worsening of hiatal hernia. When the upper portion of the stomach is 'stuck' in the diaphragm, the individual may suppress their breathing due to the pain. Because of the close proximity of the vagus nerve, a variety of other symptoms may result, leading to this condition being called the 'great mimic'.
- Confirmatory testing may include a barium swallow X-ray, or endoscopy.
- If the condition does not respond to conservative care, medical treatment involves surgical correction of the hernia.
- Visceral manipulation and AK techniques are effective non-surgical alternatives. A home remedy consists of drinking a pint of warm water first thing in the morning, then stand on your toes and drop suddenly to your heels several times. The warm water helps to relax the stomach and diaphragm, and begins to pull the stomach down. The sudden stop at the end of the heel drop helps 'adjust' the stomach to a more normal position. In a mild case, this might be enough to reduce the hernia.

Gastritis (ICD: 535)

Inflammation of the gastric mucosa. (Merck Manual, p. 245)

- Gastritis might be considered a less severe, or early manifestation of pathology which may in time progress to a gastric ulcer.
- The causes and symptoms may be similar to peptic ulcer disease. Quite often, *H. pylori* infection will be discovered. NSAID overuse will

lead to gastritis. Less commonly, Crohn's disease will manifest as inflammation of the stomach.

- The predominant symptoms are dyspepsia, epigastric pain, nausea, and upper abdominal bloating.
- Treatment must be directed at the cause.

Peptic Ulcer Disease (ICD: 533)

An excoriated segment of the GI mucosa, typically in the stomach (gastric ulcer) or first few centimeters of the duodenum (duodenal ulcer), which penetrates through the muscularis mucosae. (<u>Merck Manual</u>, p. 250)

- Peptic ulcers are most common at the first part of the duodenum (duodenal ulcer), but are also common at the lesser curvature of the stomach (gastric ulcer).
- Epigastric pain is the most common symptom. This pain may be described as 'burning' or 'gnawing'. Pain that is made worse with meals suggests gastric ulcer, whereas duodenal ulcer pain is initially relieved with eating, only to recur two to three hours after the meal.
- If vomiting occurs that appears like 'coffee grounds', this is diagnostic. Black, tarry stool also suggests an upper GI bleeding condition. Any time you suspect blood loss, perform a CBC to check for anemia.
- For many years, ulcers were thought to be a result of stress. In 1982, an Australian physician, Barry Marshall discovered that *Helicobacter pylori* is present in 95% of duodenal ulcers and 70% of gastric ulcers. Ulcers are more common in individuals with blood type O, as the bacteria have an affinity for that blood protein. Lab testing for *H. pylori* antibodies is essential.
- Antibiotic treatment, usually tetracycline, is now considered the treatment of choice for most ulcers. The bismuth metal in Pepto-Bismol has also been shown to be curative. Only 5% of *H. pylori* ulcers are located at the greater curvature of the stomach. When the ulcer occurs here, NSAID use is the probable cause. About 2-4% of patients taking NSAID's for one year develop an ulcer.
- Does stress still have a role to play in the genesis of ulcers? While the association between *H. pylori* antibodies and ulcers is high (70%-95%), approximately 25% of healthy asymptomatic individuals will also show elevated *H. pylori* antibody levels. Why don't these individuals also have a peptic ulcer? <u>The presence of bacteria does not guarantee infection</u>.
- For most people, the body's innate vitality is strong enough that the bacteria are held in check. What might happen if this individual is placed under physical or psychological stress? It is well documented that stress can suppress the immune response. With a weakened host the bacteria can now thrive. It is probably the combination of stress <u>and</u> *H. pylori* infection that causes peptic ulcers. Either alone is not sufficient to cause disease. In the words of Hans Selye, *"If microbes*

are ever present, yet do not cause disease until stress, what is the cause of disease – the microbe or the stress?"

- Please re-read the previous two paragraphs. It is the essence of how chiropractic treatment and holistic health care can benefit many visceral health problems. Just how strong is the body's innate vitality? It obviously depends upon the health of the individual, but we need to examine the numbers. At any given time the prevalence of peptic ulcer disease is about 5 million individuals, or 1-2% of the population. If the prevalence of asymptomatic infection is 25%, this amounts to approximately 70 million individuals. This means that in the United States only about one in fifteen individuals with *H. pylori* infection will go on to develop peptic ulcer disease. *Let's hear it for the innate healing potential of the body!*

Peptic ulcer prevalence vs. H. pylori infection

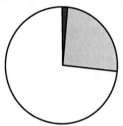

■ Peptic ulcer prevalence	5 million = 1-2%
▨ Asymptomatic H. pylori infection	70 million = 25%
□ No infection	205 million = 73%

- Upper GI problems related to long-term NSAID use are estimated to cause over 100,000 hospitalizations per year. This translates to one person every 5 minutes experiencing problems such as a bleeding ulcer from NSAID use. Of these 100,000 people, approximately 15% will **die** as a result of adverse NSAID reactions.

Mechanical Intestinal Obstruction (ICD: 560)

Complete arrest or serious impairment of the passage of intestinal contents caused by a mechanical blockage. (Merck Manual, p. 261)

- A mechanical bowel obstruction may be a surgical emergency. When the obstruction is 'strangulated' which results in vascular occlusion, infarction and gangrene can develop in as little as six hours. One of the more common causes is adhesions from previous abdominal surgery.
- The predominant symptom is severe abdominal pain, similar to what a baby experiences with 'colic'. When the obstruction is more proximal, in the small intestine, vomiting begins early. Vomiting takes longer to occur with obstruction of the large intestine. Obstipation

(total lack of bowel movements) results with complete bowel obstruction.

- Upon examination, there will initially be loud borborygmi, caused by hyperactive bowel motility. In the later stages of complete obstruction, there may be decreased bowel sounds, especially if peritonitis has set in. A KUB x-ray will disclose marked gaseous distention proximal to the obstruction.
- Initial medical management will probably involve a short period of 'watchful waiting' where the patient is NPO, or nothing by mouth. However, in most cases emergency surgery is required.
- At times the blockage will 'unkink' and not require surgery. In order to prevent future obstruction, castor oil packs are a natural remedy that has shown benefit of reducing scar tissue adhesions. For instructions, do a web search that will uncover sites such as: http://www.cayce.com/castoroil.htm

Ileus (ICD: 560.1)

A temporary arrest of intestinal peristalsis. (Merck Manual, p. 263)

- Ileus is also referred to as adynamic ileus and paralytic ileus. This condition may result from a peritoneal infection.
- While mechanical obstruction causes increased bowel sounds, adynamic ileus will cause decreased bowel sounds.
- In contrast to complete mechanical obstruction, the ability to pass gas is retained.
- This condition is more likely to respond to conservative 'watchful waiting'. Again, the patient will be NPO. Even though the individual is experiencing a great deal of pain, the doctor will be careful to not over medicate, as suppression of bowel motility is a side effect of narcotic pain medicine.

Appendicitis (ICD: 540.9)

Acute inflammation of the vermiform appendix. (Merck Manual, p. 264)

- The appendix is a three inch long extension of the proximal colon. While its' function is uncertain, it contains lymphoid tissue that may produce antibodies. If a particle of feces becomes lodged in the appendix, inflammation and infection can occur.
- Approximately one in fifteen people experience appendicitis during their lifetime. It affects males more than females, with the peak between age 10 to 15. Initially it manifests as dull periumbilical pain. As the infection progresses, the pain becomes sharp and localizes in the RLQ.
- Fever, nausea, vomiting, and anorexia are common. Rebound tenderness is likely. Muscle testing the psoas muscle or stretching the obturator muscle may aggravate the pain. Right sided rectal tenderness may be present if the appendix is located low in the pelvic bowl.

- WBC values are typically elevated above 10,000, with a shift to the left. Laparoscopic surgery with prophylactic antibiotics is the medical treatment. DDx pearl: Ask, *"Do you eat sushi (raw fish)?"* A fish roundworm can cause anisakiasis, a parasitic infection that closely mimics the symptoms of appendicitis.

Pancreatitis (ICD: 577.0)

Inflammation of the pancreas. (Merck Manual, p. 269)

- An important pancreatic function is the production of digestive enzymes. If these very powerful enzymes begin to inappropriately digest pancreatic tissue itself, severe abdominal pain can result.
- Usually, this malfunction is a consequence of alcohol abuse. In some cases, gallstones block the flow of bile, initiating pancreatic damage. The symptoms of acute and chronic pancreatitis are quite similar: severe upper abdominal pain that may radiate to the chest, back, or left shoulder. Fever, nausea, vomiting, periumbilical ecchymosis (Cullen's sign), or flank ecchymosis (Grey Turner's sign) may be associated. These skin discolorations associated with pancreatitis are caused by an accumulation of blood within the fascial planes.
- Serum amylase and lipase are elevated. With chronic pancreatitis, pancreatic endocrine function becomes impaired, manifesting the symptoms of diabetes mellitus. Obviously, the treatment of choice for pancreatitis is to eliminate the cause, alcohol.

Gastroenteritis (ICD: 005.9)

Inflammation of the lining of the stomach and intestines, predominantly manifested by upper GI tract symptoms (anorexia, nausea, vomiting), diarrhea, and abdominal discomfort. (Merck Manual, p. 283)

- Gastroenteritis may be caused by viruses, such as adenovirus or the Norwalk virus, or bacteria, such as salmonella or E coli. Gastroenteritis, also called 'stomach flu', is often caused by food poisoning. Because the condition usually resolves within a day or two, the organism causing the symptoms may not be identified.
- The predominant symptoms are nausea, vomiting, and diarrhea. While less common, a fever suggests a more significant bacterial infection.
- Upon inspection, visible peristalsis may be seen. Hyperactive bowel sounds are heard on auscultation. A CBC may show an elevated white count.
- The condition is usually self limiting, needing only supportive care. When diarrhea is prominent, bedrest with close proximity to toilet facilities is required. Electrolyte replacement (clear broth) will help with dehydration. If the diarrhea is not resolving, Kaopectate or Pepto-Bismol may help.
- If the condition persists, a stool culture and antibiotic therapy may be necessary.

Malabsorption Syndromes (ICD: 597)

Syndromes resulting from impaired absorption of nutrients from the small bowel. (Merck Manual, p. 295)

- Malabsorption syndrome is a category of conditions with a variety of causes. The pathology is a defect of digestion and absorption of food in the small intestine.
- The predominant symptoms are gas, bloating, abdominal pain, and diarrhea. With malnutrition, there may be weight loss and anemia.
- Celiac sprue, one of the more common causes, is a gluten allergy that causes inflammation of the small intestine. This inflammation interferes with the function of the microvilli. The fat that is not digested and absorbed causes pale, foul smelling stool. There is some research suggesting that early onset of osteoporosis may be caused by the anemia of celiac disease (J Assoc Physicians India 2003;51:579-584). Another journal article suggests that undetected celiac disease may be as high as 1 in 67 (NEJM 2003:348;25 2517-2524).
- Tropical sprue, presents a similar clinical picture, but is usually found in residents or individuals visiting Southeast Asia or the Caribbean. For this reason, it is thought it may be caused by a viral, bacterial, or parasitic infection.
- While Celiac sprue may manifest iron deficiency anemia, Tropical sprue displays macrocytic anemia and responds to high dose folic acid supplementation (10 mg/day), in addition to tetracycline for the suspected bacterial infection.
- New blood tests, antigliadin, antiendomysial, and anti-tissue transglutaminase (TTG) antibodies have a sensitivity and specificity for celiac disease in the range of 95%. If these tests are negative, this usually eliminates the need for an invasive tissue biopsy.

Inflammatory Bowel Disease

Crohn's Disease (ICD: 555.0)

A nonspecific chronic transmural inflammatory disease that most commonly affects the distal ileum and colon, but may occur in any part of the GI tract. (Merck Manual, p. 302)

- Inflammatory bowel disease (IBD) includes two similar conditions: ulcerative colitis and Crohn's disease. Crohn's disease is an inflammation that extends into the deeper layers of the intestinal wall. The initial description by Crohn limited the condition to the terminal ileum. While the small intestine is still the most common site for Crohn's disease, it may occur in any part of the gastrointestinal tract.
- Crohn's disease of the small intestine is called regional enteritis, and when it is found in the colon it is known as granulomatous colitis. Crohn's disease inflammation is patchy, with healthy tissue between the patches, which is sometimes referred to as a 'cobblestone' appearance.

- The condition is thought to have familial tendencies, being more common in patients of Jewish descent. The age at onset is usually between 15 and 30 years old.
- The predominant symptoms are abdominal pain and chronic, nonbloody diarrhea. With chronic malnutrition, anemia and weight loss may manifest.
- Upon examination, abdominal tenderness, especially of the right lower quadrant is likely. Associated symptoms may include iritis, photophobia, symmetric arthritis, and perianal lesions.
- A CBC will disclose anemia and the sed rate will show inflammation. The chem panel may show hypoalbuminemia and an electrolyte imbalance. Some patients with inflammatory bowel disease also experience arthropathy. When this occurs, they <u>may</u> have a positive HLA-B27.
- Medical management involves dietary and lifestyle modification. You are very capable of guiding these changes. Look in *The Encyclopedia of Natural Medicine* for specifics. If the patient does not respond to these conservative measures, they may eventually require colostomy surgery.
- Recent research (<u>JAMA</u> 12-8-2004 p. 2708-2709) suggests a possible bacterial cause of Crohn's disease and provides the rationale for taking probiotic supplements.

Ulcerative Colitis (ICD: 556)

A chronic, inflammatory, and ulcerative disease arising from the colonic mucosa, characterized most often by bloody diarrhea. (<u>Merck Manual</u>, p. 307)

- While the inflammation of Crohn's disease is patchy and extends through the entire thickness of the intestinal wall, the inflammation of ulcerative colitis affects primarily the mucosal lining, spreading in a continuous fashion. The inflammation of ulcerative colitis is most common at the colon and rectum.
- See the table on page 305 of the <u>Merck Manual</u> for more specifics on the differences between these two forms of inflammatory bowel disease.
- Both conditions cause weight loss, fever, abdominal pain and frequent diarrhea. However, with ulcerative colitis the diarrhea is usually bloody. There may be associated rectal conditions such as fissures, abscess, or hemorrhoids.
- Abdominal examination may be unremarkable except for tenderness upon palpation of the lower abdomen.
- The CBC will usually disclose anemia and leukocytosis. The sed rate will be elevated, and the chem screen may show hypokalemia and hypoalbuminemia. Definitive diagnosis requires colonoscopy with a tissue biopsy.
- Because the cause of these two conditions is similar, the management is also similar: dietary and lifestyle modification.

Irritable Bowel Syndrome (ICD: 564.1)

A motility disorder involving the entire GI tract, causing recurring upper and lower GI symptoms, including variable degrees of abdominal pain, constipation and/or diarrhea, and abdominal bloating. (Merck Manual, p. 312)

- Like inflammatory bowel disease, Irritable Bowel Syndrome (IBS) also manifests with abdominal pain and diarrhea. However, the diarrhea may alternate with periods of constipation. The condition, also called spastic colitis or mucous colitis, is common, representing 50% of all visits to a gastroenterologist. It is estimated that 15% of adults have experienced this condition.
- The condition affects females more than males and initial onset is most common in the late teens and early 20's. It is rare for this condition to develop in later life. Episodes are usually triggered by stressful life situations, such as taking exams.
- Predominant symptoms are abdominal gas and distention, lower abdominal pain that is relieved with defecation, and diarrhea alternating with constipation for three months or more. Physical examination of the stool may reveal the presence of mucous.
- These patients usually appear healthy, although if the diarrhea is marked, malnutrition may cause the individual to be thin. Physical examination may reveal nothing more than tenderness upon palpation of the left lower abdominal quadrant.
- Laboratory workup includes a CBC, sed rate, chem screen to include lipase and amylase, UA, hemocult test, stool analysis for ova and parasites.
- The results of physical and laboratory examination will be more or less normal. As such, IBS may be a 'diagnosis of exclusion'. When the inflammatory cell changes typical of IBD are lacking and there is no 'known' cause, the condition is labeled a 'functional disorder'.
- Management is supportive. Stress reduction techniques such as the relaxation response are very helpful. The individual would do well to adopt Hans Selye's aphorism, "*Always strive for your highest aim, but never put up resistance in vain.*"
- Many natural health care physicians find management of food allergies very helpful with these individuals. Supplemental fiber, such as psyllium or xanthine gum may provide symptomatic relief of acute episodes. Probiotic supplementation has been shown to help with the intestinal gas associated with irritable bowel syndrome.
- The June 14, 2001 issue of the New England Journal of Medicine (344;24:1846-1850) has an excellent review article on Irritable Bowel Syndrome.

Diverticulitis (ICD: 562.11)

Inflammation of the diverticular mucosa with attendant complications of peridiverticulitis, phlegmon of the bowel wall, perforation, abscess, or peritonitis, with or without obstruction, fistulas, and bleeding. (Merck Manual, p. 318)

- Diverticulitis is another 'disease of civilization', a direct consequence of inadequate fiber in the diet. With chronic constipation, the increased pressure that results during bowel motility causes small outpouchings (diverticula) of the mucosa through the muscular wall of the colon. When these pouches become infected, diverticulitis results.
- It is estimated that by age 60, half of us have diverticulosis. The symptoms are similar to appendicitis (severe abdominal pain, nausea, vomiting, fever), except that the side of pain is wrong (LLQ), and the individual is much older (> 40) than we expect with appendicitis.
- Upon examination, there may be a palpable mass in the left lower abdominal quadrant that is exquisitely painful. There is muscular rigidity and rebound tenderness is probable. The abdomen is distended with tympany on percussion.
- Laboratory examination will disclose an elevated white count with a shift to the left. A stool guaiac test may be positive for occult blood. With blood loss anemia may occur. A barium enema x-ray is diagnostic for diverticulitis.
- Medical management will probably include hospitalization with fluids only and IV antibiotics. If the condition is not responsive to conservative care, bowel resection surgery may be required.

Hepatitis (ICD: 070)

An inflammation of the liver characterized by diffuse or patchy necrosis affecting the acini. (Merck Manual, p. 377)

- Hepatitis is an inflammation of the liver, usually caused by a virus, however alcohol and toxins can also cause hepatitis. Hepatitis often goes undiagnosed because its symptoms are similar to flu: nausea, vomiting, fever, loss of appetite, and abdominal pain. When the production of bile is impaired, dark colored urine and jaundice occurs.
- Five types (A through E) are known, with two new variants suspected. Hepatitis A, originally called infectious hepatitis, is usually a short term illness, most commonly spread from people not washing their hands after using the toilet. Hepatitis B, originally called serum hepatitis, is usually spread via contaminated needles, although it can also be passed between partners in unprotected sex, and from mother to child before birth. In the past, when an individual tested negative for hepatitis A and B, a third type was identified. This was first called 'non-A, non-B' and is now referred to as hepatitis C. Its' transmission is similar to type B, and is thought to be a predisposing factor in liver cancer.
- Upon palpation, a liver with hepatitis may be tender and enlarged, but the edge remains soft and smooth. Jaundice of the skin, mucous

membranes and sclera will manifest. Fever and weight loss may occur, and there may be splenic enlargement.

- All cases of suspected hepatitis should receive a chem screen to assess: AST, ALT, GGT, ALP, LDH, and bilirubin. The WBC will be low normal, and atypical lymphocytes may be seen. Urinalysis will be positive for bilirubin, which is usually detectable prior to the onset of jaundice. Serologic testing is required to specify which virus is causing the inflammation.
- Medical management involves supportive care. Gamma globulin shots may help, although this is not universally agreed upon. In most cases vaccination is recommended to boost the immune response. When the condition persists for longer than six months, it is referred to as chronic hepatitis. Chronic hepatitis can lead to cirrhosis, or even death.
- Natural therapeutics, such as the herb Milk Thistle, have at times worked where the drugs have failed.

Cirrhosis (ICD: 571.5)

Diffuse disorganization of normal hepatic structure by regenerative nodules that are surrounded by fibrotic tissue. (Merck Manual, p. 372)

- Most cases of cirrhosis are the result of a lifetime of drinking alcohol. Chronic alcohol abuse causes liver parenchymal cell damage. As this tissue heals with fibrosis and scar tissue, the liver becomes non-functional. Cirrhosis is one of the leading causes of death in individuals over 65.
- The liver is a remarkably resilient organ, and can still function with 70% of its' mass destroyed or removed by surgery. However, eventually enough function is lost that symptoms manifest. Early symptoms include anorexia, malaise, weight loss, abdominal discomfort, and generalized weakness.
- Upon examination, a cirrhotic liver may be enlarged, and palpates with a smooth, firm, blunt edge. Decreased albumin production may lead to swelling in the legs and abdomen. Jaundice develops as bile products are not processed by the liver. The blockage of blood flow through the liver causes portal hypertension. This venous back pressure in turn results in splenomegaly, and enlargement of abdominal and esophageal blood vessels. Alcoholics may develop esophageal varices due to portal hypertension. A Mallory-Weiss syndrome is an upper GI bleed that may occur when esophageal blood vessels tear during coughing or vomiting.
- Laboratory examination will disclose elevated liver enzymes. Bilirubin will be increased, and albumin will be decreased. Normocytic anemia is common. As liver function is compromised, hypersplenism with attendant leukopenia and thrombocytopenia may result.
- Treatment must first be directed at the cause - stop drinking. Herbal and vitamin nutritional supplementation may help with compromised liver function.

Liver Cancer (<u>Merck Manual</u>, p. 396) (ICD: 155)

- The signs and symptoms of liver cancer may not manifest until the condition is advanced. Advanced liver cancer will present with edema in the legs or abdomen, jaundice, anorexia, fatigue, and weight loss. It is a rapid growing cancer, and is often fatal within six months of diagnosis.
- Previous hepatitis or cirrhosis is a risk factor for primary liver cancer. While primary liver cancer is common in Africa and Asia, in the US and Europe, metastatic liver cancer is 20 times more common than primary liver cancer. The liver is the most common site for metastatic disease. It is believed that the high blood flow of the liver provides a fertile environment for the growth and attachment of metastatic cancer cells. The most common primary sites are: colon, rectum, lung, breast, pancreas and stomach.
- Early symptoms may be vague and nonspecific, such as fatigue, malaise, or an unexplained fever. As the condition progresses, weight loss and abdominal pain may manifest. Upon examination, a cancerous liver palpates as enlarged, with a hard irregular border.

The following is a summary of liver palpation findings:

Condition	Size	Consistency
Hepatitis	Enlarged and tender	Soft and smooth
Cirrhosis	Enlarged	Smooth, firm, blunt edge
Liver Cancer	Enlarged	Hard, irregular border

- When an individual has a liver cancer that is a metastasis from intestinal endocrine (argentaffin) cells, these cells secrete vasoactive substances such as serotonin and histamine. This individual may experience high blood pressure, flushing, diarrhea, intestinal cramping, and bronchospasm typical of an asthma attack. This group of symptoms is referred to as carcinoid syndrome.
- Laboratory testing will disclose elevated liver enzymes. Alpha fetoprotein is a tumor marker specific for hepatocellular carcinoma. Suspected carcinoma will be confirmed by ultrasound or an MRI, and eventually a liver biopsy.
- The prognosis for liver cancer is usually grim. By the time it is discovered, it is usually advanced and rapidly fatal.

Acute Cholecystitis (ICD: 575.0)

Acute inflammation of the gallbladder wall, usually as a response to cystic duct obstruction by a gallstone. (<u>Merck Manual</u>, p. 402)

- Gall bladder attacks are usually related to gallstones, which are common, affecting 10% of the population. According to Seller, cholecystitis is the most common cause of acute abdominal pain in patients over 50. However, most gallstones are 'silent', never causing symptoms. Women are twice as likely as men to develop gallstones, and gallstones are more likely in both men and women who are overweight (Remember the four F's).

- The symptoms of severe RUQ pain, nausea, vomiting, and fever may be precipitated by eating a large, fatty meal several hours earlier. The pain may radiate to the tip of the right scapula.
- Upon examination of a patient experiencing an acute episode, the right upper abdomen will be tender to palpation. Murphy's inspiratory arrest sign is likely. The gallbladder may or may not be palpable. A fever may be present, and the pain may cause an elevated BP.
- Laboratory evaluation will likely disclose an elevated white count, possibly with a shift to the left. Liver enzymes may be slightly elevated. If the common bile duct is obstructed by a gallstone, serum bilirubin will be elevated. Definitive presurgical diagnosis will be with abdominal ultrasound, an oral cholecystogram, or a gall bladder radionuclide scan.
- Most gallbladder attacks are managed initially by 'watchful waiting'. However, if the stone becomes lodged, emergency surgery may be necessary. Laparoscopic surgery now results in less cutting, and therefore decreased scar tissue formation.
- While the 'Liver-Gallbladder flush' is not recommended in *The Encyclopedia of Natural Medicine,* many physicians find this procedure helps patients pass their gallstones. A brief discussion of this treatment was recently published in the Lancet 1999 Dec 18; 354 (9196):2171.
- Prevention is the key in gallbladder dysfunction. A low fat diet with supplemental lecithin and fiber are recommended. Allergy elimination diets may produce dramatic results. A study by JC Breneman found complete resolution of symptoms with an allergy elimination diet. Reintroducing eggs to the diet triggered gallbladder attacks in 93% of these same individuals (Ann Allergy, 1968 Feb;26(2):83-7).

Colorectal Carcinoma (Merck Manual, p. 328) (ICD: 154.0)

- Colorectal carcinoma is the third leading cause of cancer in either sex. While it can occur in young people, 90% of this cancer occurs after age 50. Routine screening is critical for early detection, as the condition may be asymptomatic until the cancer is advanced.
- Early symptoms include abdominal pain, diarrhea or a change in bowel habits, blood in the stool, anemia, and weight loss.
- Upon physical examination, a rectal mass with rolled edges and an ulcerated center may be palpable. About 50% of palpable lesions are malignant.
- Laboratory examination includes a CBC which will likely show signs of anemia. A stool guaiac test will show occult blood. Carcinoembryonic antigen (CEA) is a tumor marker for

gastrointestinal carcinoma. The condition is confirmed with fiberoptic colonoscopy.

- Prompt referral to a colorectal surgeon is indicated. Survival time varies depending upon how early the condition is found.
- A recent study (J Natl Cancer Inst 2000; 92: 1888-1896) found that people who smoke cigarettes for 20 or more years are about 40 percent more likely to die of colon cancer than are non-smokers. The study attributes 12 percent of U.S. colon cancer deaths to tobacco use.

Rectal Polyps (ICD: 569.0)

- Polyps are tumor growths on the inner lining of the colon. Most polyps are benign or hyperplastic, however adenomatous polyps are premalignant. Small polyps do not usually bleed and may go undetected. By the time blood is present in the stool, carcinoma may already be advanced.
- Polyps very near the rectum may be palpable, however flexible colonoscopy is required to adequately check the colon. The American Cancer Society recommends annual colorectal cancer screening beginning at age 50.
- Dietary prevention is key:
  o Low fat
  o Decrease intake of red meat
  o Increase intake of fruit and vegetables
  o Increase intake of soluble fiber

Hemorrhoids (ICD: 455.6)

Varicosities of the veins of the hemorrhoidal plexus, often complicated by inflammation, thrombosis, and bleeding. (Merck Manual, p. 336)

- Most people will experience hemorrhoids, essentially varicose veins of the rectum, at some point in their life. The most common cause is constipation, which induces straining at the stool.
- Internal hemorrhoids have poor pain sensation and may go unnoticed until they bleed. External hemorrhoids are painful, ranging from a dull ache to intense pain, especially with a bowel movement.
- Upon examination, visually, thrombosed external hemorrhoids present as a small blue bulge, which may bleed. Skin tags suggest previous healed external hemorrhoids. Internal hemorrhoids are visible only upon anoscopy, and may or may not be palpable with a digital rectal examination.
- Laboratory evaluation may disclose anemia if blood loss is significant.
- Thrombosed external hemorrhoids are surgically excised under local anesthetic. Internal hemorrhoids are treated by injection sclerotherapy, rubber band ligation, or electodesiccation (Keesey technique).
- As with most conditions, prevention is the key. Increase fiber and water intake, and discourage straining during bowel movements.

Anal Fissure (ICD: 565.0)

An acute longitudinal tear or a chronic ovoid ulcer in the stratified squamous epithelium of the anal canal. (<u>Merck Manual</u>, p. 337)

- When a person is constipated, the passage of hard rough stools may cause a tear in the rectal mucosa. Because of the abundance of nerve endings, these conditions are quite painful and may result in spasm of the sphincter. Obviously, the presence of bacteria in feces does not facilitate healing.
- The predominant symptom is pain with defecation. Bright red blood may be noticed on the toilet paper after bowel movements.
- Fortunately, most fissures heal without surgery. Anesthetic ointment will help with the pain. Correct the cause by increasing fiber and water intake. Stool softeners may also be helpful. Strict cleanliness after bowel movements (sitz baths) will promote healing. A sentinel skin tag may be evidence of a healed fissure.

Anorectal Abscess and Fistula (ICD: 566)

Abscess: A localized collection of pus resulting from bacterial invasion of the pararectal spaces, originating in an intermuscular (intersphincteric) space into which an anal crypt has penetrated. (<u>Merck Manual</u>, p. 338)

Fistula: A tubelike tract with one opening in the anal canal and the other usually in the perianal skin. (<u>Merck Manual</u>, p. 338)

- The anal crypts are located just proximal to the anorectal junction. When bacteria become trapped in these pockets, an abscess may form. An anal fistula develops when the abscess creates an abnormal tunnel to the surface of the skin near the rectum.
- The predominant symptoms are rectal swelling and tenderness, and when the infection is marked a fever will develop. Inflammatory bowel disease may be a contributing factor in the development of rectal abscess and fistula. Treatment normally consists of surgical incision and drainage, and antibiotics.

Pilonidal Disease (ICD: 685)

Acute abscess or chronic draining sinuses in the sacrococcygeal area. (<u>Merck Manual</u>, p. 340)

- The word pilonidal is latin for 'hair nest'. If a hair becomes ingrown, it can form a cyst similar to a sebaceous cyst. For obvious reasons, the condition is more common in men, especially men with excess body hair.
- The condition is frequently asymptomatic, however being near the rectum, an infection and abscess may develop. When this occurs, antibiotics and surgical incision are the usual treatment.

Rectal Prolapse (ICD: 569.1)

Protrusion of the rectum through the anus. (<u>Merck Manual</u>, p. 340)

- In addition to supporting the bladder and vagina, the pelvic floor musculature supports the rectum. Weakness of these muscles, especially the muscles comprising the anal sphincter, may allow a protrusion of the rectal mucosa through the anal ring.
- This condition occurs more in women, probably a consequence of over stretched musculature following childbirth. Visually it appears as a moist red rosette. Incompetence of the sphincter may allow incontinence of stool.
- The individual is given stool softeners and advised to avoid straining at stool. Surgery is the only option when the prolapse does not reduce or repeatedly prolapses.

Pruritis Ani (ICD: 698.0)

Anal and perianal itching. (<u>Merck Manual</u>, p. 341)

- Pruritis Ani is an inflammation of the perianal area that leads to intense itching. It manifests from a variety of causes, such as pinworm infection, fungal infection, or possibly food allergies.
- When an individual is overly fastidious about cleansing the rectal area with soap after a bowel movement, this removes the protective oil from the skin, and may actually aggravate the condition. It is better to clean with pure water only. After cleaning, dry the area with cornstarch powder. Topical application of cortisone cream will relieve the itching and redness.

Visceral Manipulation

While chiropractic treatment traditionally involves adjustment of spinal and extremity joints, there are techniques you can learn to facilitate healing of abdominal conditions. Dr. M.B. DeJarnette, the originator of Sacro Occipital Technique, pioneered many visceral manipulation techniques which he referred to as chiropractic manipulative reflex technique (CMRT) or "*bloodless surgery*". You will need to attend post-graduate seminars in order to learn these skills. Most chiropractic college libraries will have several several books and videos on the subject.

Study Guide Objectives

o Know the organs located in each of the four abdominal quadrants.
o Know the descriptors for the midline regions when using the nine region mapping method.
o Know the appropriate history questions for an abdominal exam.
o Why is a loss of appetite a possible cause of concern?
o Which genetic ancestry groups are most at risk for lactose intolerance?
o Know the timing of pain patterns of gastric ulcer, duodenal ulcer, and cholecystitis.
o Know the pain differences between obstruction of a viscus vs. peritoneal irritation.

- What is the significance of a rigid 'board like' abdomen?
- Know the relationship between nausea and vomiting and the onset of pain for food poisoning vs. appendicitis.
- Know the significance of discolored stools.
- Know the importance of previous abdominal surgeries.
- What patient preparation and positioning maneuvers are helpful to relax the abdominal musculature during the abdominal examination.
- What are the four terms used to describe abdominal contour?
- What is the significance of dark purple striae on the abdomen?
- What is the significance of prominent and dilated abdominal veins?
- What is the significance of a very prominent pulsation of the abdominal aorta?
- What is the significance of visible waves of peristalsis in the abdomen?
- What is the purpose of abdominal auscultation?
- In the abdomen, why is auscultation performed prior to percussion and palpation?
- When bruits are heard upon abdominal auscultation, what does this suggest?
- If you do not hear bowel sounds during abdominal auscultation, how long should you listen before you determine that bowel sounds are absent?
- What is the significance of friction rubs over the liver or spleen?
- What is the significance of a venous hum over the periumbilical region?
- What is the normal expected tone upon abdominal percussion?
- What is the normal span of the liver at the midclavicular line?
- Know the procedure used during percussion to assess for splenic enlargement.
- If splenic enlargement is detected upon abdominal percussion, how would this modify your subsequent palpation of the abdomen?
- What are two methods used to assess ascites? How are these methods performed?
- Why is Murphy's costovertebral percussion performed?
- What is the purpose of superficial abdominal palpation?
- What is the purpose of deep abdominal palpation?
- If liver enlargement is palpated, what follow-up should be performed to assess liver function?
- If your patient is in pain, where should you begin abdominal palpation?
- Which abdominal organs are normally palpable during routine examination of a healthy individual?
- If an abdominal mass is palpated, what characteristics are recorded?
- When palpating the inguinal region, what are the expected characteristics of normal lymph nodes?
- What is Rovsing's sign?
- Know how to perform the Obturator test and Iliopsoas tests.
- What is the difference between Murphy's test and Murphy's sign?
- Decreased pulses and blood pressure in the lower extremity suggest

what health condition?
- If you suspect pancreatitis, what blood tests should you order?
- If you suspect your female patient is pregnant, what test is ordered?
- What do the initials GERD stand for?
- What are the symptoms of GERD?
- What is the bacterial infection involved with most cases of peptic ulcer disease?
- What is the role of stress in peptic ulcer disease?
- What is obstipation?
- What is the difference between Ileus and mechanical intestinal obstruction?
- Know the signs and symptoms of appendicitis.
- What is the usual cause of pancreatitis?
- Know Cullen's and Grey Turner's signs and what causes these two examination findings.
- Know the differences between celiac and tropical sprue.
- Which part of the intestinal tract is the most common site for Crohn's disease?
- Which part of the intestinal tract is the most common site for ulcerative colitis?
- Which of these two conditions is most likely to manifest bloody diarrhea?
- Which of these two conditions manifests a patchy 'cobblestone' inflammation, with healthy tissue between the patches?
- Which bowel condition represents 50% of all visits to a gastroenterologist and is characterized by diarrhea that may alternate with periods of constipation?
- What are the clinical differences between appendicitis vs. diverticulitis?
- Why does hepatitis often go undiagnosed?
- Know the palpation findings for hepatitis, cirrhosis, and liver cancer.
- Which type of hepatitis is transmitted via the fecal-oral route?
- What is the usual cause of cirrhosis?
- What causes jaundice?
- Which type of liver cancer is most common in the US and Europe: primary or metastatic liver cancer?
- What is the most common cause of acute abdominal pain in patients over 50?
- Where does pain from cholecystitis often radiate?
- How common is colorectal carcinoma in relation to other forms of cancer?
- Upon physical examination, how might colorectal carcinoma palpate?
- What is the term for varicose veins of the rectum?
- Which has greater pain sensation: internal or external hemorrhoids?
- How does a thrombosed external hemorrhoid appear?
- What is the significance of a skin tag at the rectum?
- What is the difference between an anorectal abscess vs. fistula?
- What is a pilonidal cyst?
- How does rectal prolapse appear upon inspection?

12 – Male & GU disorders

Anatomy & Physiology

The male genitalia is comprised of the penis, scrotum, testicles, epididymis, and vas deferens. The seminal vesicles, bulbourethral gland, and prostate gland are considered accessory glandular structures. The shaft of the penis is comprised of three columns of cylindrical erectile tissue. The ventral corpus spongiosum surrounds the urethra and forms the distal glans penis. Dorsal and lateral to the corpus spongiosum are the two corpora cavernosum. The margin where the glans penis joins the shaft is the corona. If the male is uncircumcised, the foreskin covers the glans penis. Sloughed off skin cells and sebaceous secretions may accumulate under the foreskin to form smegma.

The scrotum is a loose, slightly muscular sac that contains the testes, epididymis, and vas deferens. The cremaster muscle contracts or relaxes as needed to keep the testes at a constant temperature. An internal septum divides the scrotal sac and separates the two testicles. The testes are ovoid, with an average size of 2 x 3 x 4 centimeters. The male testes, analogous to the female ovaries, produce spermatozoa and testosterone. After sperm are produced, they travel to the epididymis, a comma shaped structure located on the upper posterolateral surface of the testis, where they mature and remain until they are released at ejaculation. Also contained within the scrotum are the spermatic arteries, veins and vas deferens, which together form the spermatic cord.

At ejaculation, the sperm travel via the vas deferens through the inguinal canal to the seminal vesicles. The seminal vesicles are located superior and lateral to the prostate gland. The ejaculatory duct travels from the seminal vesicles through the prostate gland to the urethra. During ejaculation, the seminal vesicles supply a fructose rich fluid which nourishes the sperm, and the prostate gland provides an alkaline fibrinolysin fluid which liquefies and enhances the viability of the sperm. This fluid then travels in the urethra down the shaft of the penis, where it exits the body via the urinary meatus. Neurologically, erection is mediated via the parasympathetic nervous system, and ejaculation is mediated via the sympathetic nervous system.

The prostate gland is a bilobed structure which surrounds the urethra and neck of the bladder. The posterior surface of the prostate gland is palpable through the anterior wall of the rectum. During palpation, the normal prostate will be approximately 2.5 cm high and 4 cm wide. You should be able to palpate both the median sulcus, which separates the two lobes, and the lateral margins of the gland. Inferior to the prostate, on each side of the urethra, are Cowper's bulbourethral glands, which also secrete an alkaline fluid that counteracts the acid present in the male urethra and female vagina.

The anus is the terminal outlet of the gastrointestinal tract. The anal ring is comprised of the external sphincter under voluntary control, and the internal sphincter under involuntary control. Proximal to the sphincter is the anal canal composed of folds of mucosal tissue, the anal columns. Each anal canal is supplied by an artery and vein. If an individual strains at the stool, these veins may become enlarged to form internal hemorrhoids. The ends of the anal columns form small pockets, the anal crypts, which may become a source of infection. The anorectal junction or pectinate line is the transition area from the rectum and anal canal to the anal sphincter. The nerve sensation distal to this line is very pain sensitive, and relatively insensitive proximal to the anorectal junction.

The groin or inguinal region is very clinically significant in males. The inguinal ligament is a strong band of tissue that holds the structures between the anterior superior iliac spine and the symphysis pubis firmly in place. During fetal development the testes are located within the abdomen. Shortly before birth, the testes migrate via the inguinal canal to the scrotal sac. In the adult, this canal persists as the channel for the arteries, veins, and spermatic cord to the testes. As such this canal may become large enough for a loop of bowel to protrude through the abdomen. Inguinal hernia repair is the most common elective surgery in males.

Nature of the Patient

Females have a much shorter urethra than males. This, coupled with the close proximity of the urinary meatus to the vaginal and rectal openings, results in a much higher incidence of urinary tract infection (UTI) in females. During the development of the male fetus, the testicles migrate down the inguinal canal to the scrotum. As such, inguinal hernia is primarily a condition of males, rare in females. Conditions such as kidney stones and chronic glomerulonephritis are more likely in adults, whereas acute glomerulonephritis is primarily a condition of children. Given enough time, prostatic dysfunction will eventually manifest in all elderly males.

Key History Questions

How often do you urinate throughout the day?

- Depending upon fluid intake, most adults urinate 5-6 times per day. Frequency usually refers to <u>increased</u> frequency or polyuria. Decreased frequency is oliguria. Urgency is the feeling of inability to hold back urine. Painful urination with frequency and urgency suggests a bladder or prostate infection. When there is no pain, various causes of polyuria must be investigated.
- Polyuria with increased thirst (polydipsia) and increased hunger (polyphagia) points to diabetes mellitus. Urine and serum glucose will be elevated. Polyuria without glycosuria suggests diabetes insipidus,

or possibly a defect in renal tubular reabsorption of water, such as chronic glomerulonephritis.

- Unless there is excess fluid intake late in the evening, most people can sleep through the night without getting up to urinate. Nocturia, or the need to void urine at night suggests conditions such as prostatic enlargement or cystitis. If the person has signs of congestive heart failure (edema, dyspnea), nocturia may be due to mobilization of edematous fluid from the extremities, especially when the individual is taking diuretic medicine.

Do you have difficulty with urination?

- Dysuria, or painful urination is found with many conditions, but most commonly indicates a bladder infection.
- When a fever is also present, consider a more serious infection such as pyelonephritis or acute prostatitis.

What color is your urine?

- The presence of hematuria with dysuria suggests cystitis, kidney stones, or possibly bladder cancer. Sometimes the timing of hematuria provides clues to the origin of the blood. Initial hematuria that clears with voiding suggests bleeding at the distal structures, such as with urethritis. Terminal hematuria is when the urine flow is initially clear and then becomes discolored. In this case, the blood is probably from more proximal structures, such as the bladder or prostate gland. Kidney pathology, such as glomerulonephritis can result in 'total hematuria' where the entire flow is discolored.
- Pyuria may produce cloudy, foul smelling urine. The infection may be anywhere within the urinary tract (kidney, ureter, bladder, prostate, urethra), however bladder infection is the most likely cause.

Have you noticed any discharge from your penis?

- Urethral discharge is the cardinal sign of urethritis. The usual organism cultured is gonorrhea, however other organisms, such as chlamydia may be responsible. Infection from organisms other than gonorrhea is referred to as nongonococcal urethritis (NGU), or nonspecific urethritis (NSU). Yellow green discharge suggests gonococcal infection, while the nongonococcal discharge is mucoid and less profuse.
- Reiter's syndrome (urethritis, arthritis, conjunctivitis) may be a consequence of previous NGU infection.

Have you noticed any sores or rashes on your genitals?

- Penile sores are readily visible and have a distinctive appearance that aids diagnosis. While lesions caused by syphilis, chlamydia, and the human papillomavirus are usually painless, herpes progenitalis is typically quite painful.

Have you noticed any lumps or swelling in your scrotum?

- Testicular torsion causes a sudden onset of swelling and pain in one testicle. Ischemia may result in loss of the testicle if surgery is delayed.
- Testicular cancer is a testicular mass that does <u>not</u> transilluminate. Spermatocele and hydrocele tumors <u>do</u> transilluminate.
- A reducible scrotal mass is probably an inguinal hernia.

Are you sexually active?

- Sexual history includes current sexual activity, the number of current and previous partners, the gender of partners, satisfaction with the relationship, and STD precautions.
- While questions relating to sexual matters may be uncomfortable, this information is key to understanding the cause of many male conditions. Using neutral language and open ended questions can help facilitate communication.

Are you able to achieve and maintain an erection?

- Erectile dysfunction, or impotence, affects 10% of men at some point in life. Often the problem is psychological, especially if erections occur during sleep. Physiological causes include neurological conditions (MS, prostate surgery, diabetes), vascular compromise (atherosclerosis), and testosterone deficiency. The drug Viagra is effective in many cases of vascular erectile dysfunction.

Do you have any difficulty with your bowel movements?

- Prostatitis may cause pain with bowel movements.

What medications are you taking?

- Some drugs are toxic to kidney function. Hydrochlorothiazide blood pressure medicine works by decreasing the GFR.

Do you have any personal or family history of prostate problems?

- If you have a father or brother with prostate cancer, your risk is double the average risk of developing prostate cancer.

Examination

Explain the scope of the examination to your patient. It is normal for a male to be apprehensive about having the genitals examined. When you are confident and at ease, your professional demeanor will help to allay the tension. The external genitalia and hernia check portion of the exam are usually performed with the patient standing and the doctor seated on a stool. While the rectal portion of the examination may also be performed with the patient standing, the lateral recumbent position is more comfortable for the patient.

It is customary for the doctor to 'double glove' for the genitalia and hernia check portion of the examination, and then remove the outer glove of the dominant hand to provide a fresh clean glove for the rectal portion of the examination.

Inspect and Palpate the Penis

As you begin the genital examination, note the hair pattern. While the female hair pattern is triangular in shape, in males the hair pattern is normally diamond shaped. If the patient has a complaint of itching in the genital area, closely inspect the genital hair for the presence of scabies or lice pest inhabitants. The eggs of lice may be visible as nits on the shaft of pubic hair.

While seated in front of your standing patient, with gloved hands, inspect as you palpate the shaft of the penis. The skin should be smooth, without rash or lesions. Sexually transmitted disease (STD) often manifests as nodules, vesicles, or chancre on the shaft of the penis. The shaft of the penis should palpate without areas of stricture or tenderness. Peyronie's disease will manifest as a fibrotic hardening of the corpus cavernosum.

If the male is uncircumcised, have him retract his foreskin. When the foreskin is tight and difficult to retract, this is referred to as phimosis. If the tightened foreskin does not easily return to the extended position, this is paraphimosis. The urinary meatus should be located in the center of the glans penis. Hypospadias and epispadias refer to a congenital defect where the urinary meatus is inappropriately placed either ventrally or dorsally.

Compress the glans penis between your thumb and index finger. The urinary meatus should appear as a smooth, pink opening without evidence of stricture or discharge. If the patient complains of dysuria and a discharge is present, collect a drop on a slide for microscopic examination. Closely inspect the corona of the glans, as this is a common site for penile carcinoma. In uncircumcised males, cheesy smegma may be found between the glans and the retracted foreskin.

Inspect and Palpate the Scrotum

To provide an unobstructed view of the scrotum, have the patient hold the penis out of the way. Observe for edema or swelling of the scrotal contents. If the room temperature is cool, it is normal for the scrotum to be taut and retracted. The left testicle normally hangs lower than the right, as the spermatic cord is longer on the left.

Inspect the skin surface for rashes or sebaceous cysts. You must lift the scrotal bag to visualize the under surface. With your thumb and first two fingers, palpate each individual testicle for contour, consistency, or nodularity. If the testicles are retracted, it may be necessary to gently tug them inferior in order to palpate the entire surface of the testicle. Note the size, consistency, and surface characteristics. The normal consistency is 'firm', with a smooth, rubbery feel. The pressure used should be mild as this tissue is very pain sensitive. However, if the palpation is too light a cancerous tumor might be missed. If the testicles are insensitive to pain, this may be a danger signal for cancer.

The epididymis is a nodular, comma shaped structure on the upper posterolateral surface of the testis. This structure is softer in consistency than the testis, and should be pain free. Tenderness upon palpation suggests epididymitis. Leading from the epididymis is the spermatic cord, comprised of the spermatic arteries, veins and vas deferens. No other tumor or mass should be palpable within the scrotum. If a swelling or mass is palpated, shine a strong light behind the scrotum to transilluminate the scrotal contents. Fluid filled masses, such as hydrocele or spermatocele, will pass light and present a red glow. The testicle and solid tumors do not transilluminate. Some patients may manifest a varicocele, which palpates as a 'bag of worms'. Just as varicosities may develop in superficial leg veins, varicocele is essentially a varicosity of the spermatic vein.

Inspect and Palpate for Hernias

As you prepare for the hernia check, briefly inspect for the bulge of an inguinal hernia, which may be visible even before the patient bears down to increase intraabdominal pressure. When palpating for inguinal hernia, use your right index finger when palpating right inguinal canal, and your left index finger when palpating the left inguinal canal. Place your gloved index finger low on the scrotal sac, and slowly invaginate your finger into the scrotum and up to the external inguinal ring. You may be able to to guide your way by feeling the spermatic cord with the back of your finger. When your finger is in place, ask the patient to bear down. This will increase the intraabdominal pressure and make a hernia more palpable. If your finger is in the correct place, you will normally feel a very slight pressure on the tip of your index finger. If nothing is felt, you are probably not exactly on the external inguinal ring. Relocate your finger slightly more medially, and have the patient bear down again.

Indirect inguinal hernia, the most common type, will palpate as noticeable bulge with increased intraabdominal pressure. If the hernia presses your palpating finger anteriorly when the patient bears down, a direct inguinal hernia is the more likely cause. Perform the same inguinal hernia check for the opposite side.

Femoral hernias may be more easily detected with visualization than palpation. At the same location that you palpated the femoral pulse during your abdominal examination, inspect and palpate for the bulge of femoral hernia. Femoral hernias are the least common type of groin hernia, but the most common type in women. If the inguinal lymph nodes were not previously palpated as a part of the abdominal examination, do so now as a part of the male pelvic examination.

Inspect and Palpate the Perianal Area

The male rectal examination may be performed in a variety of patient positions: standing, knee chest, or lateral recumbent. However, the lateral recumbent position with the upper knee flexed is usually the most comfortable for the patient. Since most doctors are right handed, the patient is positioned in the left lateral position, also referred to as Sim's position. However, if you are left handed, you will probably want to palpate with your left hand, and the patient in the right lateral position.

Prior to performing the digital rectal examination, it is important to have a clean glove on your dominant hand. You can change your gloves, or most doctors find the 'double glove' procedure convenient. Place two clean gloves on your dominant hand at the beginning of the genital exam. Then when it is time to perform the rectal exam, remove the outer glove, leaving a clean glove for internal rectal palpation. This prevents external genital pathogens from being introduced into the rectum.

Inspect and palpate the sacrococcygeal and perianal areas for tenderness, rashes, lumps, rectal abscess, pilonidal cyst, or other visible pathology. Once you have removed the outer glove from your dominant hand, use your other hand for this palpation, and to spread the buttocks to visualize the anus. Have the patient bear down to inspect for rectal prolapse. If hemorrhoids or other rectal pathology are visible, the position is described using a numbers on a clock pattern, with 12 o'clock toward the symphysis pubis, and 6 o'clock near the coccyx.

Digital Rectal Palpation

With a clean glove on your dominant hand, apply KY jelly to your index finger. Place the pad of your lubricated index finger to the rectal sphincter, apply pressure, and wait for the muscle to relax. This usually takes only a second or two. While most texts advise having the patient bear down to relax the sphincter, the direct pressure and wait method is usually more comfortable for your patient. As the sphincter relaxes, slowly introduce your finger into the rectum. Rotate your finger 180 degrees, first in one direction, and then the other, to palpate the entire circumference of the rectal wall for polyps and masses. Colorectal carcinoma is the third leading cause of cancer in either sex. Many of these cancers are within the reach of the doctor's finger during the digital rectal examination. The American Cancer Society recommends that screening for colorectal carcinoma be performed every 3-5 years after age 50.

Some chiropractic techniques stress the importance of coccyx adjusting. The digital rectal examination provides the best palpation of coccyx position and mobility, however perform this palpation with care, as the coccyx may be tender. The digital rectal examination also provides the opportunity to directly palpate the tonicity of the inner surface of the piriformis muscle. This may be very clinically significant, considering that Dr. Janet Travell teaches that the piriformis syndrome is actually more common than a lumbar disc syndrome.

Prostate Palpation

Even though only the posterior wall of the prostate is palpable via the anterior wall of the rectum, most prostate cancer manifests here, making this is a very important examination in the male. With your palpating finger pointing toward the umbilicus, palpate the extent of each lateral margin as far as you can reach. With large patients you may have to exert considerable pressure down your arm to compress the buttock tissues enough to provide adequate penetration of your palpating finger. However, this pressure is exerted via the backs of your other fingers to the buttocks, with no additional pressure of your index finger on the prostate gland.

Once you have palpated the lateral margins, sweep your finger from margin to margin until you have palpated the entire surface of the prostate. Try to gauge the lateral size and how far the prostate gland protrudes into the rectum. The normal size of the prostate gland is 4 cm, with 1 cm protrusion into the rectum. Prostatic protrusion is graded:

Grade 1 = 1-2 cm protrusion
Grade 2 = 2-3 cm protrusion
Grade 3 = 3-4 cm protrusion
Grade 4 = > 4 cm protrusion

As you sweep from side to side you should readily palpate the median sulcus, and the lateral margins should be symmetric. Obliteration of the median sulcus suggests prostatic enlargement. Symmetrical enlargement is usually noncancerous, while asymmetrical enlargement is cause for concern. The normal consistency of the prostate gland is 'firm'. Various prostate conditions present characteristic findings:

Condition	Size	Consistency
Benign Hyperplasia	Nontender enlargement	Rubbery
Prostatitis	Tender enlargement	Boggy
Prostatic Carcinoma	Enlarged and irregular	Hard

Before removing your finger, assess sphincter tone by having the patient tighten around your finger. A lax sphincter may indicate neurological deficit. An overly tight sphincter may suggest stricture or spasm. Feces adherent to the gloved finger may be used to test for the presence of occult blood.

Summary of Physical Examination

Assessment of genitourinary conditions includes:

- Observation of general appearance for evidence of kidney dysfunction. A yellow brown skin without yellowing of the sclera suggests chronic uremia. Chronic kidney dysfunction may result in pale skin. Chronic hypertension due to kidney failure will cause edema.
- Measure vital signs: temperature, pulse, respiration, blood pressure. Temperature may be elevated with infection. Kidney failure will result in hypertension.
- Inspect the abdomen. Ascites and abdominal distention occur with kidney failure.
- Palpate and percuss the costovertebral angle. Murphy's kidney punch test introduces a jarring vibration to the upper urinary tract and is tender when inflammation is present.
- Percuss and palpate the abdomen. The kidneys are normally not large enough to be palpable. Polycystic kidneys are quite large. A distended bladder with urinary retention is typically painful upon palpation.
- Auscultate for bruits with the bell of your stethoscope. Renal hypertension may present with abdominal bruits over the renal arteries.
- When indicated, inspect and palpate the male external genitalia.
- Perform a digital rectal examination of the prostate gland.

Diagnostic Studies

- Routine UA
  - o Acid or alkaline urine favors the formation of certain types of kidney stones.
  - o Nitrites and leukocyte esterase are positive with bacterial infection.
  - o Kidney malfunction will cause spilling of protein in the urine.
  - o Renal tubular damage may result in glucose in the urine.
  - o Hematuria is present with kidney stones and some urinary infections.
  - o Microscopic visualization of the type of casts provides visual evidence of the anatomical location of renal disease.
- Urine culture and sensitivity (if infection is suspected).
- Sequential urine specimens may identify where along the urinary tract infection is present.
- Measurement of post voiding residual urine helps to quantify the severity of urinary retention.
- A gram stain of urinary discharge may identify the presence of gonococcal (gram negative intracellular diplococci) or nongonococcal organisms.
- Serum creatinine and BUN objectively measure kidney function.

- Prostatic Specific Antigen (PSA) will be elevated with benign prostatic hypertrophy (BPH) and prostatic carcinoma. Obviously the higher the number, the more likely the condition is cancerous.
- A KUB x-ray is considered a scout film for urological disorders, and may disclose kidney stones.
- An IVP x-ray may be required to visualize radiolucent kidney stones.
- Diagnostic ultrasound of urinary structures is often required to determine which structures require surgery.

Sample Documentation

Upon inspection, the pubic hair was free of nits and presented a normal male pattern. No lesions were visible on the glans or shaft of the penis. No hardenings or stricture were palpated in the penile shaft. The urinary meatus was patent, centrally located, and without evidence of urethral discharge. No rashes or skin lesions were observed on the scrotum. The testicles were of normal size and consistency. No varicocele or scrotal masses were palpable. No inguinal or femoral hernias were evident upon inspection or palpation. Palpation of the sacrococcygeal and perianal areas was free of lumps, lesions, or tenderness. No rashes or external hemorrhoids were visible at the anal sphincter. Sphincter tone was normal, and no polyps or masses were palpable within the rectum. The prostate gland was nontender, of normal size and firm consistency. The lateral margins were symmetric and the median sulcus was palpable. The stool was brown and a specimen was collected for hemocult testing.

Common Genitourinary & Male Conditions

Urinary Tract Infections (Merck Manual, p. 1884) (ICD: 595)

- Due to the longer route the bacteria must travel, urinary tract infection is much less common in males than females (1:50). The condition becomes more common after age fifty, usually as a consequence of prostate dysfunction. When UTI occurs in preadolescent males, a congenital stricture or anomaly is suspected. *E. coli* is the most common organism found upon bacterial culture.
- Symptoms include dysuria, frequency, urgency, nocturia, and low back pain. In addition to painful urination, the male may notice a discolored discharge on the underwear. A yellow discharge suggests a gonorrhea infection. Nongonococcal infection produces a clear to white discharge.
- Abdominal palpation may disclose suprapubic tenderness. Murphy's kidney punch test should be painfree. If not, the infection may have spread to the kidney (pyelonephritis). Examination of the external genitalia should be performed to ensure that no venereal lesions are present.
- Routine urinalysis will be positive for leucocyte esterase and nitrites. Urine culture and sensitivity testing will identify the causative organism and appropriate antibiotic. If the patient is a young,

sexually active male, STD cultures for gonorrhea and chlamydia should be performed. If STD is suspected, the patient should be counseled to avoid all sexual activity until it is confirmed that he is no longer infective.

- If the patient is elderly with symptoms of prostatitis, triple void urine specimens should be collected and sent for analysis.
- Urinary tract infections are usually cured with appropriate antibiotic therapy. Untreated UTI's may progress to pyelonephritis.
- Increasing fluid intake and cranberry juice or capsules are natural preventive measures. The herb goldenseal has a long history of documented effectiveness with microbial infection.

Urinary Calculi (Merck Manual, p. 1838) (ICD: 592.1)

- Renal calculi, or kidney stones are very common, affecting one tenth of all people at sometime in their life. Urine normally contains small amounts of dissolved solids, such as uric acid, calcium oxalate, or calcium phosphate. For reasons that are not clear, some individuals tend to form stones from these dissolved substances. Individuals with a family history of stones, or who have had previous episodes are more likely to develop kidney stones. The condition affects men more than women.
- Many stones are 'silent', passing without complication. When the stone is larger, it can become lodged in the ureter causing extreme pain. The costovertebral flank pain usually radiates to the groin region. The pain may become severe enough that nausea, vomiting, chills, and fever occur.
- Urinalysis will likely show hematuria, and possibly bacteriuria if an infection is present. Urine pH may be important. An alkaline pH favors the formation of calcium and phosphate crystals, while an acid pH may lead to uric acid or cystine crystals. Microscopic examination of the sediment will help identify the type of kidney stones present. When an infection is present, the CBC will show an elevated white count with a shift to the left. A chem screen may disclose nothing, but it should still be checked for alteration of calcium, phosphorus, and uric acid. It is unlikely that uremia (increased BUN and creatinine) will be present.
- Kidney stones usually show up on a KUB x-ray, however uric acid crystals are radiolucent, and an intravenous pyelogram (IVP) may be needed to visualize these stones.
- Most kidney stones pass within a few days and do not require surgery. A complete obstruction of the ureter can result in hydronephrosis. When the pain is persistent and severe, lithotripsy or ureteroscopic surgery may be required.
- Prevention is the key. Magnesium and vitamin B6 decrease the production and excretion of oxalates. Drink at least 2 quarts of water a day. The juice of two fresh lemons daily is a folk remedy that may prevent future stone formation.

Obstructive Uropathy (ICD: 593.4)

Structural or functional changes in the urinary tract that hinder normal urine flow, sometimes leading to renal dysfunction (obstructive nephropathy). (Merck Manual, p. 1827)

- Obstructive uropathy can be acute or chronic, and unilateral or bilateral. The condition is more common in elderly males, due to the constriction imposed by benign prostatic hyperplasia. When bilateral obstruction occurs in women, cystocele is a probable cause. When the condition is unilateral, a kidney stone is the most likely cause.
- It is important that the obstruction is dealt with, as the increased pressure on the kidney will cause hydronephrosis. With urinary stasis, urinary tract infection becomes more likely.
- Treatment must be directed at the cause. In the short term, catheterization to relieve the fluid accumulation may be necessary. Kidney stones may require ultrasound lithotripsy or surgery. Untreated obstruction will eventually cause kidney failure.

Nephritic Syndrome (Acute Glomerulonephritis) (ICD: 580)

A syndrome characterized pathologically by diffuse inflammatory changes in the glomeruli and clinically by abrupt-onset hematuria with RBC casts, mild proteinuria, and, often, hypertension, edema, and azotemia. (Merck Manual, p. 1856)

- Acute glomerulonephritis is more common in children than adults, and usually develops after a recent streptococcal infection. A few weeks after the onset of infection, the patient may suddenly experience headaches (from hypertension), abdominal pain and costovertebral angle tenderness. The face swells (periorbital edema), and the patient manifests hematuria. These symptoms last for several days, and the condition gradually improves within a few weeks.
- Depending upon how recent the prior strep infection is, the Antistreptolysin O titer may or may not be elevated. It may take as long as one month for the ASO titer to rise. Urinalysis will show hematuria and proteinuria. Microscopic examination of the sediment will show RBC casts. The CBC may show anemia. As kidney function becomes compromised, azotemia (increased serum creatinine and BUN) may manifest. If more precise measurement of kidney function is needed, a 24 hour creatinine clearance ratio will assess the glomerular filtration rate (GFR).
- The individual will likely be hospitalized for IV antibiotic therapy and symptomatic treatment of edema and hypertension. A low protein and low sodium diet will lessen the burden on the kidneys. It is possible that mild hematuria after exercise will manifest for up to two years following the infection.

Chronic Nephritic-Proteinuric Syndrome
(Chronic Glomerulonephritis) (ICD: 582)

A syndrome caused by several diseases of different etiologies, characterized pathologically by diffuse sclerosis of glomeruli and clinically by proteinuria, cylindruria, hematuria, usually hypertension, and insidious loss of renal function over years. (Merck Manual, p. 1864)

- Chronic glomerulonephritis, a condition of adults, is usually unrelated to previous acute glomerulonephritis episodes. Mild chronic glomerulonephritis may be asymptomatic, discovered when proteinuria, and possibly hematuria, is found during a routine urinalysis. When the condition is not detected early, and is no longer mild, symptoms of kidney failure manifest: anorexia, fatigue, anemia, and hypertension. The most common causes of chronic kidney disease are atherosclerosis, diabetes, and hypertension.
- When there is hematuria, the patient may notice brown, or rust colored urine. As proteinuria increases, the urine may become foamy. As with acute glomerulonephritis, there is moderate proteinuria, however the casts found in urine sediment are fine granular and waxy. As erythropoietin production becomes compromised, the CBC will show anemia. The chem screen will show azotemia.
- Treatment will be geared to the underlying cause. Because hypertension may be an effect as well as a cause of chronic glomerulonephritis, it may be difficult to control. Salt, protein and fluid may need to be restricted if the patient is in kidney failure. Dialysis will likely be required until kidney function returns or a transplant donor can be found.

Nephrotic Syndrome (ICD: 581)

A predictable complex that results from a severe, prolonged increase in glomerular permeability for protein. (Merck Manual, p. 1865)

- Nephrotic syndrome, also known as nephrosis, occurs when the glomerular filtration system of the kidney fails to retain protein. There are a variety of causes for this malfunction, such as: idiopathic minimal change disease (lipoid nephrosis), focal segmental glomerulosclerosis, or membranous glomerulonephritis. While the condition may occur at any age, minimal change disease, the most common cause of nephrotic syndrome, occurs primarily in children. Diabetes is the most common cause for nephrotic syndrome in adults.
- The kidney damage results in markedly increased protein loss in the urine (> 3.5 G / 24 hours). The excess protein in the urine may manifest as 'frothy' urine. This loss of protein in turn causes hypoalbuminemia, which produces generalized edema. The edema is typically mobile, manifesting as puffy eyes when recumbent, and swelling of the ankles after standing for a while. Fluid accumulation in the lungs may cause shortness of breath, with crackles heard upon auscultation.

- Urinalysis will disclose marked proteinuria, and microscopic examination of the sediment will show fatty, granular, hyaline casts. A 24 hour specimen collection of urine will contain greater than 3.5 grams of protein. The chem screen may disclose an underlying fat metabolism problem (increased cholesterol and triglycerides). Serum albumin will be decreased, and uremia may be present.
- If the cause is treatable, which is usually the case with children, the prognosis is good. Many times the condition responds to corticosteroid medicine. In adults, when nephrotic syndrome is due to some other underlying pathology, such as an immune disorder, the prognosis is less favorable, and the condition may progress to end stage renal disease.

Acute Renal Failure (ICD: 584.0)

Clinical conditions associated with rapid (days to weeks), steadily decreasing renal function (azotemia), with or without oliguria. (Merck Manual, p. 1841)

- Acute renal failure has three main causes:
    o Prerenal azotemia may occur with disorders having decreased renal perfusion, such as uncontrolled diarrhea or hemorrhage (fluid depletion), and cardiomyopathy (low cardiac output).
    o Intrinsic renal damage may result from drugs or other nephrotoxins, such as streptococcal infection.
    o Postrenal azotemia is seen with conditions that block urine outflow, such as ureteral or bladder obstruction.
- Symptoms reflect the underlying causes.
    o Patients with fluid depletion will manifest thirst, decreased urine output, dizziness and orthostatic hypotension.
    o Patients in cardiac failure with low cardiac output will have orthopnea and paroxysmal nocturnal dyspnea.
    o Acute glomerulonephritis manifests as with the triad of hematuria, edema, and hypertension.
    o Prostatic obstruction is a common cause of postrenal azotemia, and manifests as urinary frequency, urgency, and hesitancy.
- Upon examination, the patient may manifest oliguria or anuria. Generalized fluid retention and swelling is likely.
- While the 24 hour creatinine clearance ratio is the usual method of assessing glomerular filtration rate and kidney function, in the emergency setting, immediate clinical decisions will likely be made using serum creatinine. Microscopic examination of urinary sediment may help diagnose intrinsic renal disease. Additional testing will be geared to identifying the underlying cause of kidney failure.
- Emergency dialysis has greatly decreased the mortality previously associated with acute renal failure. If the patient is young and otherwise healthy, such as with acute glomerulonephritis, the

prognosis is good. However, with older patients having cardiomyopathy, the prognosis is poor.

Chronic Renal Failure (ICD: 585)

The clinical condition resulting from chronic derangement and insufficiency of renal excretory and regulatory function (uremia). (Merck Manual, p. 1845)

- Chronic renal failure is a pattern of symptoms that manifest when kidney function is compromised from a variety of causes, such as diabetes, hypertension, polycystic kidney disease, or nephrotoxic drugs. While it can occur in young people, it is predominantly a condition of adults and shows no sex predilection.
- The edema that manifests may reflect an underlying hypertensive condition. Uremia may produce pruritis, dry skin, and a metallic taste in the mouth. Compromised erythropoietin production by the kidney may cause pallor, anemia, and fatigue.
- The CBC may manifest normochromic, normocytic anemia and thrombocytopenia. As kidney function becomes compromised, the chem panel will likely show increased BUN, creatinine, triglycerides, potassium, phosphorus, and uric acid.
- When kidney function worsens, the individual must receive hemodialysis or peritoneal dialysis, which will need to be continued indefinitely until a compatible kidney donor is found for transplantation.

Polycystic Kidney Disease (ICD: 753.13)

Inherited disorders characterized by many bilateral renal cysts that increase renal size but reduce functioning renal tissue. (Merck Manual, p. 1903)

- Polycystic kidney disease is an autosomal dominant condition that affects about one in 1,000 people. Initially the condition is asymptomatic. The earlier the condition manifests the poorer the prognosis.
- When the condition becomes symptomatic, the individual may notice blood in the urine, excessive urination at night, flank pain, and abdominal pain or tenderness. As kidney function becomes more compromised, hypertension develops that is difficult to control.
- Urinalysis may show pyuria, even in the absence of infection. The hematocrit and RBC count may be either decreased or increased depending upon how the cysts affect erythropoietin production.
- Abdominal ultrasound, CT, or MRI will confirm the presence of multiple cysts on the kidneys. About 50% of people with polycystic kidney disease also have cysts on the liver.
- There is no medical treatment for polycystic kidney disease. As kidney function continues to decline, the individual will eventually require dialysis and kidney transplantation. Up to 10% of patients

with polycystic kidney disease have an associated cerebral aneurysm. As hypertension becomes more pronounced, at least half of these individuals will experience a rupture of this aneurysm by age 50.

Benign Prostatic Hyperplasia (BPH) (ICD: 600)

Benign adenomatous hyperplasia of the periurethral prostate gland, causing variable degrees of bladder outlet obstruction. (Merck Manual, p. 1829)

- Prostate dysfunction is very common in males over fifty. The saying goes, "*It is not if you are going to have trouble, but when you are going to have trouble with your prostate.*" It is estimated that 95% of men over age 80 have BPH.
- While the hyperplastic tissue is benign, the growth of tissue can still result in significant urinary obstruction. Symptoms include frequency, urgency, and a sense of incomplete emptying of the bladder. Nocturia and back pain may manifest.
- Upon examination, abdominal palpation may disclose a distended bladder. Digital rectal examination (DRE) of the prostate will manifest smooth, symmetrical enlargement with a rubbery nontender consistency. The median sulcus may be less palpable.
- A CBC and routine UA should be performed to check for infection. If urinary retention has been long standing, a chem screen to assess kidney function would be a wise precaution.
- A PSA should be performed. Some labs recommend that you draw the blood sample before the DRE, as prostatic massage might cause a false elevation of the PSA. Ravel recommends that if the DRE is performed first, the blood specimen should be drawn within one hour, to minimize this effect. BPH can cause an elevated PSA, although this number will usually be less than 10 micrograms/liter. When the PSA is greater than 10, carcinoma is much more likely.
- Medical management of BPH usually involves the drug Proscar. If the condition is pronounced, or does not respond to conservative care, transurethral resection of the prostate (TURP) will be performed.
- Natural therapeutics are very effective with BPH. Zinc, essential fatty acids, and the amino acids glycine and glutamic acid are documented to help with BPH. The herb Saw Palmetto was actually found to be more effective than the drug Proscar in the treatment of BPH.

Prostatitis (Merck Manual, p. 1831) (ICD: 601)

- Infection of the prostate gland may be either acute or chronic. Typically it is usually caused by an upward migration of a urethral infection. While the organism may be nonbacterial, such as *Chlamydia*, it is more commonly caused by *Escherichia coli*, *Proteus*, or *Enterococcus*.
- Symptoms may include signs of infection (fever, chills, malaise), in addition to urethral discharge, dysuria, and a dull pain in the perineal area, or low back pain. If the condition is chronic, the systemic

symptoms of infection may be subtle or absent. In addition to dribbling, and hesitancy, the male may have testicular pain and painful ejaculation.

- With acute prostatitis, signs of a fever may be present. The prostate will be very tender upon palpation, and will be slightly enlarged, and and manifest a 'boggy' consistency. Chronic prostatitis may be relatively asymptomatic, and the prostate may be only mildly tender upon palpation.

- Lab testing includes a triple void urine specimen (initial, mid stream, after prostatic massage) for culture and antibiotic sensitivity. A routine CBC and UA are also indicated. If the condition is chronic, kidney function may be compromised, and a chem screen to include BUN and creatinine is needed.

- Referral for antibiotic treatment is indicated, with monthly urine cultures until infection is no longer present.

Prostate Cancer (Merck Manual, p. 1918) (ICD: 185)

- Prostate cancer is the second leading cause of cancer in men, causing as many deaths in men as breast cancer does in women. The condition is rare before age 50. Symptoms include frequency, urgency, dysuria, and low back pain. While at least 90% of low back pain is due to mechanical causes, you must always be alert to possible organic causes for your patient's pain.

- Upon digital rectal examination a hard nodule may be palpable on the prostate. The lateral margins may be asymmetric, and the median sulcus less palpable.

- A CBC should be performed. If the cancer has metastasized, anemia may occur. Serum acid phosphatase and alkaline phosphatase will also be elevated with metastasis.

- While some consider the PSA (Prostatic Specific Antigen) test to be controversial, it actually has a higher predictive value than mammography. This test should be used by all doctors interested in preventive health care as PSA serum levels begin to rise two decades before the clinical detection of cancer (NEJM, 2003;349:299).

- Additional diagnostic testing includes transrectal ultrasound to visualize the tumor and a bone scan to quantify the extent of metastasis. When a tumor is biopsied, the Gleason scoring system is the grading method used measure the severity and progression of prostate cancer.

- Prostate cancer treatment is also controversial. Many consider 'watchful waiting' preferable to surgery, radiation, and hormonal therapy (JAMA, 269(20):2650-8 1993 May 26).

Urinary Incontinence (ICD: 788.3)

The involuntary leakage of urine. (Merck Manual, p. 1815)

- Urinary incontinence is never normal, however incontinence may be due to functional, rather than anatomic causes. The condition is quite common in women, affecting 26% of women during their reproductive years, and 30-40% of post menopausal women.

- Stress incontinence occurs when the individual coughs, laughs, or sneezes and dribbles a small quantity of urine. Women who have had children, are more at risk, due to the weakening of the pelvic floor musculature. Atrophy of vaginal tissues with menopause, also predisposes to stress incontinence. Males with prostate dysfunction may also experience dribbling.

- Urge incontinence manifests as an inability to delay urination. For whatever reason, the sphincter is unable to remain closed until reaching the bathroom. Infection or allergies may make the sphincter hypersensitive, and conditions such as MS or stroke may result in decreased sphincter tone.

- The detrusor muscle is the external muscular layer of the bladder. When the bladder fills, stretch of this muscle normally triggers a synergistic relaxation of the sphincter muscle. Diabetic neuropathy, spinal cord injury, prostatic obstruction, and some drugs may interfere with this function and cause overflow incontinence.

- Functional causes of incontinence are transient and reversible. Enuresis may have psychological elements, but subluxation and management of food allergies may be key to resolution of the problem. Constipation or fecal impaction exert mechanical pressure on the urethra resulting in temporary overflow incontinence. Urinary tract infection will make the sphincter hypersensitive and result in transient urge incontinence.

- Treatment must be directed at the cause. The patient should undergo routine urinalysis to check for infection. If infection is present, a urine culture will identify the causative organism and appropriate antibiotic. Kegel pelvic floor exercises may help with outlet incompetence. If overflow incontinence is suspected, a post voiding catheterization will quantify residual urinary retention. Normally less than 50 ml will result. If greater than 200 ml is found post voiding, the urologist may instruct the patient in self catheterization to deal with residual urinary retention.

Neurogenic Bladder (ICD: 596)

Vesical dysfunction resulting from a congenital abnormality, injury, or disease process of the brain, spinal cord, or local nerve supply to the urinary bladder and its outlet. (Merck Manual, p. 1825)

- As a chiropractor, neurogenic bladder is something you must never fail to recognize. The consequences of missing this diagnosis can be catastrophic to your patient's health and your career. When bladder innervation is dysfunctional, a hypotonic or hypertonic bladder may result.

- A flaccid hypotonic bladder will be distended and result in overflow incontinence. If the condition is chronic, urinary tract infection is common. The nerve compression of a cauda equina syndrome may manifest as neurogenic overflow incontinence.

- A spastic hypertonic bladder may manifest as urge incontinence or spontaneous emptying of the bladder.
- All patients under your care for a lumbar disc syndrome should be instructed to notify you immediately, should they begin to experience urinary retention or incontinence.

Erectile Dysfunction (ICD: V41.7)

The inability to attain or sustain an erection satisfactory for coitus. (Merck Manual, p. 1836)

- Erectile dysfunction is the medical term for what is commonly referred to as 'impotence'. Erection requires psychological stimulation, intact neurological sensation, as well as adequate arterial circulation to the penis. A deficit in any one of these can inhibit the ability to maintain an erection.
- Males normally achieve 5-6 erections per night while asleep. If the male is able to achieve an erection while asleep, the disorder may be psychological. Erectile dysfunction in young males is most often the result of 'performance anxiety'.
- As males age, testosterone levels decline, which in turn causes a diminished libido. Occasionally the problem is due to alcohol intoxication. As Shakespeare wrote, "*Alcohol provokes the desire, but it takes away the performance.*"
- Conditions such as diabetes and MS can damage nerve sensation. It is not uncommon for prostate surgery to damage the nerve supply to the penis.
- The older the male, the more likely the impairment is physical, rather than psychological. Atherosclerosis of the penile arteries may restrict blood flow to the penis. Impotence is a side effect of many cardiac drugs.
- The urological workup may be brief or quite involved. At a minimum the evaluation will include a chem screen, CBC, and UA. Assessment of pituitary and thyroid function may be indicated. Specialized testing that assesses penile circulation and nerve function may be required to quantify the deficit.
- Medical treatment will likely take three avenues:
  o Psychological counseling
  o Medical management (including drugs such as testosterone and Viagra)
  o Surgery (penile implants)
- The herb *Yohimbine* is actually an FDA approved 'drug' for the treatment of impotence. The herb *Ginkgo biloba* promotes vasodilation and is often beneficial with circulatory conditions.

Priapism (ICD: 607.3)

Painful, persistent, and abnormal erection, unaccompanied by sexual desire or excitation. (Merck Manual, p. 1833)

- Priapus was the Greek god of fertility. Priapism is the name given to prolonged, painful erection not associated with sexual stimulation. While sickle cell anemia and spinal cord injury can cause this condition, the drug Viagra will also cause this condition. Medical referral is indicated, as permanent damage to the erectile tissue of the penis may result if the condition persists for more than a few hours.

Peyronie's Disease (ICD: 607.89)

Fibrosis of the cavernous sheaths leading to contracture of the investing fascia of the corpora, not unlike Dupuytren's contracture, resulting in deviated and painful erection. (Merck Manual, p. 1833)

- For reasons that are not clear, men over 45 may develop fibrotic hardening in the corpus cavernosum. During erection the penis will bend toward the side of the fibrotic tissue. The condition may be painful, and if severe will make intercourse impossible. Vitamin E supplementation may help mild cases, but severe Peyronie's disease will probably require surgery.

Phimosis and Paraphimosis (Merck Manual, p. 2229) (ICD: 605)

- Phimosis refers to a constriction of the terminal foreskin making it difficult or impossible for the foreskin to retract. When the tightened foreskin retracts but will not return to the extended position, paraphimosis results. If paraphimosis restriction is cutting off blood circulation to the glans, an emergency surgical circumcision is required.

Hypospadias and Epispadias (Merck Manual, p. 2228) (ICD: 752.6)

- A congenital defect may manifest as an inappropriately placed urinary meatus. When the opening is displaced ventrally toward the scrotum, this is hypospadias. Less commonly, the opening may be displaced dorsally, referred to as epispadias.

Genital Herpes (ICD: 054.10)

Infection of the genital or anorectal skin or mucous membranes by either of two closely related herpes simplex viruses (HSV-1 or HSV-2). (Merck Manual, p. 1337)

- Genital herpes, also known as herpes progenitalis and venereal herpes, is usually caused by the HSV2 virus, very similar to the HSV1 virus that causes oral herpes. It is very common, affecting about one in four adults, although most of these individuals do not realize they are infected. The initial outbreak is usually the most severe. Approximately 40% never experience a second attack. The virus remains dormant and the individual may experience recurrent attacks, especially at times of stress, for the remainder of life. The lesions present as a cluster of small vesicles that are usually painful. Within a few days the vesicles burst, leaving small shallow ulcers that heal within a few weeks. All sexual contact should be avoided when the lesions are present, as they are highly infective.

Penile Cancer (Merck Manual, p. 1920) (ICD: 187)

- Penile carcinoma is rare, occurring primarily in uncircumcised males. It presents as a nontender ulcer on the corona of the glans penis that is similar in appearance to syphilitic chancre or genital warts. A biopsy is required to determine if the lesion is cancerous. Surgical excision of the lesion does not usually interfere with urinary or sexual function.

Disorders of the Scrotum

Cryptorchidism (Merck Manual p. 2229) (ICD: 752.5)

- In the fetus, the testicles grow within the abdomen. Soon before birth the testicles descend into the scrotum. Approximately 3% of male babies have an undescended testicle. The condition is more common on the right, and the infant will present with an empty half of the scrotum. Many of these will correct spontaneously within a month of birth. If the testicle still has not descended at one year, surgery should be considered. When the testicle remains in the abdomen, infertility is more likely and early detection of testicular cancer becomes impossible.

Small Testis (Merck Manual, p. 2239) (ICD: 758.7)

- Adult testes normally range between 4-5 cm long. When they are less than 3.5 cm long they are considered small. Small soft testes suggests testicular atrophy from a variety of conditions, such as cirrhosis, hypopituitarism, or as a consequence of estrogen therapy. Very small testis (less than 2 cm long) with normal firm consistency may be due to Klinefelter's syndrome (hypogonadism caused by XXY chromosomal inheritance).

Testicular Torsion (Merck Manual, p. 2230) (ICD: 608.2)

- The testes are normally anchored within the scrotal sac. When this is not the case, the testicle may rotate enough to cut off blood supply to the testicle. It is most common during the teenage years. Symptoms include sudden onset of pain, and possibly nausea and vomiting. Upon palpation, the scrotum and cord may be swollen and elevation of the testicle may increase the pain. If not corrected surgically within a few hours, the testicle will die.

Orchitis (Merck Manual, p. 2326) (ICD: 604)

- Orchitis is an inflammation of an entire testicle. While the most common cause is mumps, it may also be a consequence of an STD infection. The testis will be swollen and tender to palpation. Tissue edema may make palpation of the epididymis difficult. There may be an associated hydrocele that transilluminates. Antibiotics are indicated for STD infections. Mumps is a self limiting viral condition that needs only supportive therapy.

Varicocele (Merck Manual, p. 1834) (ICD: 456.4)

- Varicocele is a tortuous dilation of the spermatic veins. It is more common on the left and is usually discovered in early adolescence. It palpates as a 'bag of worms' that diminishes when the young man moves from the standing to the supine position. The poor blood drainage is thought to increase testicular temperature, which may lead to infertility. Treatment is surgical ligation of the spermatic vein.

Spermatocele (Merck Manual, p. 1834) (ICD: 608.1)

- Spermatocele is a fluid filled mass in the epididymis. It palpates as a small (the size of a pea), painless, movable lump, located above and behind the testicle. Being fluid filled, it passes light with transillumination. When it is large it may appear similar to hydrocele and is surgically removed.

Hydrocele (Merck Manual, p. 1834) (ICD: 603.9)

- The testicle is bathed in fluid to allow it to move freely. If this fluid accumulates in excess, a hydrocele (water tumor) manifests. When seen in infancy it usually resolves spontaneously. In older males, it may develop as a consequence of trauma or infection. The mass palpates as a painless swelling, that transilluminates, and feels 'heavy' to the patient. The ability to palpate above the mass distinguishes this condition from a scrotal hernia. The physician may choose to aspirate the fluid with a needle, which confirms the diagnosis. If the fluid reaccumulates, surgical removal of the sac may be necessary.

Epididymitis (Merck Manual, p. 1835) (ICD: 604)

- Epididymitis is usually a consequence of an STD infection. In older men epididymitis may accompany prostatitis. Tuberculosis is another cause of chronic epididymitis.
- The scrotum is enlarged and tender. Palpation is extremely tender, however the pain may be somewhat relieved by raising the testicle (as contrasted to increased pain with elevation of testicular torsion). Urination may be painful and a discharge may be present. If the infection is pronounced a fever may be present.
- Routine urinalysis will disclose pyuria. Urine culture to identify the causative organism and antibiotic sensitivity testing will be conducted. The CBC will likely show leukocytosis.
- The antibiotic of choice depends upon the organism identified. Appropriate antibiotic treatment is usually curative. If the condition

becomes chronic and spreads to the testis (orchitis), infertility may result.

Testicular Cancer (Merck Manual, p. 1920) (ICD: 186)

- While testicular cancer is rare overall (1% of all male cancer), it is the most common form of cancer in males age 20-34. When detected early, the cure rate approaches 100%, which highlights the importance of testicular self examination (TSE). Early testicular cancer appears as a painless nodule on or within the testicle. As the neoplasm grows, the nodularity spreads where it may replace the entire testicle. The cancerous testicle will be larger than the normal side, and the patient may remark that it feels 'heavy'. Surgical removal of the cancerous testicle is usually curative, and does not affect fertility if the remaining testis is viable.

Hernias (Merck Manual, p. 1834)

Scrotal Hernia (ICD: 550)

- Embryologically, the testicles develop within the abdomen. Later they migrate through the inguinal canal into the scrotum. The persistence of this canal provides for the spermatic cord, as well as arterial and venous circulation to the testes. When this opening is too large, a loop of bowel may protrude through into the scrotum. Usually scrotal hernias are 'indirect', passing through both the internal and external inguinal rings. Most hernias are 'reducible', easily pushed back into the abdominal cavity. When incarcerated or not reducible, or when they continually recur, surgical repair is indicated. Ninety percent of all hernias occur in men, and hernia repair is the most common surgery performed on men.

Indirect Inguinal Hernia (ICD: 550)

- Indirect inguinal hernias is the most common type, comprising 60% of all hernias. The condition is often congenital, affecting 1-2% of infant males. The hernia passes down the inguinal canal and exits at the external inguinal ring. Upon examination, the hernia presses the tip of the palpating finger.

Direct Inguinal Hernia (ICD: 550)

- Direct inguinal hernia is less common, usually acquired from obesity or heavy lifting. The hernia does not pass through the inguinal canal, but exits 'directly' through the external inguinal ring. The hernia presses the palpating finger anteriorly when the patient coughs or bears down.

Femoral Hernia (ICD: 553.0)

- Although located in the inguinal region, femoral hernia is not an inguinal hernia. It is the least common groin hernia, and occurs primarily in obese women who have had several pregnancies. A femoral hernia is visualized as well as palpated. It presents as a bulge lateral and inferior to the external inguinal ring, at the site of the femoral pulse.

Study Guide Objectives

o   Know the anatomy of external and internal male genitalia.
o   Which structures are considered to be accessory glandular structures?
o   What structure forms the glans penis?
o   What is smegma?
o   Know the function of the cremaster muscle.
o   Know the structures that produce and provide transport for sperm.
o   Why is the pH of Cowper's bulbourethral gland secretions important?
o   What is the approximate size of the normal prostate gland?
o   Know the neurological control (voluntary vs. involuntary) of the external and internal anal sphincters.
o   Where are the testes located during fetal development?
o   Which sex is more likely to experience a urinary tract infection? Why?
o   Which kidney condition is primarily a condition of children?
o   What does nocturia suggest?
o   What is 'total hematuria' and what conditions cause it?
o   What does a yellow green urethral discharge suggest?
o   What does the triad of urethritis, arthritis, and conjunctivitis suggest?
o   Which STD infection causes painful genital lesions?
o   Which testicular masses pass light upon transillumination?
o   What are three causes of erectile dysfunction? The drug Viagra is used for which type of erectile dysfunction?
o   What is a side effect of hydrochlorothiazide blood pressure medicine?
o   What is the purpose of 'double gloving' during the male genital examination?
o   What is the difference in genital hair pattern in males vs. females?
o   What is the difference between phimosis and paraphimosis?
o   What is the difference between epispadias and hypospadias?
o   Why is it important to inspect the corona of the glans penis?
o   What is the normal consistency of the testicles?
o   What is the significance of decreased pain sensation of the testicles?
o   Where is the epididymis located?
o   If a structure within the scrotum palpates as a 'bag of worms' what does this indicate?
o   What is the most common type of groin hernia in males? in females?
o   What is Sim's position?
o   What is the third leading cause of cancer in either sex?
o   According to Dr. Janet Travell, what low back condition is more common than a lumbar disc syndrome?
o   Which surface of the prostate gland is palpable via digital rectal examination? How is this significant in relation to prostate cancer?

- If the median sulcus of the prostate gland is not palpable, what does this suggest?
- What does asymmetrical enlargement of the prostate gland suggest?
- Know the size and consistency palpation findings for a normal prostate gland, benign prostatic hyperplasia, prostatitis, and prostatic carcinoma.
- Both jaundice and uremia cause yellowing of the skin. How does each of these two conditions affect the sclera of the eye?
- In males, why does urinary tract infection become more common after age 50?
- Which type of kidney stones are radiolucent and do not show up on a routine KUB x-ray? How are these stones visualized?
- What are the nutritional measures used to prevent the formation of kidney stones?
- What is the most likely cause of unilateral obstructive uropathy?
- In males, what causes bilateral obstructive uropathy?
- What is the older terminology for nephritic syndrome? In what age category is this condition most common?
- What type of infection usually causes nephritic syndrome?
- What is azotemia?
- What is the older terminology for chronic nephritic-proteinuric syndrome?
- What are the three most common causes of chronic kidney disease?
- What does brown or rust colored urine indicate?
- What does foamy urine indicate?
- Why do some kidney diseases cause anemia?
- What kidney condition is characterized by massive proteinuria (> 3.5 grams in 24 hours)?
- When this condition occurs in adults, what is the most common cause?
- Why does a patient with kidney disease manifest generalized edema?
- Know the three main causes of acute renal failure.
- Know the difference between prerenal azotemia vs. postrenal azotemia.
- Acute glomerulonephritis manifests with the triad of _____, _____, and _____.
- What is the significance of itchy, dry skin, and a metallic taste in the mouth?
- What kidney condition is inherited, affecting about one in 1,000 people?
- Up to 10% of individuals with this inherited condition have what associated abnormality, which is of concern to the chiropractor who may want to adjust their neck?
- Approximately how common is benign prostatic hyperplasia (BPH) in elderly males?
- What is the lab test used to assess function of the prostate gland?
- What is the herb that has been found to be more effective than the drug Proscar in the treatment of BPH?

- Which test has a higher predictive value in the detection of cancer: the PSA test or breast mammography?
- What is the name of the scoring system used to grade the severity and progression of prostate cancer?
- Why are post menopausal women more at risk for stress incontinence?
- What is overflow incontinence and what condition is it a danger signal for?
- What is the medical term for impotence?
- What is Peyronie's disease?
- Genital herpes is usually caused by which virus?
- What are the consequences of not correcting an undescended testicle?
- What is Klinefelter's syndrome?
- What is the most common cause of orchitis?
- A fluid filled mass in the epididymis referred to as _____.
- What is the most common form of cancer in males age 20-34?
- What is the most common form of scrotal hernia?
- Know the differences between the three types of groin hernias.

13 – Female & GYN disorders

Anatomy & Physiology

The structures of female external genitalia are collectively referred to as the vulva. Overlying the symphysis pubis is a hair covered fat pad called the mons pubis. Inferior to the mons pubis are the labia majora and labia minora. The area encircled by the labia minora is the vestibule. The clitoris, a small pea shaped expansion of erectile tissue located superior to the union of the labia minora, contains sensory nerve fibers very similar to those found on the male penis. The urethral meatus is located in the superior portion of the vestibule. Inferior to this opening are Skene's paraurethral glands. The vaginal orifice occupies the inferior portion of the vestibule. The openings of Bartholin's vestibular glands are lateral and inferior to the vaginal orifice. These glands secrete the clear lubricating fluid that is needed during sexual intercourse. The area between the vestibule and anus is the perineum.

The vagina, the first part of the internal genitalia, is a long tubular canal positioned between the urinary bladder and rectum. As such, the anterior wall is referred to as the vesicovaginal septum and the posterior wall is referred to as the rectovaginal septum. The vaginal walls greatly expand during childbirth, and the folds in this expansile tissue are rugae. At the end of the vagina, the uterus is positioned at a right angle toward the anterior. The cervix is the inferior portion of the uterus that is visible at the terminal end of the vagina. The cervical os is where the vaginal squamous epithelial tissues meet the uterine columnar epithelium. Pap smear specimens are collected at this squamocolumnar junction. When viewed from the anterior, the uterus is a pear shaped structure attached only at the inferior neck of the uterus. The superior fundus of the uterus is freely movable. As such, the uterus may easily become malpositioned in a retroflexed or retroverted position. Adnexa is the collective term for the ovaries and fallopian tubes lateral and superior to the body of the uterus. The ovaries produce female hormones, in addition to the eggs which will become an embryo when fertilized by sperm. The fallopian tubes provide the passage way from the ovaries to the superior body of the uterus.

Nature of the Patient

Vaginitis may be related to a lack of estrogen, either in prepubertal or postmenopausal females. Bacterial vaginosis is the most common cause of vaginal discharge in postpubertal females. When bacterial vaginal infection occurs in young girls prior to menarche, sexual abuse should be investigated. While pelvic inflammatory disease can occur at any age, it is most common among sexually active teenagers. Cervical cancer is most common between 30 and 50 years of age. Uterine fibroid tumors become progressively more common in the later child bearing years.

Key History Questions

Tell me about your menstrual periods?

- *When was the first day of your last menstrual period (LMP)?* Amenorrhea can be either primary (lack of menarche in a woman at least 16 years of age), or secondary (cessation of menses in a woman who has previously experienced normal menses). Pregnancy is the most likely cause of secondary amenorrhea. When a woman of childbearing age experiences amenorrhea, an hCG pregnancy test should be performed. Menstrual cessation can also occur in women involved in intensive athletic activity, or with severe caloric restriction (anorexia). If the cause is still not identified, endocrine studies may be required.

- *How old were you when you began menstruating?* Most women begin menstruating between 12 and 14 years of age. Early menarche <u>may</u> be a sign of excess estrogen production, which is a breast cancer risk factor. Late menarche <u>may</u> indicate low levels of estrogen, which is an osteoporosis risk factor.

- *How frequent are your periods, and how long to they last?* While the average cycle is 28 days, the normal range may be as short as 18 days or as long as 45 days. Women living in a dormitory may experience 'menstrual synchrony'. The duration of flow averages from 3 to 7 days.

- *How heavy is your flow?* Menorrhagia (heavy menstrual bleeding), or bleeding longer than eight days may be a sign of uterine fibroids or hormonal excess. About one third of the 600,000 hysterectomies performed each year are to treat menorrhagia. Heavy menstrual flow is documented in terms of the number of pads or tampons used per hour or day. Prolonged uterine bleeding will cause iron deficiency anemia.

- *Do you experience cramping or pain with your period?* Dysmenorrhea is common, affecting the majority of women at some time. It is thought that vasoconstriction causes uterine muscle hypoxia, which in turn leads to the production of pain causing prostaglandins. Supplemental magnesium may help. All cases of dysmenorrhea should receive a pelvic examination to rule out more serious conditions, such as ectopic pregnancy, uterine fibroids, or endometriosis.

Have you ever been pregnant?

- Obstetric history includes:
    - Gravida - the number of pregnancies
    - Para - the number of live births
    - Abortions - includes miscarriage and elective abortion

How often do you have a gynecological checkup?

- Gynecologic history includes documentation of previous GYN examinations, Pap smear test results, as well as previous surgeries such as dilation and curettage (D & C), tubal ligation, or hysterectomy.
- *Do you recall your mother ever mentioning taking DES hormones while she was pregnant with you?* Prenatal exposure to diethylstilbestrol (DES) hormones can cause cervical and vaginal abnormalities.

Have your periods slowed down or stopped?

- Menopause or cessation of menses normally occurs between age 45 to 55. The natural decrease in estrogen production can result in 'hot flashes', night sweats, nervousness, fatigue, mood swings, and vaginal dryness and itching. While the studies regarding the safety and efficacy of estrogen replacement therapy (ERT) are not conclusive, many women obtain relief from the symptoms of menopause with supplemental ERT. Herbal estrogen precursors, such as Wild Yam (Dioscorea) may help the body to produce more estrogen.

Do you have any difficulty with urination?

- Women have a much shorter urethra than men. This, coupled with the close proximity of the urinary meatus to the vaginal and rectal openings, results in a much higher incidence of urinary tract infection (UTI) in women. Dysuria warrants a urine dipstick measurement for bacteria. If nitrate and leukocyte esterase are positive, a urine culture will identify the pathogenic organism.
- While hematuria usually indicates kidney pathology, a bladder infection sometimes causes blood in the urine.
- With childbirth and aging, the tone of the muscles that support the bladder decreases. The additional pressure on the sphincter when a woman sneezes, coughs, or laughs may result in 'stress incontinence'. Kegel pelvic muscle exercises can strengthen the muscles near the urethra.
- Sudden loss of urine when not coughing or laughing may be a sign of more serious pathology, such as cystitis, or rarely a neurogenic bladder (overflow incontinence).

Do you have you any vaginal discharge?

- The vagina normally secretes a small quantity of clear to slightly cloudy, non irritating discharge. Monitoring the slippery feel of this normal mucus is the basis of the ovulation method of birth control.
- The color and character of the discharge may suggest an infection causing organism:
  - Trichomonas - Frothy, greenish yellow, foul smelling discharge.
  - Candida - Thick, white, 'cottage cheese' like discharge.

- o   Gardnerella - Thin, gray white discharge, with a 'rotten, fishy' odor.
- *Do you use a vaginal douche? If so, how often?* Frequent douching can raise the vaginal pH, which may favor bacterial infection.
- *Do you use feminine hygiene spray?* These sprays may cause contact dermatitis.
- *Do you wear nylon underpants or pantyhose?* Garments that do not breathe well may contribute to vaginitis. Vaginitis may result in painful intercourse (dyspareunia).

Are you sexually active?

- Sexual history includes current sexual activity, the number of current and previous partners, the gender of partners, satisfaction with the relationship, and methods of contraception and STD (sexually transmitted disease) precautions.
- While questions relating to sexual matters may be uncomfortable, this information is key to understanding the cause of many female conditions. Using neutral language and open ended questions can help facilitate communication.

What medications are you taking?

- Oral contraceptives can deplete some of the B vitamins (B6, folic acid), and increase the risk of clot formation, especially if the woman is a smoker.
- A woman who is is pregnant or trying to conceive should stop drinking and smoking, and be cautious about taking medicine. Even OTC medicine, such as aspirin or cough syrup, can harm the fetus.

Do any female problems run in your family?

- A woman with first degree relatives (mother, sister, daughter) with breast, endometrial, or ovarian cancer have an increased risk for these cancers.

Examination

The pelvic examination is a very intimidating examination procedure for a woman. While little can be done to moderate the invasiveness of the procedure, you should always respect her modesty, and expose sensitive areas only as needed during the examination. Using the examination as a teaching experience helps to dissipate some of the tension. Always tell the patient what you are about to do before you do it. Proper patient positioning will help your patient to observe your hands and the instruments during the examination:

- Raise the head of the table to elevate her head and shoulders
- Have your patient place her heels in the stirrups, with the angle and length adjusted to ensure she is not tensing her muscles

- Have her slide toward the foot of the table until her pelvis is at the edge of the table
- Cover her knees and torso with a sheet, but push the drape down between the legs so your face and hands are visible
- Hand her a mirror so she can observe the progress of the examination

Be sure to have your patient empty her bladder prior to the examination. Wear gloves during the examination. If you 'double glove' on your dominant hand, this will allow you to merely remove the outer glove when performing the rectovaginal examination, rather than having to change gloves. The instruments and your hands should be warm. Before you touch the external genitalia, use the back of your hand against the inner thigh to begin with a 'neutral touch'.

External Genitalia

In order to adequately visualize the structures, inspection and palpation of the external genitalia are performed together. Observe the pattern of hair distribution. If scabies or lice are suspected, inspect the pubic hair for nits. Inspect and palpate the labia majora for swelling or inflammation. With the fingers of one hand, spread the labia majora to inspect the labia minora and clitoris. The labia minora are normally dark pink and moist. Palpation should be free of tenderness. Clear vesicles may be a sign of genital herpes infection.

Gently insert your index finger into the introitus and with a slight superior pressure draw your finger anteriorly to 'milk' the urethra for possible discharge. Urethral discharge is usually caused by infection. Tenderness with this motion may indicate inflammation of Skene's paraurethral glands. Palpate the inferior lateral portion of the external vaginal wall between your thumb and index finger. Swelling or tenderness in this area suggests a Bartholin gland cyst. Have your patient bear down as if pushing a bowel movement. Observe for uterine prolapse or urinary incontinence.

Internal Speculum Examination

If cytological specimens are to be collected, do not use gel lubricant as it has bactericidal effects that may interfere with cell analysis. Lubricate the speculum with water only. Warm running water also serves to take the chill off the speculum. After explaining to your patient the next portion of the examination, and first using a neutral touch, insert the index and middle fingers of your nondominant hand into the vagina. Exert a downward pressure on the posterior vaginal wall to relax the pelvic floor muscles. Use the index and middle fingers of your dominant hand to hold the blades of the speculum closed. While holding the speculum at an oblique angle, gently insert the speculum at a downward angle. As you remove the fingers of your nondominant hand, continue with a downward pressure of the speculum, which helps to avoid pressure on the sensitive urethra. As you continue insertion, gradually rotate the speculum until the blades are horizontal.

After the speculum is inserted to the length of the vaginal canal, spread the blades at the handle and rotate the thumbscrew clockwise to secure them. Then squeeze the handle with your thumb to spread the distal end of the blades. If the blades are positioned at the correct angle and depth, you should be able to visualize the cervix. If the cervix is not seen, you may have to slightly withdraw and reposition the speculum. With the cervix in view, rotate the second thumbscrew clockwise to lock the distal end of the blades open. Inspect the color, size, position, and surface characteristics of the cervix. Note the quantity and characteristics of discharge present on the cervix and in the 'vaginal pool'. Using tools and procedures supplied by your lab, obtain and prepare the appropriate Pap smear specimens. After specimen collection, rotate both thumbscrews counterclockwise to unlock the blades. As you withdraw the speculum, observe the tissues of the vaginal wall between the speculum blades. Let the blades approximate, but be careful to not pinch the vaginal tissues. When you are near the end of the vaginal canal, again rotate the blades to an oblique angle to avoid pressure on the sensitive urethra.

Bimanual Examination

Bimanual palpation is performed with the doctor standing. Place lubricant on the index and middle fingers of your dominant hand. Again with a downward pressure, insert your two palpating fingers into the vagina. Your fourth and fifth fingers are curled against your palm, and your thumb is abducted to avoid any pressure on the urethra or clitoris. Your nondominant hand is placed over the lower abdomen. Place your two intravaginal fingers on either side of the cervix. The normal consistency of the cervix is 'firm'. Attempt to move the cervix from side to side. If this motion is painful, suspect pelvic inflammatory disease. With your abdominal hand superior to the symphysis pubis, bring both hands toward each other to attempt to palpate the uterus. If palpable, the body of the uterus should also have a firm consistency. Shift your abdominal hand laterally to palpate the adnexa. The ovaries and fallopian tubes are not usually palpable. Adnexal tenderness may indicate pelvic inflammatory disease (PID). Repeat the palpation for the opposite adnexal area.

Rectovaginal Palpation

Change gloves, or remove the outer glove from your double gloved hand, to avoid introducing possible vaginal organisms into the rectum. Lubricate your index and middle fingers. With your middle finger, apply gentle pressure to the anal sphincter. As the musculature relaxes, introduce your middle finger into the rectum and your index finger into the vagina. Press your two fingers together to gently assess the integrity of the rectovaginal septum. Using bimanual palpation, it is possible that you will now palpate a retroverted uterus that was not previously palpable.

Withdraw your index finger from the vagina, and gently rotate your middle finger 180 degrees, first in one direction and then the other, to check the entire circumference of the rectum for polyps or carcinoma. As you palpate, assess sphincter tone. A lax sphincter may indicate neurological deficit. When the sphincter is tight, scarring from previous rectal disease may be present. After palpation is complete, feces adherent to the gloved finger may be used to test for the presence of occult blood.

It is not uncommon for doctors to omit the rectal portion of the pelvic examination in young women in their teens or twenties. However, as a woman approaches 40 years of age, it would be unwise to omit the rectal portion as colorectal cancer is a significant cause of cancer death in both men and women.

Summary of Physical Examination

- Observation of general appearance
  - o Normal sexual development should approximate Tanner's Sexual Maturity Rating scales.
  - o When a young woman of short stature with webbing of the neck is late entering puberty, suspect ovarian dysgenesis secondary to Turner's syndrome.
  - o Skin and hair that are coarse and dry suggest hypothyroid tendencies, which may cause menorrhagia.
  - o Hirsutism points to an excess of androgenic hormones.
- Gynecologic examination
  - o Inspection and palpation of the external genitalia may provide evidence of urethral discharge, or inflammation of Bartholin's or Skene's glands. STD infection may manifest as chancre or condylomata growths near the vagina.
  - o Internal speculum examination provides the opportunity to observe the characteristic lesions that <u>may</u> occur with the various causes of vaginitis. However, definitive diagnosis of the infective organism requires laboratory examination. A woman should receive a Pap smear examination annually or every other year depending upon her clinical risk factors.
  - o Bimanual palpation allows the physician to detect uterine malposition, as well as benign and possibly malignant tumors. Cervical motion or adnexal tenderness is highly suggestive of infection, or possibly ectopic pregnancy.
  - o Rectovaginal palpation checks the integrity of the rectovaginal septum, as well as searching for rectal polyps and carcinoma.

o If not performed as a part of the routine abdominal examination, inguinal lymph nodes should be palpated for enlargement.

Diagnostic Studies

- Cytological examination of specimens collected during the speculum examination may include:
    o pH of vaginal secretions (> 4.5 predisposes toward bacterial and trichomonas infection)
    o KOH (candida and bacterial vaginosis)
    o wet mount (Trichomonas and bacterial vaginosis, PID)
    o Candida culture (expensive)
    o Herpes culture (expensive)
    o Thayer-Martin culture (gonococcal infection)
    o VDRL (Syphilis)
    o HIV test
    o PCR *Chlamydia* test (less expensive & quicker turnaround time than a *Chlamydia* culture)
- CBC & UA
    o The presence of urine nitrites and leukocyte esterase indicates bacterial infection. Culture and sensitivity testing should be performed when infection is present.
    o Hemoglobin and hematocrit (anemia due to menorrhagia)
    o The WBC differential may provide evidence of infection
- Prothrombin Time (PT) and Partial Thromboplastin Time (PTT) may help determine if bleeding abnormalities are due to clotting disorders.
- Serum chemistry examination may include:
    o FSH (increases with menopause and ovarian failure)
    o LH (LH/FSH ratio > 3 is diagnostic for polycystic ovarian syndrome)
    o Estradiol (low with menopause)
    o Beta hCG pregnancy test
    o Progesterone (low levels are a confirmatory test for ectopic pregnancy)
    o TSH may confirm hypothyroid tendencies, a possible cause of amenorrhea.
    o Prolactin should be ordered when galactorrhea not associated with pregnancy occurs.
- Tumor markers
    o CA-125 (endometrial & ovarian carcinoma)
- Vaginal and pelvic ultrasound will be performed on all suspected pelvic tumors.
- Dilation and Curettage (D & C)
    o Abnormal uterine bleeding that is not responsive to conservative care will probably require scraping of the lining

of the uterus. Removed tissues are sent for laboratory cytology testing.
- Hysteroscopy and laparoscopy
  - o Direct visualization of the lesion allows for collection and biopsy of suspect tissue.
- When carcinoma is found, a CT, MRI, or bone scan may be performed to investigate possible metastasis.
- CT or MRI of the head, if a prolactin secreting pituitary adenoma is suspected.
- Bone densitometry will quantify the extent of osteoporosis in a postmenopausal woman.

Sample Documentation

Upon inspection, the pubic hair was free of nits and presented a normal female pattern. No swelling or inflammation of the external genitalia was present. The urethral meatus was patent without evidence of discharge. Straining did not elicit uterine protrusion or urinary incontinence. Internal speculum examination disclosed pink and moist vaginal walls without bulging or lesions. A scant, clear, mucoid discharge was present in the vaginal pool. The cervix was midline with a nulliparous os. Tissue specimens were collected from the squamocolumnar junction and vaginal pool. Bimanual palpation disclosed a smooth, firm cervix that was not painful to motion. The uterus was midline, slightly anteverted, and of normal size and consistency. The ovaries were not palpable and no tenderness was elicited upon palpation of the adnexa. Rectovaginal examination disclosed normal sphincter tone. The rectovaginal septum was intact and no polyps or masses were palpated. The stool was brown and a specimen was collected for hemocult testing.

Common Gynecological Conditions

Premenstrual Syndrome (ICD: 625.4)

A condition characterized by nervousness, irritability, emotional instability, anxiety, depression, and possibly headaches, edema, and mastalgia, occurring during the 7 to 10 days before and usually disappearing a few hours after the onset of menses. (Merck Manual, p. 1932)

- Premenstrual syndrome (PMS) is very common, affecting an estimated 20-90% of all women during their child bearing years. For approximately 20% of these women, the symptoms are severe enough that it produces significant impairment of their activities of daily living. *Mittelschmerz* is a term that refers to severe midcycle pain that occurs at ovulation.
- Although PMS may be broad enough to include more than 150 symptoms, diagnosis should include at least one of the following symptoms during the five days before the onset of menses:

Somatic	Affective
breast tenderness	depression
abdominal bloating	angry outbursts
headache	irritability
swelling	anxiety
	confusion
	social withdrawal

- While the cause is unknown, it is thought to be related to an increased ratio of estrogen to progesterone.
- Medical management is symptomatic, diuretics for fluid retention and analgesics for pain. For some women, the exogenously supplied hormones in oral contraceptives seem to lessen their symptoms. However, for others it is ineffective or may worsen their condition, as depression and water retention are side effects of birth control pills.
- Natural therapeutics offer the greatest hope for management of this condition. Intervention should be multifactorial and comprehensive:
  - Exercise - Exercise has been shown to reduce breast tenderness, fluid retention, and depression in women with PMS.
  - Tobacco - The proinflammatory toxins in tobacco will worsen PMS symptoms.
  - Dietary changes - A diet low in fat and meat seems to help reduce symptoms. Many women following a vegetarian diet experience relief of symptoms. Caffeine and sugar increase symptoms for many PMS sufferers and should be eliminated from the diet. Salt intake should be minimized as this contributes to fluid retention. Soy products contain phytoestrogens and should be used liberally, provided the woman does not have a soy allergy. Food allergy should be investigated and properly managed.
  - Nutritional supplementation - B vitamins, especially B6 helps to reduce PMS symptoms. Magnesium helps to relax tense muscles and nervousness. Vitamin E and GLA help to reduce premenstrual breast tenderness. Several herbs, such as licorice and wild yam are thought to be herbal precursors to female hormones.

Primary Dysmenorrhea (functional dysmenorrhea) (ICD: 625.3)

Cyclic pain associated with ovulatory cycles without demonstrable lesions affecting reproductive structures. (Merck Manual, p. 1933)

- While there are a few women who can say they have never experienced menstrual cramps in their life, they are in a definite minority, as just about all women experience dysmenorrhea at some time during their reproductive years. 10-15% of women experience dysmenorrhea severe enough that it disrupts their daily activities.

- Symptoms include a crampy lower abdominal pain that usually starts 12-24 hours prior to the onset of menses. The pain may be intermittent or a dull constant ache that may radiate to the lower back and thighs. The pain is usually worst on the first day of menses and gradually resolves over the next two to three days.
- Associated symptoms may include headache, fatigue, bloating, or even nausea and vomiting.
- Functional dysmenorrhea is thought to be caused by excessive prostaglandin release, which in turn leads to ischemia and hypercontractility of the uterus.
- Physical examination will be negative for overt pathology found with secondary dysmenorrhea.
- As with PMS, medical management is symptomatic. If the woman desires birth control, oral contraception is considered the treatment of choice. By suppressing ovulation, there is a marked reduction in prostaglandin synthesis and uterine muscle cramping. The following article is quite thought provoking: *Nuisance or natural and healthy: should monthly menstruation be optional for women?* (Lancet, 2000 Mar 11;355(9207):922-4).
- When contraception is not indicated, nonsteroidal antiinflammatory drugs (NSAID's) are used to decrease pain and inhibit prostaglandin synthesis.
- Magnesium is an antispasmodic and may alleviate menstrual cramps. EPA fish oil, bromelain, and the herb ginger are safe nutritional alternatives to NSAID medicine for regulation of prostaglandin synthesis.
- Chiropractic treatment, such as Logan Basic Technique, is often very effective for dysmenorrhea.

Secondary Dysmenorrhea (acquired dysmenorrhea)

Pain with menses caused by demonstrable pathology. (Merck Manual, p. 1933)

- Secondary dysmenorrhea is more common in older women and the pain is not limited to just before the onset of menses. Additional symptoms such as painful intercourse (dyspareunia) or menorrhagia will likely be present.
- Physical examination may disclose a mucopurulent vaginal discharge, cervical motion tenderness, and possibly ovarian enlargement and tenderness. Vaginal ultrasound or laparoscopy may be required for definitive diagnosis.
- Secondary dysmenorrhea is caused by organic pathology, such as endometriosis, uterine fibroids, or pelvic inflammatory disease, which must be identified and treated appropriately.

Amenorrhea (ICD: 626.0)

Absence of menstruation - either because it never began or later ceased. (Merck Manual, p. 1933)

- For most young women, menstruation usually begins around age 12 or 13. When menarche has not begun by age 16, this is referred to as primary amenorrhea. While menarche may be delayed in very thin or athletic young women, delay beyond 16 years of age requires that hormonal imbalances be investigated.
- Turner's syndrome is a genetic abnormality manifesting in about one in 4,000 live female births. In addition to a short stature and webbing of the neck, a predominant feature of Turner's syndrome is ovarian dysgenesis, with consequent lack of secondary sexual development.
- Once menarche has commenced, cessation of regular menses for any cause is secondary amenorrhea. The most common cause of secondary amenorrhea is pregnancy. Exercising more than 20 hours a week has been shown to suppress ovulatory hormones. Anorexia and extreme weight loss may also cause amenorrhea.
- Polycystic ovarian syndrome (PCO) manifests as abnormally high testosterone levels which suppress ovulation. In addition to increased facial hair, oligomenorrhea or amenorrhea will manifest.
- If galactorrhea is present in addition to amenorrhea, a prolactin secreting pituitary tumor should be investigated.
- Laboratory workup of secondary amenorrhea may include:
    o Beta hCG pregnancy test
    o TSH and T4
    o Serum prolactin
    o FSH (if ovarian failure is suspected)
    o LH/FSH ratio (if polycystic ovaries are suspected)
    o Cortisol and DHEA (if an adrenal tumor is suspected)
- Medical treatment of amenorrhea depends upon the cause. Polycystic ovarian syndrome is often successfully managed with birth control pills.

Menopause (ICD: 627.2)

Physiologic cessation of menses due to decreasing ovarian function. (Merck Manual, p. 1942)

- Estrogen is a vital body hormone. It affects bone growth, heart and circulatory function, as well as its stimulatory effect on breast and female reproductive tissue.
- At about age 50 for most women, the decline in ovarian function results in a variety of physiological effects. For some women, this change is gradual enough that their symptoms are mild. For others, this period of change produces severe symptoms, such as:
    o Hot flashes
    o Night sweats
    o Vaginal dryness leading to painful intercourse
    o Nocturia and urge incontinence
    o Anxiety, nervousness, irritability
- Upon examination, the vaginal mucosa may be thin, dry, and friable (lacking normal elasticity). The vaginal mucosa may appear pale, with

abraded areas that bleed easily. The vaginal discharge may be blood tinged.

- Laboratory evaluation will disclose low estrogen and elevated FSH. FSH values > 40 mIU are considered diagnostic for menopause.
- Medical management normally includes estrogen replacement therapy. Every medical intervention must be evaluated on a risk vs. benefit basis. However, many physicians feel that the benefits to the cardiovascular and skeletal systems, as well as the relief of symptoms, outweigh the increased statistical risk of cancer. If estrogen replacement therapy is begun, estrogen patches provide a more stable sustained delivery than oral forms such as Premarin.
- Many nutritional substances, such as Vitamin C, Vitamin E, essential fatty acids, and herbal phytoestrogens exert a tonic effect on the female reproductive system.

Premature Ovarian Failure (premature menopause) (ICD: 256.3)

Disorders in which women < 40 yr present with symptoms and signs due to estrogen deficiency and have high levels of circulating gonadotropins (especially FSH) and low levels of estradiol. (Merck Manual, p. 1939)

- Most women undergo menopause between age 45-55, with a mean age of 51. When menopause occurs under age 40 it is considered premature. This phenomenon occurs in 1% of women age 30-39.
- Laboratory evaluation of hormonal status will disclose low estrogen and elevated FSH.
- While the cause of premature ovarian failure is unknown, it is thought that autoimmunity and genetics play a role.
- Medical management involves hormone replacement therapy (HRT) to compensate for the lack of endogenous estrogen.

Abnormal Uterine Bleeding (ICD: 626.2)

Excessive duration (menorrhagia) or amount (menorrhagia, or hypermenorrhea) of menses or both; too-frequent menstruation (polymenorrhea); non-menstrual or intermenstrual bleeding (metrorrhagia); or postmenopausal bleeding (any bleeding > 6 mo after the last normal menstrual period at menopause. (Merck Manual, p. 1939)

- For about 25% of the women with abnormal uterine bleeding, organic pathology can be identified. When all possible organic causes have been eliminated, the condition is referred to as dysfunctional uterine bleeding (DUB).
- Organic causes which should receive appropriate medical care may include:
  - Endometriosis
  - Uterine fibroids
  - Ovarian cysts
  - Atrophic vaginitis
  - Uterine or cervical carcinoma

- o Ectopic pregnancy
- o Miscarriage, or threatened abortion
- o Pelvic trauma, or complications from an intrauterine device (IUD)
- o Hematological clotting disorders

Dysfunctional Uterine Bleeding (functional uterine bleeding) (ICD: 626.8)

Abnormal uterine bleeding not associated with tumor, inflammation, or pregnancy. (Merck Manual, p. 1941)

- Dysfunctional uterine bleeding is usually triggered by a rise of estrogen, unopposed by progesterone. Because 90% of the time it is associated with anovulation, it is also referred to as anovulatory uterine bleeding.
- Hormonal fluctuations which cause dysfunctional uterine bleeding are more common at the beginning and end of a woman's reproductive years.
- The menstrual cycle will be irregular. There may be episodes of heavy bleeding, usually without pain, as well as episodes of amenorrhea.
- A complete pelvic examination, with a Pap smear should be performed, however the results will be normal when organic pathology is absent.
- A CBC should be performed to assess anemia, and a beta hCG pregnancy test is indicated. Measurement of FSH, LH, and thyroid function help to assess hormonal function. Vaginal ultrasound may be needed to rule out pathology.
- Most cases of dysfunctional uterine bleeding are successfully managed with oral contraceptive pills. If the bleeding continues, a dilation and curettage (D & C) may be performed to scrape the inner lining of the uterus.

Endometriosis (ICD: 617.0)

A nonmalignant disorder in which functioning endometrial tissue is present outside the uterine cavity. (Merck Manual, p. 1956)

- Endometriosis is a common condition, affecting 10-20% of adult women. Endometriosis is a major cause of infertility, and has a much higher prevalence in women unable to conceive.
- The tissue that lines the inside of the uterus normally sloughs off once a month during menstruation. For reasons that are not clear, sometimes endometrial tissue is found outside the uterus, within the fallopian tubes or abdominal cavity. Because this tissue is still sensitive to monthly hormonal variation, it becomes engorged with blood once a month. However, lacking the normal vaginal outlet, a cyst may form, with eventual scarring and adhesions.
- Symptoms include heavy menstrual bleeding (menorrhagia), perimenstrual pain, and painful intercourse (dyspareunia). A common

concern of women with endometriosis is the inability to conceive, or infertility.

- Speculum examination will likely be normal. Bimanual palpation may elicit tenderness, and small nodular masses may be found on the posterior fundus and adnexa. Definitive diagnosis requires laparoscopic visualization and biopsy of the lesions.

- If the condition is mild, initial management will be hormonal therapy (birth control pills) which suppresses menstruation. For more severe cases, laparoscopic surgery may be performed to remove as many of the abnormal tissue implants as possible. When these more conservative measures fail, a total hysterectomy is the treatment of last resort, provided the woman can accept the outcome of no future child bearing.

- For less severe cases, herbal phytoestrogen precursors, such as wild yam and black cohash may help to normalize hormonal function and provide symptomatic relief. Chiropractic and acupuncture techniques may provide substantial relief of perimenstrual pain.

Uterine Fibroids (leiomyomas, myomas, fibromyomas) (ICD: 218.9)

Benign uterine tumors of smooth muscle origin. (Merck Manual, p. 1959)

- Leiomyomas, or uterine fibroids are the most common pelvic tumor in women. One guideline teaches that 30% of 30 year old women, 40% of 40 year old women, and 50% of 50 year old women have uterine fibroid tumors.

- While the cause is not known for certain, they are more common in women with high levels of estrogen. Again for reasons that are not clear, African American women are three times more likely to have fibroid tumors of the uterus.

- The most common symptom these women experience is heavy, possibly continuous menstrual bleeding. Pelvic pain and painful intercourse are also common. If bleeding is marked, iron deficiency anemia will result.

- Upon examination, the uterus will present with irregular, firm, painless nodules in the uterine wall. The tumors may be microscopic in size, or grow to the size of a grapefruit. Vaginal ultrasound will likely be performed to confirm the size and location of the tumor.

- For mild cases, medical management will include NSAID medication to decrease the pain and possibly even the blood loss. Gonadotropin releasing hormone agonist medication may be used to suppress ovarian estrogen production.

- Severe cases will require surgery. If the woman is motivated to continue having children, a myomectomy, surgical removal of just the fibroid tumors is an option. Otherwise, the doctor will likely recommend a total hysterectomy. By age 70, approximately one half of women in the US have received a hysterectomy, many of which are performed to treat fibroid tumors.

- The American College of Obsetricians and Gynecologists has established criteria for what conditions warrant a hysterectomy. A recent study (Obstet Gynecol 2000 Feb; 95(2):199-205) found that 76% of hysterectomies were inappropriate due to a *"lack of adequate diagnostic evaluation and failure to try alternative treatments before hysterectomy."*
- Natural therapeutics aimed at normalizing estrogen function may provide benefit. The declining estrogen levels that occur with menopause usually causes existing tumors to shrink, although if the woman is also taking estrogen replacement hormones, this will complicate that outcome.

Endometrial Cancer (Merck Manual, p. 1960) (ICD: 182)

- While fibroid tumors are the most common pelvic tumor, endometrial carcinoma is the most common pelvic cancer, more common than cervical carcinoma. Endometrial carcinoma accounts for 13% of all cancer in women.
- Increased estrogen levels are thought to stimulate hyperplasia of endometrial tissue. As such, risk factors include: obesity, early menarche, late menopause, and tamoxifen or unopposed estrogen replacement therapy.
- The condition is usually detected when the physician is searching for the cause of dysfunctional uterine bleeding. The woman may experience intermenstrual bleeding, or a woman who has passed through menopause may experience vaginal discharge or bleeding. The older the woman, the more likely that postmenopausal bleeding is carcinoma.
- Bimanual palpation discloses an enlarged uterus. While a Pap smear may be positive, an endometrial biopsy is required.
- Hysterectomy is the usual medical treatment. If the surgery is performed when the cancer is still confined to the uterus (stage 1), the five year survival rate is 80-90%. Fortunately, the majority of endometrial cancer is detected while it is still in stage 1.

Ovarian Cancer (Merck Manual, p. 1962) (ICD: 183.0)

- Ovarian cancer is the second most common gynecologic cancer, and the fourth highest cause of cancer death in American women. While it can occur in younger women, most cases occur after menopause. About one in seventy women will develop ovarian cancer during her life.
- When ovarian cancer is detected early, the five year survival rate is 90%. Unfortunately, most ovarian cancer is not detected early. The survival rate for advanced ovarian cancer (stage III and IV) is about 25%.
- Early ovarian cancer is essentially asymptomatic. By the time symptoms such as abdominal discomfort, urinary urgency, painful

intercourse, or a change in bowel habits develop, the cancer has already spread.

- While it is not known what causes ovarian cancer, we do know that the condition is more common in affluent industrialized countries. It is thought that a high fat diet, delayed childbearing, and the use of oral contraceptives may play a role.
- Bimanual palpation will disclose a solid, fixed, poorly defined mass. Vaginal ultrasound will be ordered. However, definitive diagnosis will require microscopic examination of a tissue biopsy. If the biopsy is positive, surgery is required. If the cancer has spread beyond the ovary, chemotherapy will also be recommended.
- Approximately ten percent of ovarian cancer is familial. Women at high risk should strongly consider periodic testing with the CA-125 'tumor marker'.

Cervical Cancer (Merck Manual, p. 1964) (ICD: 180)

- Cervical carcinoma is the third most common gynecologic cancer in women.. While it can occur in women in their 20's, the peak incidence is 30-50 years of age, and shows increased incidence among women of African American or Hispanic origin.
- The cervical os is a transition area between two different types of cells. These cells can undergo malignant transformation. The Pap smear is performed to detect this cellular dysplasia. It is estimated that 95% of women with cervical carcinoma have infection with the human papilloma virus, thus the rationale for the Pap smear.
- Symptoms of cervical cancer include dyspareunia, intermenstrual bleeding or bleeding after intercourse, and a vaginal discharge, possibly dark or blood streaked.
- Speculum examination may disclose an enlarged cervix that bleeds easily. Bimanual palpation may or may not be tender. Further confirmatory testing may include colposcopy or a cervical cone biopsy.
- Some research suggests that many abnormal Pap smears are indicative of folic acid deficiency, rather than true cervical dysplasia, especially if the woman is taking oral contraceptives.

Ovarian Cyst (Merck Manual, p. 1947) (ICD: 620.2)

- Ovarian cysts are common. As the egg matures in the ovary, it develops within a cyst like structure. Upon ovulation, this follicle bursts and the egg is released. When this fails, an ovarian cyst may result. Ovarian cysts vary from benign to those requiring surgery.
- A symptomatic ovarian cyst may present with menstrual irregularities, pelvic pain, and possibly symptoms similar to pregnancy, i.e. morning sickness and breast tenderness. Many ovarian cysts resolve spontaneously in 2-3 months without treatment.
- Examination may vary from normal, to a nontender palpable adnexal mass, to a very painful adnexal mass. When the symptoms are mild,

birth control pills may help regulate the cycle and suppress the formation of cysts. Severe ovarian cysts may require surgery. In any case, medical referral is indicated to ensure that ovarian cancer is not present.

- Polycystic ovarian syndrome, also known as Stein-Leventhal syndrome, is a similar but more serious disease, related to an excess of androgenic hormones. Symptoms that should alert you to the possibility of polycystic ovarian syndrome include:
  - o amenorrhea or oligomenorrhea
  - o infertility
  - o obesity
  - o hirsutism

Genital Herpes (ICD: 054.1)

*Infection of the genital or anorectal skin or mucous membranes of either of two closely related herpes simplex viruses (HSV-1 or HSV-2). (*Merck Manual, *p. 1337)*

- According to the CDC, about 25 million Americans have genital herpes. Treatment is especially important for a pregnant woman, as the infection can be transferred to the baby at birth.
- The symptoms are similar to oral herpes or cold sores, small vesicles that itch and become painful. There may be associated fever, fatigue, and lymphadenopathy. Within a few days the blisters break, leaving small painful ulcers.
- Healing occurs within one to two weeks, however the virus remains in the body for the remainder of life. Recurrent outbreaks, which are likely to occur at times of stress, are generally shorter and milder.
- Antiviral drugs, such as Acyclovir, or nutritional supplements, such as Monolaurin, can decrease the severity and duration of the outbreak.

Lower Genital Tract Disorders (ICD: 616.1)

*Infections and other inflammatory disorders affecting the vaginal mucosa and sometimes the vulva, commonly producing a vaginal discharge. (*Merck Manual, *p. 1948)*

- Vulvovaginitis is one of the most common gynecological complaints. It may be the result of a contact allergy, infection, or from vaginal atrophy that results with declining hormonal function.
- When a young woman enters puberty, the vaginal pH becomes more acidic, which helps to protect against infection. Infection prior to puberty is usually due to fecal bacteria, such as *E. coli*, or possibly a contact allergy to chemicals such as bubble bath soap. Due to the higher pH, Candida infection is less likely in young girls. When gonorrhea infection is found, sexual abuse must be investigated.
- After menopause, the decline of estrogen stimulation predisposes toward atrophic vaginitis. The vaginal discharge is alkaline and scant.

Upon examination, the vaginal epithelium is thin and pale. Estrogen replacement therapy, and topical vaginal creams containing estrogen are very effective.

- In women of childbearing age, the vaginal pH is 3.2 to 4.5. This pH is the consequence of the *Lactobacillus acidophilus* 'normal flora' of the vaginal tract. Candida yeast is also a normal inhabitant, in <u>small</u> quantities, of the vaginal membranes. When the beneficial acidophilus bacteria are missing, usually a consequence of antibiotic therapy, an overgrowth of candida yeast can result. It is estimated that 75% of all women experience vaginal candidiasis at least once in their life. Symptomatically, the woman may experience vaginal itching and burning. A thick 'cottage cheese' like discharge is apparent upon vaginal examination.

- When the *Lactobacillus acidophilus* are lacking, the vaginal pH will rise. The higher pH favors the growth of certain bacteria. Bacterial vaginosis is a vaginal infection with *Gardnerella vaginalis*. Bacterial vaginosis accounts for about 60% of all vulvovaginal infection. While the organism is usually sexually transmitted, it has been cultured in young women not yet sexually active. Approximately one half of women with this infection are asymptomatic. Some women may experience 'constant wetness', with a musty or fishy odor. Vaginal examination discloses a gray white discharge adherent to the cervix and vaginal walls. Antibiotic treatment is indicated. Previous bacterial vaginosis infection may contribute to infertility or ectopic pregnancy.

- Trichomoniasis is a sexually transmitted disease (STD) caused by the flagellated protozoa *Trichomonas vaginalis*. Symptomatically, the woman may experience vaginal itching, painful urination and notice a frothy, yellow green, foul smelling vaginal discharge. Upon speculum examination, the cervix and vagina may exhibit a red granular 'strawberry' appearance. Treatment of both partners with the drug Flagyl is indicated.

- Chlamydia is the most common STD in the US. Early identification is important, as untreated chlamydia infection can lead to pelvic inflammatory disease (PID) and infertility. About one third of infected women are asymptomatic. Consequently, current guidelines suggest that sexually active women be screened yearly, especially if they have multiple partners and unprotected sex. The condition mimics and may coexist with gonorrhea infection. The woman may experience increased urinary frequency and painful urination. Speculum examination may be normal or disclose a mucopurulent vaginal discharge. If the condition has progressed to PID, cervical motion may cause tenderness (Chandelier's sign). Antibiotic treatment of both partners is indicated.

- Gonorrhea is an STD caused by the *Neisseria* gonococcus. Because as many as 80% of women who contract gonorrhea are asymptomatic, it may go undetected. Untreated, it can cause PID and eventually sterility. If the infection spreads to other parts of the body, arthritis, skin lesions, endocarditis, and even meningitis may result. When symptomatic, vaginal discharge and dysuria are the most common symptoms. Gynecological examination may disclose vaginal inflammation, an abscess of Bartholin's or Skene's glands, and pain with adnexal or cervical motion. A gram stain is positive in only 50% of infected females, therefore a GC culture is indicated. Again, antibiotic treatment of both partners is essential.

Summary of vaginal discharge characteristics

Candidiasis	thick 'cottage cheese' like discharge
Gardnerella	gray white discharge 'constant wetness', with a musty or fishy odor
Trichomoniasis	frothy, yellow green, foul smelling discharge 'strawberry' flea-bitten appearance to cervix

Pelvic Inflammatory Disease (ICD: 614.9)

Infection of the upper female genital tract, including endometritis (infection of the uterine cavity), salpingitis (infection of the fallopian tubes), mucopurulent cervicitis (infection of the cervix), and oophoritis (infection of the ovaries). (Merck Manual, p. 1954)

- Pelvic inflammatory disease (PID), is the most common complication of STD. It occurs when a vaginal infection spreads to the uterus, and eventually to the fallopian tubes and ovaries. While PID is usually a consequence of *Chlamydia* or *Gonorrhea* infection, it may be a complication of an intrauterine device for birth control (IUD).
- While PID can occur at any age, it is most common among sexually active teenagers. The condition presents with lower abdominal pain, stomach cramps, fever, and chills, in addition to a purulent malodorous vaginal discharge.
- The symptoms of PID are very similar to appendicitis. Abdominal palpation may elicit rebound tenderness. For this reason, women with suspected appendicitis should receive a pelvic examination. Speculum examination may disclose cervical inflammation with a yellow discharge.
- CDC guidelines for the diagnosis of pelvic inflammatory disease requires all of the following:
  - o Lower abdominal tenderness
  - o Adnexal tenderness
  - o Cervical motion tenderness
  - o Absence of a competing diagnosis
- Laboratory evaluation should include a CBC with differential, hCG pregnancy test, ESR, C-reactive protein, and culture for chlamydia and gonorrhea infection.
- Antibiotic treatment of the STD infection is required. Chronic or recurrent infections may require IV antibiotics. If an IUD is present, it

should be removed. Women with previous PID have an increased risk of infertility and tubal pregnancy.

Ectopic Pregnancy (ICD: 633)

Pregnancy in which implantation occurs outside the endometrium and endometrial cavity- ie, in the cervix, uterine tube, ovary, or abdominal or pelvic cavity. (Merck Manual, p. 2055)

- During conception, the egg and sperm unite in the fallopian tube. The fertilized embryo then travels down the tube to implant in the uterus. If this process is impeded, usually due to scar tissue from previous PID infection, the embryo begins development outside of the uterus. In most cases of ectopic pregnancy, implantation occurs within the fallopian tube, hence the commonly used term tubal pregnancy.
- Approximately 1% of all pregnancies are ectopic. While at least one half of these women have a history of previous PID infection, intrauterine devices and birth control pills also increase the risk of ectopic pregnancy.
- Initially the woman will experience the signs of a normal pregnancy, i.e. amenorrhea, morning sickness, and breast tenderness. However, after about six weeks the increased embryo size will begin to cause severe abdominal pain, and possibly vaginal bleeding. If rupture and hemorrhage occurs, the woman may manifest signs of shock, i.e. decreased BP, clammy skin, pallor, tachycardia.
- Upon examination, unilateral lower abdominal and pelvic pain will be evident. Cervical motion will be painful, and a unilateral painful adnexal mass will be palpable. An hCG pregnancy test should be performed and will be positive.
- Ectopic pregnancy is a surgical emergency. When the condition is detected early, the fallopian tube may be saved. If the tube ruptures, it is surgically removed along with the embryo. Without surgery, ectopic pregnancy is usually fatal.

Dyspareunia (ICD: 625.0)

Painful coitus or attempted coitus. (Merck Manual, p. 1985)

- Dyspareunia is a symptom, referring to painful sexual intercourse, rather than an anatomical pathology. While the condition is primarily a female complaint, men may experience ejaculatory pain when prostatic or urethral infection is present.
- Psychological factors may contribute to the condition, especially if previous sexual experiences have been painful. However, dyspareunia can usually be traced to an inflammatory condition, or a lack of vaginal lubrication.
- Causes that must be identified and appropriately treated include:
  - o Atrophic vaginitis
  - o Bacterial vaginitis
  - o Candida yeast infection

- o   Endometriosis
- o   Uterine fibroid tumors
- o   Cervical carcinoma
- o   Genital herpes infection
- o   Pelvic inflammatory disease
- o   Gonococcal or nongonococcal urethritis
- Treatment must be directed at the cause. However, if no pathology is present other than a lack of vaginal lubricant, water soluble KY lubricant will provide symptomatic relief.

Abnormalities of the Pelvic Musculature

Cystocele (ICD: 618.0)

- The bladder rests on the pelvic floor musculature. With multiple vaginal childbirth deliveries, this support is weakened. A cystocele, sometimes referred to as a 'dropped bladder', is a protrusion of the bladder through the anterior wall of the vagina. The woman may experience stress incontinence and protrusion with bearing down. Kegel pelvic muscle exercises may help mild cases, however 'bladder suspension' surgery may be required.

Rectocele (ICD: 618.0)

- Rectocele is when part of the rectum protrudes through the posterior wall of the vagina. Constipation may be associated with this condition. Straining with a bowel movement may cause further protrusion. Because the uterus helps anchor the vagina, rectocele sometimes develops following a hysterectomy.

Uterine Prolapse (ICD: 618.4)

- Uterine prolapse is a third condition related to weakening of the pelvic floor musculature. It may occur in conjunction with either or both of the previous conditions. Kegel exercises and avoidance of straining with a bowel movement may help, but severe prolapse will require either a uterine resuspension or hysterectomy surgery.

Pregnancy (ICD: 650)

- Obviously pregnancy is not an abnormal condition. It is however, a condition you must be able to recognize. Pregnancy is the most common cause of amenorrhea in a woman who was previously menstruating. Additional signs include nausea (morning sickness), breast tenderness, and weight gain. Speculum examination will disclose bluish discoloration of the vaginal and cervical tissue (Chadwick's sign) 6-8 weeks after conception.

Study Guide Objectives

- o   Know the anatomy of the external and internal female genitalia.
- o   What is the term for the region lateral to the uterus?

- Know the functions of the female reproductive structures.
- Know the difference between primary and secondary amenorrhea.
- What is the most common cause of secondary amenorrhea?
- Know the significance of early menarche or late menopause.
- Know the significance of late menarche or early menopause.
- Know how to record the obstetric history.
- What is the normal age range for menopause?
- Know the color and characteristics of the vaginal discharge caused by different infections.
- What are the patient positioning measures needed prior to the female pelvic examination?
- What does tenderness near the urethral meatus indicate?
- What does tenderness at the posterior lateral region of the vestibule suggest?
- Why is it usually advised to not lubricate the vaginal speculum used in the internal vaginal exam?
- Know the proper method of speculum insertion.
- Know how and where Pap smear specimens are collected.
- What is the doctor position for performing the vaginal bimanual examination?
- What is the normal consistency of the cervix?
- What does adnexal tenderness suggest?
- What is the purpose of the Tanner's rating scale?
- What is hirsutism and what does it suggest?
- Know the pathologic changes that occur with the various female conditions discussed.
- What is mittelschmerz?
- Know the difference between somatic and affective PMS symptoms.
- What dietary changes are recommended for women with PMS?
- What is the difference between primary and secondary dysmenorrhea?
- What are some of the causes of secondary dysmenorrhea?
- How does polycystic ovarian syndrome affect menstrual flow?
- Know the changes that occur with menopause.
- What is the most common cause of vulvovaginal infection?
- At what age would menopause be considered premature ovarian failure?
- Know the definition of menorrhagia, hypermenorrhea, polymenorrhea, and metrorrhagia.
- Know the organic causes of abnormal uterine bleeding.
- What is endometriosis and what other health problem does it cause?
- Know the synonym terms for uterine fibroid tumors.
- Know the risk factors for endometrial cancer.
- Why does ovarian cancer have such a poor survival rate?
- What type of cancer does the Pap smear detect?
- What nutritional supplementation is recommended for an abnormal Pap smear?
- Know the symptoms of polycystic ovarian syndrome.

o   When a young woman enters puberty, how does the vaginal pH
    change?
o   In women of childbearing age, what creates the normal vaginal pH?
o   What is Chandelier's sign?
o   What is the usual cause of pelvic inflammatory disease (PID)?
o   Know the CDC guidelines for the diagnosis of PID.
o   Women with previous PID have an increased risk of what conditions?
o   What is the consequence of untreated ectopic pregnancy?
o   What is dyspareunia and what are the causes?
o   What are the differences between cystocele and rectocele?
o   Know the changes that occur in the female reproductive structures
    with pregnancy.
o   What is Chadwick's sign?

14 – Vascular & Lymphatic System

Anatomy & Physiology

The arteries are vessels that carry blood from the heart to the tissues of the body. As a result, they must be strong and yet flexible enough to handle the high pressure exerted when the heart contracts. The heartbeat creates a wave of pressure or pulse that can be palpated at various points on the body. The pulses most easily felt are close to the surface and easily compressed against adjacent bony tissue. The primary arteries accessible to palpation are:

- Temporal - in front of the ear as it passes over the zygoma bone
- Carotid - in the groove between the trachea and SCM muscle
- Brachial - over the antecubital fossa as the artery pass medial to the biceps tendon (or at the medial arm in the furrow between the biceps and triceps muscles)
- Ulnar - at the medial anterior wrist
- Radial - at the lateral anterior wrist medial to the styloid process
- Femoral - in the groin, at about the medial one third of the inguinal ligament
- Popliteal - in the popliteal fossa
- Posterior tibial - posterior to the medial malleolus of the ankle
- Dorsal pedis - on the dorsum of the foot between the first and second ray

The abdominal aorta is a central, rather than a peripheral artery, but it is accessible to palpation, and is evaluated during the abdominal examination.

When there is blockage of arterial circulation, the tissues supplied may experience ischemia. Partial blockage may produce pain and pallor in the impaired tissues. Complete blockage may cause infarction or cellular death.

While arterial circulation is a high pressure system, venous circulation is low pressure. Many of the veins run parallel to the arteries, but are usually closer to the surface of the skin. Because the veins lack a 'pump' to propel the blood back to the heart, a combination of factors aid in venous return:

- The veins contain one way check valves that allow blood to flow toward the heart, but close when gravity causes blood to flow away from the heart.
- The veins are surrounded by skeletal muscle. As the muscles contract, this 'milks' the flow of blood toward the heart.
- The abdominal veins lack skeletal muscle to serve this pumping function. However, with each inspiration of the lungs, the

diaphragm draws down which causes decreased intrathoracic pressure and increased abdominal pressure. Increased abdominal pressure serves a similar function to the skeletal muscle in the extremities.

The walls of the veins are thinner than arterial blood vessels. They are larger diameter and have the ability to stretch and accept more blood volume as needed. However, when they stretch too far, the intraluminal valves may no longer close properly and become 'incompetent'. This results in pooling of blood, primarily in the legs, producing varicose veins.

The lymphatic system is another low pressure system that functions similar to venous circulation. Lymphatic ducts start out as small capillaries that collect fluid from interstitial tissues. These vessels become progressively larger and form ducts. The flow of lymph toward the heart uses the same mechanisms that propel blood to the heart.

Lymph nodes are found at various locations along the course of lymph duct drainage. The nodes contain white blood cells that fight foreign invaders that may be found in the fluid returning to the heart. With infection, the nodes proximal to the infection may become enlarged, inflamed, tender and more palpable. The locations of head and neck, and axillary lymph nodes have already been discussed. Epitrochlear lymph nodes are found superior to the medial elbow. Inguinal lymph nodes are found in the groin region and drain the legs, external genitalia, and lower abdominal wall. The inguinal nodes are divided into a superior group that is more horizontal, and an inferior group that is more vertical.

Most of the lymphatic drainage of the body is to the thoracic duct which drains into the left subclavian vein. The right lymphatic duct drains nodes coming from the right lung and pleura, the right thorax, the right arm and shoulder, and the right side of the head and neck. Because the supraclavicular lymph nodes are found very near the terminal point of lymphatic drainage, they deserve careful attention. Enlargement of the left supraclavicular node, also known as Virchow's sentinel node, may be the first sign of abdominal malignancy.

In addition to conserving fluid and plasma proteins that leak from the capillaries, the lymphatic system aids with the absorption of lipids from the gastrointestinal tract. The lymphatic system also includes a group of related organs that help mediate the body's immune response to foreign invaders.

The spleen located in the left upper abdominal quadrant has four main functions:

- Stores red blood cells
- Destroys old red blood cells

- Filters microorganisms from the blood
- Produces antibodies

The palatine and pharyngeal tonsils help to combat infection that may arise from organisms that enter the body via the nose and mouth.

The thymus is a small gland that lies anterior and superior to the heart. T-lymphocytes take their name from this gland. This gland is quite large at birth and gets progressively smaller as we age. While most texts state that the thymus gland has 'no function' in the adult, natural care physicians often find that supplementation with thymus glandular helps to enhance the body's immune response.

Peyer's patches are essentially lymph nodes of the abdominal lymphatic ducts.

History

Do you experience leg pains or cramps?

- What is the quality of your pain?
  - Acute arterial occlusion may have a throbbing quality.
  - Pain from chronic arterial occlusion produces claudication symptoms, i.e. cramping, numbness, tingling, and the leg may feel cold.
  - Acute venous disease (thrombophlebitis) produces intense, sharp deep muscle pain.
  - Chronic venous insufficiency produces an achy tired feeling in the leg.
- What makes your pain worse? Prolonged standing interferes with venous return of blood to the heart, which increases the pain of chronic venous insufficiency. If exercise and activity worsen the leg pain, this suggests claudication (pain with walking), associated with diminished arterial blood flow. If possible, you should quantify the distance the individual can walk before pain begins. This serves as a marker to assess treatment effectiveness.
- Does anything lessen your pain? Lying down with the limb elevated facilitates venous blood return and lessens the pain of venous insufficiency. The claudication pain of arterial insufficiency decreases very quickly with a couple of minutes of rest with the leg in a dependent position (sitting or standing).

Have you noticed any skin changes on your arms or legs?

- Arterial insufficiency produces pale extremities. If the condition is long standing, the skin may be thin and shiny, with ulcers over bony prominences, such as the toes or malleoli.
- Chronic venous insufficiency produces thickened skin that may have a brownish discoloration. Backflow of blood past incompetent valves may produce dilated, tortuous veins.

- Do you have any sores on your feet or leg? Leg ulcers occur with both chronic arterial and chronic venous insufficiency. Venous ulcers have bleeding uneven edges, whereas arterial ulcers tend to have well defined edges with no bleeding.

Have you noticed any swelling in your legs?

- 'Pitting' tissue edema is associated with venous insufficiency. 'Non-pitting' edema suggests blocked lymphatic drainage. Heart, liver, or kidney disease can also cause pitting edema in the legs.

Do you have any swollen glands or lymph nodes?

- Is the person taking any drugs? Some drugs, such as dilantin, antibiotics, and some blood pressure medicine can cause lymphadenopathy.
- Is the lymph node enlargement local or generalized? Focal lymphadenopathy points to an infection from the region that drains into the node. Diffuse lymphadenopathy suggests systemic causes such as infectious mononucleosis, Hodgkin's disease, etc.

Examination

Inspect the hands and fingers. Note skin color, texture, underlying turgor, and the presence of edema or digital clubbing. Press down on the fingernail and note the time it takes for the color to return. Normally the blood flow refills in less than a second. Capillary refill times greater than two seconds suggest poor arterial blood flow. Palpate the radial pulses. When it is convenient, palpate both sides simultaneously. This will save you time, and provides an instantaneous side by side comparison. If no pallor or other signs of vascular deficit are noticed, it is not usually necessary to palpate the ulnar pulses. If any numbness or tingling is present in the hands, you should palpate both radial and ulnar pulses.

Pulse amplitude is graded on a numerical scale:

0	=	Absent
+1	=	Decreased, or weak, sometimes called 'thready'
+2	=	Normal
+3	=	Increased
+4	=	Very increased, or bounding

Palpate the brachial pulse. On a routine exam, if the distal pulse is strong, we often make the assumption that the more proximal pulses are also intact. Again, it depends upon the reason for the exam. If the arms and hands are asymptomatic, it is probably not necessary to palpate the more proximal pulses. However, if the distal pulse is weak, or if arm symptoms are present, it would be wise to palpate all pulses in the arm. After palpating the brachial pulse, palpate for enlargement of the epitrochlear lymph nodes.

Inspect the feet and toes. Observe the thickness and color of the skin, the presence of edema or abnormal venous patterns, absence of hair, and the condition of the nails. Palpate skin turgor and temperature. Check for capillary refill time of toenails. Palpate the dorsal pedis and posterior tibial pulses. The popliteal pulse may be hard to feel, and is ordinarily not attempted unless peripheral pulses are deficient. The popliteal lymph nodes are not normally palpable, unless there is an infection more distal in the leg. The femoral pulse is easily palpated. Inguinal lymph nodes and femoral pulses are usually palpated as a part of the abdominal examination.

When you check for edema, press the skin for a few seconds. When you release your fingers, the underlying tissue should rebound right away, otherwise 'pitting' edema is present, which is also graded on a numerical scale:

+1 = Mild - slight indentation
No perceptible swelling of the leg

+2 = Moderate - slightly deeper than +1
Indentation disappears rapidly (seconds)

+3 = Deep pitting - leg looks swollen
Indentation remains for a short time (minute)

+4 = Very deep pitting - leg is very swollen
Indentation remains a long time (minutes)

Spleen palpation is performed during the abdominal examination.

Sample Documentation

The skin of the upper and lower extremities was a normal pink color, without evidence of cyanosis, erythema, or skin lesions. The extremities were of normal size, without atrophy or edema. Radial, brachial, femoral, posterior tibial, and dorsal pedis pulses were strong (+2) and symmetrical. No lymphadenopathy was palpable in the inguinal or epitrochlear regions.

Vascular and Lymphatic Conditions

Hodgkin's Disease (ICD: 201)

Localized or disseminated malignant proliferation of tumor cells arising from the lymphoreticular system, primarily involving lymph node tissue and the bone marrow. (Merck Manual, p. 955)

• Hodgkin's disease was first described in 1832 by Thomas Hodgkin, a London pathologist. It is a cancer of the lymphatic system. This lymphatic cancer can localize in lymph nodes in the neck, axilla, or groin. However, the condition can also spread to the chest lymph nodes and spleen.

- The condition is comparatively rare, with approximately 7,000 new cases annually in the US. While the condition can occur at any age, it is most common in young adults, and more common in males. Symptomatically, the individual may notice a lump or swelling in their neck, groin, or axilla. Other symptoms include fever, night sweats, weight loss, fatigue and severe itching. When the intrathoracic lymph nodes are affected, the individual may experience a cough, shortness of breath, or possibly chest pain.
- Upon examination, the doctor may palpate an enlarged spleen in addition to enlarged lymph nodes that palpate as rubbery or matted. However, in many cases the individual experiences no symptoms and the condition is discovered as the result of a chest x-ray that is performed for non-specific symptoms.
- As the condition progresses, anemia and lymphocytopenia may manifest. Definitive diagnosis requires the presence of Reed-Sternberg cells (unusually large multinucleated white blood cells) in a lymph node biopsy.
- As with most forms of cancer, prognosis depends upon the stage or extent the cancer has spread. Prior to 1960, the survival rate was less than 40%. Since 1990, this survival rate has doubled to over 80%. The primary methods of medical management are radiation in the early stages, with chemotherapy for advanced or recurrent cancer.
- Autologous bone marrow transplantation involves collection of the patient's own white blood cells, chemotherapy to destroy the bone marrow, followed by reintroduction of the non-cancerous cells. This regimen is said to be successful 50% of the time, although many of these individuals subsequently develop leukemia after the 5th year of their "cure".

Non-Hodgkin's Lymphomas (ICD: 200)

Malignant monoclonal proliferation of lymphoid cells in sites of the immune system, including lymph nodes, bone marrow, spleen, liver, and GI tract. (Merck Manual, p. 958)

- Non-Hodgkin's lymphoma (NHL) refers to lymphatic cancer that does not meet the pathological definition of Hodgkin's lymphoma. Perhaps because it is a catch-all category for all remaining lymphomas, non-Hodgkin's lymphoma is much more common, approximately eight times more common than Hodgkin's lymphoma.
- The incidence of non-Hodgkin's lymphoma has doubled since 1970. One reason for this increase may be that HIV infected individuals are at increased risk of developing lymphoma.
- The signs, symptoms, and treatment of non-Hodgkin's lymphoma are similar to Hodgkin's lymphoma. Definitive diagnosis requires the biopsy of lymph node tissue.
- While the five year survival rate for non-Hodgkin's lymphoma has also risen since 1960, it is less survivable (50%) than Hodgkin's lymphoma.

- Burkitt's lymphoma, a lymphatic cancer endemic to central Africa, is the most aggressive form of lymphatic cancer. It is thought to be related to Epstein-Barr virus (EBV) infection. It primarily affects the jaw region and is usually fatal.

Infectious Mononucleosis (ICD: 075)

An acute disease due to Epstein-Barr virus, characterized by fever, pharyngitis, and lymphadenopathy. (Merck Manual, p. 2336)

- Infectious mononucleosis or 'mono' is a very common disorder. It is caused by the Epstein-Barr virus (EBV) that belongs to the herpes group.
- Many people have become infected in childhood, with the infection being mistaken for the common cold or flu. While the condition can occur at any age, the peak incidence is among young adults. Because the virus can be spread via saliva, it is sometimes referred to as the 'kissing disease'. Approximately 80-90% of adults have antibodies to the EBV, indicating that they may have experienced prior infection. Chronic EBV infection may be implicated in chronic fatigue syndrome.
- The symptoms are similar to flu: fever, sore throat, headache, fatigue, malaise. The condition often causes lymphadenopathy, especially in the cervical region. Older pathology texts note the importance of the lymph nodes by commenting on an alternative name for infectious mononucleosis: 'glandular fever'. Some individuals may experience periorbital pain and edema.
- Upon physical examination, lymph nodes usually palpate as symmetrically enlarged, firm, mobile, and tender. Splenomegaly or occasionally hepatomegaly may manifest.
- Several lab tests are available to assess infectious mononucleosis. The monospot test is a heterophile agglutination test (the Paul-Bunnell test was an early heterophil agglutination test). If the monospot test is negative, the infection may be due to cytomegalovirus (CMV). A CBC with differential count will likely disclose an elevated white blood count with lymphocytosis. Microscopic examination of the blood smear will disclose large atypical lymphocytes (Downey cells). The serum can also be tested for the presence of EBV antibodies. Assessment of liver enzymes and a throat culture for strep infection would also be prudent (30% of infectious mononucleosis patients also have a strep throat infection).
- Infectious mononucleosis is a 'self-limiting' condition. Most people recover from the acute phase within a few weeks. Nutritional immune support and chiropractic treatment may facilitate recovery. Because of the possibility of splenomegaly, the individual is advised to avoid strenuous or contact sports for several months. Because of the possibility of Reye's syndrome, children with flu-like symptoms should not be given aspirin.

Human Immunodeficiency Virus Infection (ICD: 044.9)

Infection caused by one of two related retroviruses (HIV-1 and HIV-2) resulting in a widespread range of clinical manifestations varying from asymptomatic carrier states to severely debilitating and fatal disorders related to defective cell-mediated immunity. (Merck Manual, p. 1312)

- HIV is a viral infection that in most cases eventually progresses to acquired immune deficiency syndrome (AIDS). AIDS was first recognized when in the early 1980's homosexual men began contracting rare conditions such as Kaposi's sarcoma and *Pneumocystis carinii* pneumonia.
- While AIDS continues to show a male predominance, it is transmissible to females via sexual contact. Worldwide an estimated 43% of all HIV infections are among women. Infants born of HIV infected mothers are at risk of contracting the virus. For this reason, the obstetrician may elect to deliver the baby via cesarean section.
- After unprotected sex, the other main risk factor is sharing of IV drug needles. Hemophiliacs have need to take blood products after an injury. These products were not screened for HIV prior to 1985, and many of these individuals subsequently contracted HIV.
- AIDS may present initially with flu-like symptoms similar to mononucleosis. The following symptoms are 'red flags' that should alert you to the possibility of AIDS:
    - long term fatigue for no apparent cause
    - lymph nodes swollen for over six months
    - fever that lasts for more than ten days
    - night sweats
    - unexplained weight loss
    - severe persistent diarrhea
    - purplish or discolored lesions on the skin or mucous membranes that do not heal
- Laboratory testing involves an enzyme linked immunosorbent assay (ELISA) test. If the ELISA test is positive, it should be followed up with a Western Blot test. HIV destroys the body's immune system primarily by infecting helper T cells. As such, the helper T lymphocyte (CD4) count is used to monitor the progression of the disorder.
- Medical management involves antiviral drugs such as AZT and 3TC.
- Individuals with HIV are often interested in alternatives, and may present in your office seeking natural methods of boosting immunity.

Peripheral Arterial Occlusion (ICD: 443.9)

Occlusion of blood supply to the extremities by atherosclerotic plaques (atheromas), a thrombus, or an embolism. (Merck Manual, p. 1784)

- Peripheral arterial occlusion is usually caused by fatty deposits on the intima of arteries. This restricts the flow of blood to structures supplied by those vessels. When these tissues experience a lack of oxygen, symptoms such as intermittent claudication can occur. The individual experiences a cramping muscle pain in the legs while walking, which is relieved when they stop to rest. About ten percent of individuals over age 70 experience symptoms of peripheral arterial occlusion.

- The condition is typically chronic, however if a thrombus breaks loose and becomes lodged, the individual may experience sudden throbbing pain. The location of the pain may identify the location of the blockage, with no symptoms proximal to the blockage. Leriche's syndrome is a 'saddle thrombus' blockage of the bifurcation of the aorta into the two iliac arteries, resulting in severe bilateral lower extremity vascular occlusion.
- Upon examination, arterial insufficiency typically manifests as decreased or absent pulses. The skin is pale, has a cool temperature, and may be thin with a loss of hair. Buerger's test may show 'elevation pallor, dependent rubor'.
- Other tests include Doppler ultrasound and measurement of sequential leg blood pressure readings. An ankle brachial blood pressure index (ABI) less than 1.0 indicates occlusive vascular disease. When this index is less than 0.6 the individual may have ulcers that do not heal, and places the individual at risk for gangrene and amputation of the limb.
- Conservative management is essentially the same as for coronary atherosclerotic disease.

Thromboangitis Obliterans (Buerger's Disease) (ICD: 443.1)

An obliterative disease characterized by inflammatory changes in small and medium-sized arteries and veins. (Merck Manual, p. 1788)

- Thromboangitis obliterans a specialized form of peripheral arterial occlusion. While the symptoms are similar, the etiology is different from atherosclerotic arterial occlusion. This condition occurs primarily in men, age 20-40, who are smokers. While men of this age may have the beginning of atherosclerotic changes, there are undoubtedly other contributing factors.
- The inflammatory nature of the condition is highlighted by the fact that the condition is not seen in people who do not smoke. Obviously, correction of the cause requires the individual to stop smoking. If they do not quit, they are vulnerable to the same dire consequences that occur with atherosclerotic occlusive disease.

Raynaud's Disease and Phenomenon (ICD: 443.0)

Spasm of arterioles, usually in the digits and occasionally in other acral parts (eg, nose, tongue), with intermittent pallor or cyanosis. (Merck Manual, p. 1790)

- Raynaud's disease in some ways is the opposite of Buerger's disease. It primarily affects young women, rather than men, and affects the digits of the upper extremity, rather than lower extremity vascular occlusion.

- The symptoms are the result of vasospasm of the small arterioles of the fingers resulting in impaired blood flow. Initially the fingers turn white from the lack of blood, then blue as the blood gradually returns, then red when the blood vessels undergo full dilation.

- Raynaud's disease may be secondary to connective tissue disease, such as scleroderma, rheumatoid arthritis, or systemic lupis erythematosis. As such, an arthritic lab panel might prove helpful in the management of this condition.

- Vasospasm attacks may be precipitated by stress, smoking or exposure to cold. Keeping the fingers warm with gloves often helps, and if your patient is a smoker, they must quit. Approximately 26% of patients with Raynaud's also experience migraine headaches (Degowin & Degowin, p. 423). As such, management of allergies may be indicated.

Acrocyanosis (ICD: 443.9)

Persistent, painless, symmetric cyanosis of the hands and less commonly, the feet, caused by vasospasm of the small vessels of the skin. (Merck Manual, p. 1791)

- Acrocyanosis is similar to Raynaud's disease in that it causes a bluish discoloration of the hands. It differs from Raynaud's in that the fingers do not manifest the white or red skin discoloration phases. Paradoxically, the cold fingers may sweat profusely.

Erythromelalgia (ICD: 443.9)

A rare syndrome of paroxysmal vasodilation with burning pain, increased skin temperature, and redness of the feet and, less often, the hands. (Merck Manual, p. 1791)

- In contrast to the arterial vasospasm of Raynaud's and acrocyanosis, erythromelalgia is caused by vasodilation. The increased blood flow causes swelling, redness, and a burning pain in the feet. The condition has similarities to inflammatory arthritis and may respond to anti-inflammatory therapies.

Venous Thrombosis (ICD: 453.9)

The presence of a thrombus in a vein. (Merck Manual, p. 1792)

- Phlebitis is inflammation of a vein. If a blood clot subsequently forms, this is referred to as thrombosis. These conditions typically occur together and are referred to as thrombophlebitis. If this blood clot detaches and travels to another site, it is referred to as a thrombotic embolus. If the embolus travels and lodges in the lungs, it is a pulmonary embolus. Pulmonary embolus is the leading cause of mortality in people who are hospitalized, with approximately 200,000 deaths annually.

- Rudolph Virchow commented, "*Phlebitis dominates all pathology*". While we now have more specifics of the pathophysiology, the mechanisms he identified in 1846 still hold true: venous stasis, vessel wall injury and a hypercoagulable state.
- As such risk factors include: prolonged immobility (bedrest, sitting for extended period of time), injury (recent trauma or surgery), and smoking or taking medicine such as birth control pills that promote platelet aggregation.
- Thrombophlebitis usually affects superficial veins, and may occur in conjunction with varicose veins. Deep vein thrombosis is less common. However, because the deep veins are larger, these blood clots are potentially larger and more dangerous.
- Symptoms of superficial phlebitis include local pain that may be burning or throbbing. A tender cord may be palpable and visible beneath the surface of the skin. The most common location for deep venous thrombosis (DVT) is the calf. The leg may be swollen and edematous. Homans' test is useful to differentiate calf tenderness caused by thrombophlebitis vs. sciatic nerve pain.
- Superficial thrombophlebitis may resolve with warm moist compresses and bed rest, with the limb elevated until the inflammation resolves. Deep vein thrombosis is more serious and may require hospitalization and anticoagulant therapy to prevent pulmonary embolism.
- Natural health care prevention involves multifactorial reduction of all the above risk factors.

Arterial and venous insufficiency can present with similar findings, which may also mimic neurogenic claudication. The following is a summary chart from a British Medical Journal article (Burns P, Gough S, Bradbury A. Management of peripheral arterial disease in primary care. *BMJ* (2003) 326:584-587):

Characteristic	Intermittent claudication	Venous claudication	Nerve root pain
Quality of pain	Cramping	"Bursting"	Electric shock-like
Onset	Gradual, consistent	Gradual, can be immediate	Can be immediate, inconsistent
Relieved by	Standing still	Elevation of leg	Sitting down, bending forward
Location	Muscle groups (buttock, thigh, calf)	Whole leg	Poorly localized, can affect whole leg
Legs affected	Usually one	Usually one	Often both

Varicose Veins (ICD: 454)

Elongated, dilated, tortuous superficial veins (usually in the legs) with incompetent valves, permitting reversed flow. (<u>Merck Manual</u>, p. 1794)

- One-way check valves in the veins normally prevent a retrograde flow of blood. When venous pressures are high, the vessel baloons out to where the valve cusps no longer meet. This permits blood to flow in the direction of gravity.
- Superficial varicosities present as bluish, ropelike cords beneath the skin. Varicose veins are usually located on the lower leg, but may also present as hemorrhoids or varicocele. The condition is common, affecting 10-20% of the population, women more than men.
- Risk factors include pregnancy, obesity, and occupations that involve standing for hours at a time.
- Prevention is the key with varicose veins, as once the damage is done, it can be stabilized, but reversal of the condition is unlikely.
- Conservative management involves nutritional support to strengthen the integrity of the vascular wall. Elastic compression stockings help to compress the venous blood back towards the heart. Obviously maintenance of normal blood pressure and body weight are recommended.
- In extreme cases, surgical vein stripping (which is actually ligation and removal of the entire superficial vein) may be recommended.
- Varicose veins that are chronic and severe may progress to chronic venous insufficiency. With this condition, the decreased flow of blood back to the heart can lead to pitting edema. The skin becomes thick and 'brawny'. Skin ulceration is common, especially at the medial ankle. In contrast to arterial insufficiency, pulses are normal, unless the individual has concomitant arterial pathology.

Lymphedema (ICD: 457.1)

Accumulation of excessive lymph fluid and swelling of subcutaneous tissues due to obstruction, destruction, or hypoplasia of lymph vessels. (<u>Merck Manual</u>, p. 1798)

- The lymphatic ducts allow for return of interstitial fluid back to the heart. If these ducts become blocked, the interstitial lymph fluid will accumulate. This blockage may be due to congenitally small lymph ducts, infection (lymphangitis), or a complication of surgery such as mastectomy where axillary lymph nodes have been removed.
- Symptomatically, the individual experiences a painless feeling of fullness in the limb. In contrast to the pitting edema seen with congestive heart failure, lymphedema produces non-pitting edema. Another distinction is that while CHF edema is bilaterally, symmetry is unlikely with lymphedema. With chronic lymphedema the skin may become thickened and harder than usual.

- If the patient has an infection, obviously this will probably require antibiotic treatment. If there are non-infectious structural blockages to lymph flow, physical therapy of intermittent pneumatic compression (IPC) help to reduce limb swelling.
- Intermittent pneumatic compression (IPC) is a physical therapy modality that has proven benefit for peripheral vascular disease. When you have a patient with lymphedema or venous insufficiency, you should investigate non-surgical alternatives for your patient. The Chattanooga Group is a chiropractic supplier that manufactures an excellent IPC unit.

Lymphangitis (ICD: 457.2)

Acute inflammation of the subcutaneous lymphatic channels, usually caused by S. pyogenes. (Merck Manual, p. 795)

- Lymphangitis may develop as a consequence of a wound such as an animal bite. Initially, the wound may appear to be mild. Then days later a red streak, which is warm and painful, appears proximal to the apparently healed animal bite.
- The infective organism is typically a strep or staph infection. If the infection spreads to the bloodstream, systemic symptoms such as fever, chills, headache, and myalgia may manifest.
- Prompt referral for antibiotic therapy is necessary, as untreated systemic infection can prove fatal.

Study Guide Objectives

o   Know the pulse sites accessible to examination.
o   Which vascular condition causes pain and pallor in the extremities?
o   What factors are responsible for venous return to the heart?
o   What causes the intraluminal valves in the veins to become incompetent?
o   How is lymphatic fluid propelled toward the heart?
o   Know the organs related to the lymphatic system.
o   Know the mechanisms and pathways of lymphatic drainage.
o   What is the significance of Virchow's sentinel node?
o   Know the functions of the spleen.
o   What are Peyer's patches?
o   Know the appropriate history questions for examination of the peripheral vascular and lymphatic system.
o   What is claudication and what circulatory condition causes it?
o   What circulatory condition causes thickened skin with brownish discoloration?
o   What conditions cause pitting vs. non-pitting edema?
o   Know the difference between focal vs. diffuse lymphadenopathy and the causes of each.
o   Know the grading scale for pulses.
o   Know the grading scale for pitting edema.
o   Know the pathologic changes that occur with the various vascular

and lymphatic conditions discussed.

o   Reed-Sternberg cells are associated with what condition?

o   Know the virus that causes infectious mononucleosis.

o   The heterophil agglutination test is used to detect what condition?

o   What two rare conditions manifest as a consequence of AIDS?

o   Know the 'red flag' symptoms that should alert the clinician to the possibility of AIDS.

o   What is Leriche's syndrome?

o   What condition manifests 'elevation pallor and dependent rubor'?

o   What is the significance of a decreased ankle brachial blood pressure index (ABI)?

o   Buerger's disease occurs primarily in what age and sex category?

o   Raynaud's disease occurs primarily in what age and sex category?

o   What are the differences between acrocyanosis and erythromelalgia?

o   Know the three mechanisms of phlebitis identified by Rudolph Virchow in 1846.

o   What are the risk factors for phlebitis?

o   What test is used to differentiate calf tenderness caused by thromboplebitis vs. sciatic nerve pain?

Index

288

289

290

About the Author

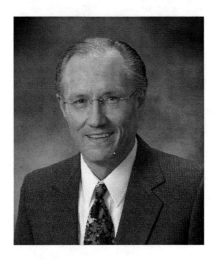

Dr. Edward Brown is a 1981 magna cum laude graduate of Western States Chiropractic College. He practiced in Oregon for 18 years prior to moving to Texas to begin teaching at Parker College of Chiropractic.

Dr. Brown has extensive postgraduate training, which includes certification as a diplomate of the American Board of Chiropractic Internists (DABCI), and a fellow of the International Academy of Clinical Acupuncture (FIACA).

Dr. Brown has served as:

- Chair, Department of Diagnosis & Clinical Applications at Parker College of Chiropractic

- Vice President of the American Board of Chiropractic Internists

- Part III National Board of Chiropractic Examiners test committee member

Prior to becoming a chiropractor, Dr. Brown graduated magna cum laude from the University of Utah, with a BS in Social Science, and was elected to the Phi Beta Kappa and Phi Kappa Phi national honor societies. Prior experience in the health field includes working as an EMT and a US Air Force Aeromed tech.

Dr. Brown helped to start the *Natural Medicine* forum on CompuServe, and has a special interest in computer-assisted diagnosis, artificial intelligence, and all phases of integrating computer technology into natural health care.